Life, Liberty, and the Pursuit of Healthiness

Also by Dean Edell, M. D.

Eat, Drink, and Be Merry

Life, Liberty, and the Pursuit of Healthiness

Dr. Dean's Commonsense Guide for Anything That Ails You

DEAN EDELL, M.D.

with

MELISSA HOUTTE

HarperCollins*Publishers*

HarperCollins books may be purchased for educational, business, or sales promotional use. For information, please write: Special Markets Department, HarperCollins Publishers Inc., 10 East 53rd Street, New York, NY 10022.

FIRST EDITION

Designed by Nicola Ferguson

Printed on acid-free paper

Library of Congress Cataloging-in-Publication Data
Edell, Dean.
Life, liberty, and the pursuit of healthiness : Dr. Dean's commonsense guide for anything that ails you / Dean Edell with Melissa Houtte.—1st ed.
p. cm.
ISBN 0-06-057723-1
1. Medicine, Popular.   I. Houtte, Melissa.   II. Title.

RC81.E24 2004
610—dc22   2003061095

04 05 06 07 08 NMSG/RRD 10 9 8 7 6 5 4 3 2 1

Dedicated to my listeners and viewers,

who have made me a better doctor.

Acknowledgments

Creating a book is a curious and amazing process for me, especially a book that is based on so many conversations with people I will never meet, but to whom I am indebted because they found the time to write or call me. Thank you all for sharing your observations, your personal experiences, and your worries. While I cannot always be the bearer of good news—that is the nature of medicine—I hope I have helped you, because you have helped me educate many people and, hopefully, save lives.

HealthCentral.com, the Web site that has showcased many of the questions asked on my radio show in recent years, also played a significant role in the development of this book. The HealthCentral team of writers, editors, and producers created a product that was essential to the shaping of the manuscript.

My family's support—especially that of my wife, Sharon—is also a key factor in making this book possible. When deadlines loom, it is always nice to know that once the microphones have been turned off and the computer is shut down, I will find wisdom, humor, and understanding at home.

This book would not be possible without my radio show, and the show wouldn't be possible without the daily support of Heather Hamann, who talks to many more callers than I do, and who knows when I've goofed—and has no problems telling me so.

I continue to be indebted to Susan Maruyama of Round Mountain Media, whose tenacity and publishing savvy made my first book possible and who then stayed on my case to get the second one off the ground. Susan's the one who introduced me to Melissa Houtte, my editing/writing partner whose enthusiasm and energy were highly contagious. Melissa is an award-winning newspaper and magazine journalist who asks good questions and hates medical scams just as much as I do. So we were a good team—even when I announced I was moving offices during the middle of the project.

Thanks also to Brianne Miller for a bunch of book title ideas, including the one you see here, to Kathryn Bing-You, for her copy editing talents, and to Megan Newman and Camille DeAngelis of my publisher, HarperCollins. This is my second book with Megan and I could not ask for a more lively, supportive, and intelligent relationship.

Contents

Introduction

We live in the greatest place on Earth. I am reminded of this every day on my radio show, when I spend an hour talking to people about the most amazing—and sometimes shocking—subjects. We have few limitations. The government, religion, sex, politicians, and medical practices are all fair game, as they should be. Despite our country's problems—and I don't want to minimize those—we do have the proverbial life, liberty, and pursuit of happiness.

But we—you and I—have created a kind of chaos because of where we live. Our freedom—freedom to do business, freedom to make personal choices, freedom to say whatever we want—has allowed us to have the best and worst that society has to offer. And nowhere is that more evident than in the world of health and medicine.

If I have to be sick anywhere, I'd rather be sick here. But that doesn't mean everything is perfect; and many Americans have become riddled with doubt or confusion about the state of medicine in America. Sometimes it really can be difficult to determine what is best for you and your family. It seems that everyone has an opinion about the best path to good health.

I am reminded of a letter I received not too long ago, one that symbolizes the craziness that we all have to sort through.

"Dear Radio Host," it began, like so many of the commercial pitches I get every day from product and personality promoters—most of which go right into my wastebasket.

This promotion was straightforward but instantly suspect: "How to protect yourself against West Nile fever without toxins." Mosquito season was on the way, and this "expert" was seizing the moment.

OK. We have a disease that has killed hundreds of Americans who've been bitten by mosquitoes, and the best protection, according to all medical experts, is to use a potent repellent and take other protective measures when outdoors during mosquito season. But this guy had better ideas, and he wanted the opportunity to talk about them on my show.

Over my dead body. But I kept reading.

Instead of using traditional repellents, according to this letter, we should all go to the kitchen for "natural substances for killing the virus fast." Aha. "Natural"—the word that's launched multimillion-dollar supplement companies, alternative grocery chains, and endless lines of beauty products. If it's "natural," it's got to be good for you, right? Well, tobacco and certain wild mushrooms are natural and look where they'll get you. The cemetery.

The West Nile fellow's natural repellent ideas were imaginative, to say the least, and my favorite made me want to plan a trip to Italy. In short, he seemed to suggest that before heading outdoors we all smear ourselves with a combination of spaghetti sauce and honey. Yes, you read it right.

I knew some talk show somewhere would soon have him on as a featured guest, because he claimed thousands of past bookings on radio and television programs. And people would hear him and not know just how ridiculous his advice was, and somewhere unfortunate little kids would spend a summer outdoors looking like giant meatballs. Hopefully, that would be the only damage done by his advice.

How did the most sophisticated, technologically advanced country on earth get to the point where fears can be manipulated like this? Why are so many of us gullible? Why are some of us convinced that conspiracy is behind much of legitimate modern medicine and health science?

I don't have a simple answer to these questions. I sincerely believe that most of us want to do the right thing for ourselves, but the pursuit of healthiness is not a straightforward matter. Far from it. One day the newspaper headlines and morning talk shows trumpet news of research showing that margarine is good for you. A few months later, oops, it now appears it will kill you. Carbohydrates go from being the healthiest foods on earth to a hidden menace in cakes and cookies, a quick path to a coronary. Chocolate is the devil or it's the answer to everything from toe fungus to baldness. Who wouldn't be confused by the ceaseless information overload—even if every story were thoroughly and accurately reported? Which they frequently aren't.

And sometimes, science has been known to cut a wide swath through an issue—estrogen is a good example—before we fully know what's right and what isn't. Early research doesn't always tell us everything we need to know, but occasionally our society is so desperate for a solution that doctors and patients grab at whatever seems best at the moment.

When women began calling my show twenty years ago with their first estrogen therapy questions, lots of good doctors had already bought into this treatment. I couldn't see the proof that menopausal women would benefit from it, but that was one opinion—and I can't blame women who went with their doctor's advice. These were smart physicians who wanted nothing more than to help their patients—we just didn't see the research quite the same way.

It took a long time for studies to get to hard answers on estrogens, but we now know that not only do they do no good but also that they may actually promote killers like heart disease and Alzheimer's. If doctors are confused about something this profound, how can the public fail to be confused—and fearful?

Unfortunately, some of the very liberties we so cherish in this culture have now become a source of danger to our health. The promotion of health has become a huge business that sometimes veers out of control. Yes, we have amazing new medications, medical tests, and technology that save many lives. But the bad apples in the industry—and medicine is an industry—have no qualms about cashing in on our anxieties.

We are told we can fight cancer, protect our memory, and improve our sex life, and almost everything seems to come with a "guarantee." The manufacturers and marketers often hide behind the right to free speech, but they can make Pinocchio look like a saint in need of a nose job. Tiny tight buns, bulging bosoms, and six-pack abs are not just an 800 number away. Remember: Nothing good or lasting comes that easily.

In spite of our ever-increasing longevity and strides toward better health, we are a society of the worried well. We often rush to emergency rooms and doctors' offices for the most minor ailments. While images of terrorism, bio warfare, and SARS swirl around us, we freak out about the mercury in our fillings, the mold in our basement, the trans fats in our Oreo cookies. The incongruities are humorous, but they are also unsettling.

At a deeper level, I see worries that border on paranoia, and those could endanger all of us. I have talked to people who think there is a medical conspiracy that will prevent cancer from ever being cured. One in five Americans—20 percent—believes that an AIDS vaccine already exists but is being kept secret from the public. And over 40 percent of us don't know that all vaccines first must be tested on human volunteers before being made available to the public.

The panic about childhood vaccines shows itself on my show at least once a week, and some people are nearly hysterical in their belief that these protective substances cause autism. Why don't more of us remember the horrible diseases that have all but disappeared because of these vaccines? And why don't we want to believe the scientific proof that infants are showing the earliest signs of autism months before they are exposed to any vaccines?

I still remember the women with breast implants who picketed the San Francisco television station where I broadcast, because of my view that breast implants did not cause disease. But science be damned. By the time implants were exonerated, billions of dollars had been paid out by juries that were overwhelmed by slick lawyers and questionable experts. I hate that, but do I still believe in our justice system? You bet, though changes are in order.

"Junk science"—the use of marginal or faulty research presented by people with initials after their names—has destroyed many otherwise reliable companies and products. In most legal situations, a high standard is required for evidence presented in courtrooms. But when it comes to health and science issues, we lower the bar. How else to explain the fact that one recent lawyers conference on how to cash in on the mold panic was promoted as "Mold Is Gold."

And our society's penchant for lawsuits has taken a new turn. We are abdicating our responsibility to take care of ourselves. We are too fat because McDonald's forces us to eat their fries. We have lung cancer because the tobacco companies made us smoke. Blaming others for our poor health habits means we have given up the control to improve them. That scares me.

With all the voices out there vying for your attention, no wonder you're calling me with questions about stress and anxiety like never before. I want to help, but you have to believe you can help yourself. You can regain control, you can feel more optimistic about the future, but it won't happen overnight, and it requires hard work.

My approach in *Life, Liberty, and the Pursuit of Healthiness* is to educate by example and focus on the health issues of most concern to you. To do that I've drawn on a familiar yet untapped resource: You.

Over the past twenty-five years I have probably answered fifty thousand questions on the air. You have been my greatest teacher, and now I want to return the favor by providing the latest information I can find on issues that you have most consistently brought to the fore. These questions are the ones that we all face at different points in our lives and that dominate our collective health consciousness.

You may recognize yourself or a friend on one of these pages, because we've kept the questions real, with all their quirks and idiosyncrasies. While you may not be dealing with exactly the same problem, we've packed the answers with information that we hope will be beneficial to all.

Sometimes you will find clear-cut, black-and-white responses, but not always, because medicine doesn't have all the answers—and the questions keep changing. No two headaches or stomachaches are the same. That's what makes life and medicine both interesting and, at times, a bit scary.

As you sort through the chapters, looking for a specific topic or just browsing, please remember two points that I believe are critical to moving healthcare in the right direction.

One: Science and objective thinking are our only allies against fear, superstition, and hype. It's much healthier to be skeptical than fearful, but don't ignore hard facts. And if you don't have the facts, ask for them.

Two: Doctors will get off their pedestals when patients get off their knees. We are your partners. We want you to get well. We need your help. So, let's get on with it.

Life, Liberty, and the Pursuit of Healthiness

Chapter 1

There's a Reason We're Fat

My philosophy about food is simple: Enjoy what you eat.

Eating is one of the most fundamental pleasures in life, and yet many folks see it as a chore or, at the other extreme, a luxury they can't afford. That's too bad, because there's research supporting the idea that enjoying what you eat is an aspect of healthy living—and it has nothing to do with whether you're eating caviar or homemade soup. For me, eating pleasurably translates into a bowl of linguini marinara or a handful of macadamia nuts; I make them work in my diet because they make me happy.

I've noticed that the dietary guidelines of many countries include a message about the joy of eating. Britain has a slogan "Enjoy Your Food," the Vietnamese advise eating meals that are "delicious," and Norway concludes: "Food and Joy = Health." Unfortunately, in the United States, the slogan might be "Do They Have Drive-thru?" or "We Don't Have Time to Sit Down for Dinner." Our society is paying dearly for such habits, in both our health and our relationships.

Eating well does take some effort, but American cities have more well-stocked grocery stores than ever before, not to mention a diversity of restaurant experiences offering everything from pad thai to spicy tuna rolls to carne asada. If you are bored by food, you have no one to blame but yourself. If you're intimidated by it, afraid of it, or confused by it, just keep reading. A little food knowledge could have a good effect on your appetite.

The taste, texture, and appearance of food all combine for a pleasurable eating experience. But, studies show, the look and taste of cuisine can also make what you eat more nutritious and healthy. Your body's digestive system reacts positively to a happy meal (no, I'm not talking about McDonald's) by releasing juices that absorb more nutrients. But take that meal off the plate and put it in a blender before it's consumed, and there's less absorption of certain nutrients.

Of course, very few of us would put a chicken breast and mashed potatoes into the Osterizer for a meal on the run. But we are doing some strange things, because we have become obsessed with—and often misinformed about—eating for maximum good health.

What is the best diet for a healthy life? That's not easy. It's like asking, "What's the best way to make love?" If you look all over the world, and study eating habits throughout history, you will find different solutions. Eskimos and our forebears through the Ice Age ate lots of meat and fat and seemed to do just fine. In other parts of the world, people who depended heavily on carbohydrates in the form of plants and nuts lived healthy lives, too.

But somewhere along the line, we've been sold this idea that there must be a "best" food—that the world is made up of good foods and bad foods, and if only we could find the good ones, we'd live forever. Forget it.

This "moral nutrition" concept has created more anxiety and misinformation than anything I can think of. Human beings, it turns out, are capable of surviving and being healthy on a variety of diets. The critical word here is "variety." For example, we know the French eat more fat than we do, yet they do not succumb in the same numbers to the heart disease and obesity that we have in the United States. How can that be? Well, they eat a more diverse mix of foods, and so their bodies receive a broader assortment of micronutrients.

The "French Paradox" actually can be found throughout the Mediterranean, where the majority of fat consumed is olive oil. A recent study of the Greek diet found that an emphasis on fruits, vegetables, grains, nuts, fish, and olive oil—as well as wine at most meals—lowered death rates from cancer and heart disease.

Of course, people eating traditional diets in the Mediterranean may have other behaviors that explain their healthiness, from less stress to more exercise.

And, let me repeat: No individual food group conferred benefits—it's the total diet.

I know too many people—and maybe this is true in your own family—who consistently eat the same limited diet week in and week out. And who go to the same restaurants when they eat out and order the same thing. Yet, if they become concerned about their weight, or their children's weight, they look for a miracle food—or a diet plan—to fix things. We've all done that, but it almost never works—or lasts for very long.

In the sixties, I tried vegetarianism, and most of my kids are still vegetarian. But I'm not, and I'm much more relaxed about my diet. While I generally eat what I want, the things I want to eat come from many cuisines—and I eat much differently than I did as a child, when I ate my breakfast cereal with heavy cream every day and even put sugar in my Coca-Cola because it wasn't sweet enough. Nowadays, parents would be demonized for allowing such behavior.

But I'm not sure we're much better off, food-wise, than when I was a child. The problem in America is not only what we're not eating, but the amount of what we are eating—and that's a critical issue that nutrition research is finally addressing. One of the newest pieces of research, from the University of North Carolina, looked at portion sizes for a variety of popular foods. Disturbingly, they found that between 1977 and 1996, portions both at home and in restaurants increased for everything but pizza. And some of those increases were staggering: A homemade hamburger jumped from 5.7 ounces to 8.4 ounces. Did you serve a half-pounder last weekend without even knowing it?

Equally unsettling was a recent report from the American Institute for Cancer Research. In a survey of one thousand adults, 69 percent said they finish their meals most of the time or all of the time, even when the portions are large.

Eating more food than your body needs is not only unhealthy but also promotes obesity. We want to have our cake—and a second piece, too. Why has this happened? Three Harvard University researchers argue that technology has made eating all too easy for us, from the not-so-healthy French fries that weren't always so easily attainable to the now-popular habit of grazing among many tempting snacks—and eating more than we realize.

No matter how much we may enjoy a day that starts with a stack of pancakes and sausage and ends with a big steak, fries, chocolate cake, and a couple of glasses of wine, you can't do that every night and not see—and feel—the effects. But if the day starts with two pancakes and half a grapefruit and ends with a small steak—and spinach salad and black beans and one glass of wine—you have already begun to make an impact. Smaller portions. Food diversity. A priority on making the meal a pleasure to eat. These are all much more important than finding the "right" diet plan, because there isn't one that's been proven to deliver long-term success.

The way we prepare our foods also is critical. Many studies have shown that when you reduce the amount of sugar, salt, and fat in a variety of well-prepared meals, people don't notice it. And, unfortunately, we are not a nation known for taking our time—and taking pleasure—in preparing food for its sensuous qualities. So our blood pressure is a problem, and so is our weight.

As a vegetarian, I ate fabulous dishes without the meat that I once thought was necessary for a satisfying meal—and I still have many meals during the week that don't include meat. Going a big step further, one of the most intriguing restaurants in the United States, Roxanne's in Northern California, uses no dairy, wheat, or soybeans—and everything is raw. Folks have waited months for a chance to sample innovative dishes, which work because the chef understands that how the food is prepared and presented is critical to a pleasurable meal.

I've always felt that one of the skills that many children could benefit from—and which might make their early food experiences more positive and adventurous—is learning how to cook. The five-year-old who participates in making a fresh batch of from-scratch pancakes will know the difference when she's served something of lesser quality—and she's much more likely to willingly eat the food she's made herself.

Unfortunately much of the marketing in the food, diet, and nutrition industry works against us making intelligent decisions for ourselves and our children. On billboards, in magazines, and on television, we are being sold the newest low-fat food or diet du jour—and it's frequently billed as the short path to good health. This not only affects the decisions of adults but also shapes the thinking of our children for decades to come. We need to fight this every time we go to the grocery store or consider a stop at a fast-food restaurant.

At the same time, and I don't want to confuse you about this, we need to balance our thinking about a core element of good diet and nutrition: body weight. Our nation's rising obesity rates are the subject of almost nightly news reports—and the issue is a critical one as it relates to children.

Yet, many people worry about their body weight because of how they look to themselves. This is a relatively recent phenomenon; in other times, people with a little fat on their bones were considered healthier—and better off. After all, it was a matter of pride that we could obtain enough food for our body to be able to store fat. Fat also was considered beautiful. The tombs from the Tang dynasty of China tell us that, and so do the paintings of Peter Paul Rubens, from which we still have the marvelous descriptive, "Rubenesque."

I hate to challenge the current advice you hear from experts, but you are not automatically a medical basket case if you are overweight. Yes, if you have hypertension or diabetes—two diseases that can be related to obesity—you are at a high risk for poor health, and you need to make some changes. But that is not an issue in everyone who is overweight, and, more important, these diseases have a strong genetic component. The primary concern may be fitness and not obesity.

No study has ever shown that if you weigh 200 pounds and you lose 50 pounds you become as healthy as a person who weighs 150 pounds to start with. As a matter of fact, it's upsetting to find that most of the major studies show us that significant weight loss is bad for you. Yes, if you lose weight your blood pressure should come down, and your diabetes should improve, but, in overall statistics, the results of weight loss are disappointing—possibly because we are focusing too much on the numbers, i.e., what we see on the scale.

People who are overweight as a group have worse health statistics because their fitness levels—how efficiently their heart and lungs perform—may be lower. There is lots of research to support the fact that if you are relatively fit and fat you're going to be OK. But don't assume you are fit just because you walk a mile every day; you need to talk to your doctor about specifics.

It gets more complicated when you factor in the fact that a lot of fitness is genetic and sometimes skewed by gender, too. One Belgian study of twins and their parents determined that almost all aerobic capacity—good or bad—in girls could be linked to heredity. Another study of twins, in Finland, established a direct genetic link for men between exercise and weight loss—doing the same exercise, men will all burn the same number of calories, but they will *not* all lose the same amount of weight.

Perhaps most important—and a fact that is kept secret by the diet industry—is that we all have different genes when it comes to obesity. It's naïve to assume that if every human on earth ate the exact same diet we would all weigh the same. And yet that is what the diet industry would have you believe, which leads to an amazing amount of frustration. People constantly tell me, "I'm only eating 1,500 calories a day and I'm not losing weight," while other folks will lose weight while eating more calories.

Enter the protein versus carbohydrate diet debate, which seems to draw more attention among Americans than international politics. This battle dates back one hundred years, when high-protein diets were first proposed, and we've gone back and forth ever since. It's not rocket science to figure out that there are only two basic diets: high carbohydrate, which means you don't have a lot of room for proteins and fats, or high fat and protein, which means you don't have a lot of room for carbs.

But you won't find any research spanning forty or fifty years that confirms the benefits of either approach, because few people follow one diet that long. I listen to the Atkins high-protein followers complaining they want something crunchy, and are desperate for bread and pasta and cakes, while those trying to stick to ultra-low-fat diets wind up craving meat and fat. Such extreme denial doesn't make sense for a lifetime, does it?

I promise that you will be much happier and healthier if you remember two simple things: One, there's no such thing as an unhealthy food, just unhealthy diets. And two, if you burn more calories than you take in, you are going to lose weight.

That's probably the best advice going, not only for our waistlines but because we know that reducing our caloric intake will help fight heart disease and some cancers and will prolong longevity. The solution for every individual is different, but it doesn't have to be complicated, though the questions I hear on my show and which you'll see in this chapter often deal with confusion about the most basic nutrition facts. The more we know about food and its relation to our bodies, the easier it is to stay fit and healthy.

That's the foundation of my advice for healthy eating. However, if there are two things that stand out among the many calls I get every week, it is just how few fruits and vegetables are finding their way into our diets—and how much we want to use supplements to take care of that problem. This is short-sighted, unhealthy, and expensive.

For those of you who depend on supplements to make up for a lousy diet—because you don't have time to eat or you see food as a nuisance—it's time to reassess your priorities. What could be more important than taking care of your body? As for diet pills, you are telling yourself that you can't do it on your own. But sooner or later you are going to stop taking the pills and you will probably gain back whatever weight you have lost. It is much healthier to find a permanent lifestyle solution. That means committing to regular exercise and eating in a way that you enjoy, in a manner that you can stick to for the rest of your life. If you decide you are going to be fat—and always eat as much as you want—then you at least need to be active. That's your best antidote. Or you can let the roulette wheel spin and take your chances. It's your choice.

Diet Plans and Eating Regimens

Q: I have about 140 pounds to lose. How do I find the best weight-loss clinic? I'm not interested in the short-term, magic pill. I want the plan that has the best success rate for overall weight loss, the one that gets people to keep the weight off the longest and is the safest.

A: The first point to explore is how the plan will support you through the long haul. Ask yourself, "What will my eating habits be after I lose the weight?"

The program that recognizes that sustained weight loss means a permanent change in the way you eat, and helps you maintain the change, is a first-rate program. I have no problem with any of the franchise, nonpharmacological, nonmedicinal weight-loss groups as long as they do this for their members.

Any plan that you can't stay with physically and emotionally for the long term is doomed. We don't have any useful data on diet clinics, because they are not required to be accountable. Also, because of demographic variables like genetics and ethnicity, data wouldn't give an accurate picture.

You certainly can't stay on pills or shots for any length of time. Some clinics use injections that are placebos. Many years ago I actually worked in one for a time. The placebos were effective for a while, because the dieters had to come in every day to face the music and be weighed. Also, their friends were in the waiting room spooning out the encouragement. But when the placebos and daily visits stopped, so did the weight loss.

Some weight-loss centers use real drugs—amphetamines; those can be addictive or kill you. So, please, scratch those from your list of options.

Being fit is critical. Being overweight doesn't automatically mean your are unfit. We are finding that you can be fit and healthy and overweight. Fat people who are fit fare better than do thin people who are unfit. A lot of data supporting this comes from the renowned Cooper Clinic in Dallas.

Bariatrics is a branch of medicine that specializes in weight loss. I object to any doctor doling out medication to someone who is only ten pounds overweight, but someone like you, with a lot of weight to lose, may benefit from consulting with a specialist, especially if your weight is causing serious health problems.

Many bariatric physicians argue that since it's appropriate to put people on lifelong medication for chronic conditions like high blood pressure, why not give overweight people lifelong appetite suppressants. In my opinion, they can make a case for taking that risk only if the excess weight is a serious health threat.

Ultimately, you have to ask yourself if you are committed to losing the weight and making the needed changes to keep it off. You alone know the answer.

Q: I know that you speak out against the Atkins diet, and all high-protein/low-carbohydrate plans. My wife's doctor told her to try that diet, because she has diabetes. The results have been miraculous. Her blood sugar has dropped way down. How can you be opposed to that?

DID YOU KNOW?
ARE YOU A PEAR OR AN APPLE?

Your body shape may tell you more than your realize. And, if you are overweight, you may have yet another reason to tackle those extra pounds. A study of more than forty thousand middle-aged female nurses found that those who are apple-shaped (their waist-to-hip ratio is more than .76), or who had waists of more than thirty inches, had a higher risk of heart disease than those women who are pear-shaped (waist-to-hip ratios of less than .76). How do you figure the ratio? It's simple; divide your hip measurement into your waist measurement. Example: a thirty-inch waist and forty-inch hips mean a ratio of .75.

A: A high-protein/low-carbohydrate diet will lower your blood sugar because you're not eating any sugar. That's something we've known for a long time.

But what does her doctor propose to do about the fact that these high-protein diets are extremely high in fat? Fat is the enemy of diabetics, because they have extraordinarily high rates of heart disease, stroke, and vascular problems. When her blood sugar goes down, you may think she's being helped, but a major killer of people with diabetes is heart disease.

One of the main fears of the medical community has been that the good accomplished by decades of teaching people to eat complex carbohydrates like pasta and of moving them away from all the greasy fat would be wiped out by a couple of talk shows. Now everyone's afraid of carbohydrates and running back to fat.

We need objective science to justify what's being peddled to the public. We have bushels of evidence on diets that doctors and nutritionists can recommend for good health. Radical diets like this should not be recommended for someone with a chronic disease like diabetes, without proof that it is safe and effective. We should insist that just as planes don't leave the ground unless they are tested, we won't gobble diets that aren't proven, especially over the long term.

The breakdown of carbohydrates does raise the blood sugar. The body needs sugar. Even most diabetics can handle it under a doctor's care and with medication.

Right now, the majority of nutritionists and dietitians oppose Atkins. With real evidence of its value, their opinions will change, and so will mine. But a couple of short-term studies don't overturn decades of good research.

Q: I have a diet book with a plan for weight loss that's based on eating specific combinations of food. It was written in 1952 and is republished every year. What do you know about it?

A: Throw the book away. If your doctor based your health care on a 1952 medical journal, you would run the other way. But when it comes to fad diets, the older they are the more confidence they seem to inspire.

The idea that the way food combines during digestion has anything to do with nutrient absorption and weight gain is nutritional nonsense. This notion continues to make the rounds in different packages—the Beverly Hills Diet is one of those.

In many foods, nature itself combines carbohydrates, proteins, and fats.

Your body uses an amino acid as an amino acid whether it came from corn or a hamburger. If you are like most Americans, your diet has room for improvement. Instead of using a vintage diet plan, keep a complete log of everything you eat for a week and see how you're doing. Does it include a variety of foods and ample amounts of fruits and vegetables? At the same time, write down everything you did to keep fit that week. If you're honest with yourself, you should be able to spot some changes you can make that will improve your overall health.

Q: **About a year ago, I lost 100 pounds on the Atkins diet and went down from 460 to 360 pounds. Then I quit, because I kept hearing how harmful that diet is, but now I've gained back all the weight. What's the biggest harm, my weight or the diet? I'm forty-five, and my cholesterol and blood pressure have always been normal.**

A: Most people assume that being overweight automatically means having high cholesterol and high blood pressure, but that isn't so.

You've asked a question to which we really don't have the answer. Not only that, but I will add another question. Is losing weight and gaining it back doing more harm than staying where you are?

When all the pieces don't add up to a clear picture, our best guide is to go by what research has shown so far. As you know, the Atkins diet is a high-fat, high-protein diet. Well, most nutritionists will tell you that too much protein is unhealthy, and the majority of research says that if you eat a lot of fat, you're more likely to wind up with heart disease than the next guy is. This isn't automatic, though.

Oddly enough, if you were sixty-five instead of forty-five, you would be at a point statistically where the weight would no longer have much of an effect on

QUIZ

Which alcoholic beverage has the most calories?
A) 12-ounce can of light beer   B) 1 ounce of 80-proof whiskey
C) 1 ounce of 100-proof whiskey   D) 3.5 ounces of white wine
E) 3.5 ounces of red wine
(A: light beer, with 134 calories; B is the lowest, with 65 calories.)

longevity. Excess weight does not have much of an impact on life span if a person gets beyond middle age into the senior years.

Because you are still in your middle years, and you are at a weight that is likely to be damaging to your health, my suggestion is that if you truly enjoy the foods allowed on Atkins that you get back on the diet and lose the weight—as long as you do it under the care of a physician who is monitoring your cholesterol levels and cardiovascular profiles.

Then your challenge will be to switch to a diet on which you can maintain your weight loss without threatening your health with too much fat and protein. Also, you might want to ask your doctor if another diet plan would be better for you. In an analysis of the diet of 2,681 dieters who had maintained at least a thirty-pound weight loss for a year or more, less than one percent followed a diet similar to the Atkins plan, according to researchers with the National Weight Control Registry. Most of them followed a high-carbohydrate, low-fat diet to maintain the weight loss.

Q: Recently I was at a luncheon where someone said he couldn't eat the meal because he was a vegan. Someone else at the table thought he was talking about a religion, but I asked, and the vegan explained his no-animal-products food restrictions. Is this healthy?

A: Vegetarianism isn't as simple as it once was. Since the sixties, when vegetarianism made a roaring comeback—it dates back to 1846—a few subtypes have sprung up. Some can be humorous; most of my kids have been vegetarians, and one of them is a McDonald's vegetarian. That means he'll eat a Big Mac, but that's it. Otherwise, his diet is all dairy and vegetables.

Vegans are not supposed to eat any dairy, meat, fish, or fowl—no animal by-products of any sort. Basically the risk vegans take is to miss out on vitamin B12—it's only found in meat and dairy—which many vegans get with a supplement. You can be healthy as a vegan, but you have to be smart about how you eat. You have to know how to combine different kinds of proteins to get all the amino acids that are necessary. Only meat and dairy products contain all the amino acids that are necessary to produce proteins in the human body. But a complete protein can be had by combining something like corn and beans: what one lacks in amino acids, the other will have.

While veganism is not a religion, the fervency with which some cling to this program certainly sounds like radical fundamentalism at times. Vegans have a much higher rate of eating disorders, and if your children adopt this diet, it's wise to keep track of their dietary habits.

I've known several teenagers who were vegans, but, sooner or later, they found it a nuisance to follow—or it just became too difficult to pass up a chocolate milk shake and a cheeseburger. Or they met a nice boy or girl who loved nothing more than to cook them roast chicken with lots of mashed potatoes.

Q: My daughter is fourteen months old and she doesn't walk yet, in fact she doesn't even pull herself up. The pediatric neurologist says that my child has hypotonia (lack of muscle tone), and has scheduled her for an MRI.

Our family is vegetarian, but we are not vegans. We eat dairy products. The baby loves dairy and eats a lot of it. The neurologist said we have to start immediately feeding the baby meat, because the fatty acids in meat help to create the myelin that she's missing. My pediatrician said that she's never heard of this.

I've been a vegetarian for fifteen years, but I'd feed my baby a steak tonight if I thought it would help her. What do you think?

A: Since she's not walking at fourteen months, your baby is a little late, but she is still on the curve. But, as you know, not pulling herself up by now is a sign that she is delayed in one of the normal markers of growth.

I doubt very much that being a vegetarian is part of your little girl's problem. I assiduously follow the literature on vegetarianism because of my interest in it, and I've never heard of this.

It is true that fatty acids are necessary for the growth of nerves, but, to my knowledge, the fatty acids in dairy products are similar to the fatty acids in meat. Dairy products contain plenty of complete proteins.

Health-conscious parents sometimes do their children the disservice of feeding them low-fat diets. Among those children, we do find a higher than normal rate of inadequate nutrition. Kids need fat.

Vegans do sometimes have protein and certain vitamin B12 deficiencies. But even among vegans that happens rarely, and when it does, it doesn't cause hypotonia.

I am not eliminating the possibility that your baby's diet could be deficient; a child may have protein or calorie malnutrition, but because she eats a lot of vegetables her folks assume she's healthy.

In general, though, doctors are not very knowledgeable on the finer points of nutrition. I advise you to consult with a registered dietitian. Talk to him or her about the type and amount of food that your baby eats, just to be sure she isn't missing any vital nutrients. Since she is a lacto-ovo vegetarian, I doubt that she is.

In the meantime, you must, of course, follow through with the neurological evaluations to get to the bottom of this.

Q: I'm seventy-five, and I'm suffering from lumbar pain in my lower back and hips, so I knew I had to lose weight, among other things, and get some exercise. For the past ninety days, I've had just one meal a day at noon—anything I want, vegetables, meat, even a little candy sometimes. Then I eat nothing else for another twenty-four hours, and only drink coffee. I've lost twenty-six pounds in ninety days. Is this an effective way to lose weight?

A: I eat only one meal a day and I can do that fairly easily. I don't think people through the centuries always sat down and said oh, it's lunchtime, and ate by the clock, like we do. And I think one good meal a day has probably satisfied people in the past, while others found it difficult. The less you have to think about what you eat, the more likely you are to stick to a diet and lose weight.

If you've found a regimen that is easier than worrying at each particular meal about what you should and shouldn't eat, then more power to you. Just make sure to make that one meal count—try to get in all your servings of fruits and vegetables. Also, be careful not to lose more weight that you need

DID YOU KNOW?
KNOW YOUR COW!

The leanest cuts of the cow are the parts that get the most exercise when the animal moves. The lean cuts also have more protein, vitamins, and minerals, because there are more nutrients in muscle than in fat. If your steak does have fat on it, trim it before you cook it, not afterwards: One study at Texas A & M University found that a pre-trimmed strip steak had 19 percent less fat than one that was trimmed of its fat after broiling.

DID YOU KNOW?
TOO MUCH VITAMIN A IS NOT A GOOD THING

Too often, people assume that you can't get too much of a good thing. Wrong. Consuming a lot of fat-soluble vitamins, like D and A, for instance, can make you very sick. In addition, too much vitamin A can cause headaches, blurred vision, vomiting, and liver and bone problems. A Swedish study in 2003 confirmed that those with the highest levels of vitamin A in their blood are more likely to break a bone in old age. Vitamin A is found in fish liver oil, liver, kidneys, and milk, and sometimes it is added to dairy products. It is an important vitamin for good health, but excessive consumption (25,000–50,000 international units (IU) per day or more) is not a good thing. The Recommended Daily Intake is 5,000 IU.

to. Now, true confessions: If I'm on a cruise or other family vacation, and I'm confronted with three meals a day—or a buffet—I can pack it away with the best of 'em.

Q: I've been on Xenical for ten months. I've lost more than fifty pounds and the side effects aren't as bad as everyone says they are. I think it has been effective for me as behavior modification. How long can I safely stay on it?

A: You are right on target. If taking Xenical results in weight loss, it is due to its behavior modification function. Xenical is a prescription drug that blocks the absorption of fat, but only to a certain degree. Double blind studies have shown that it does help people to lose some weight, but not a lot.

In other words, if you've lost fifty pounds, it's because you've stuck to an appropriate diet, and avoiding the side effects of Xenical is what kept you on the diet. If you take Xenical and try to get away with eating a lot of fat, you may pay for it with an oily discharge and fecal incontinence. So Xenical kind of forces you to be an honest dieter in the way Antabuse keeps alcoholics off the sauce—it makes them sick if they drink.

We don't know what the long-term effects of Xenical are, but it is not intended for long-term use. One concern is that along with flushing fat from the body, Xenical may also flush fat-soluble vitamins and nutrients. You might develop deficiencies of vitamin A, E, D, or K. So I advise you to take those vitamins, even though the Xenical may flush the pills out, too.

The threat of vitamin loss is one reason you can't stay on this drug forever. The other is that at some point you have to face the fact that the way to maintain the weight you want is to create healthy eating habits and stick to them for life. I think that time is now.

You've already lost fifty pounds because you stuck with your diet, not because of the Xenical or an appetite suppressant. So maybe you don't need the stuff anymore. Talk to your doctor about the next steps.

Q: I'm having some problems losing weight. I gave birth to my second child about ten months ago, and I can't lose the last twenty pounds I put on during the pregnancy. I've been on a 1,000-calorie diet and exercising for months, and out of desperation, I just recently lowered my calorie intake to about 500 a day. How harmful is it to dip down to that level? I am so frustrated.

A: You're headed down the wrong path! If, miraculously, you can stick to a 500-calorie-a-day diet and you lose your weight, what are you going to do then? When you go on a severe diet like this, what adjustments do you think your body is going to make? It's going to figure, "I'm going to lay down fat more efficiently for every calorie that she's eating because this woman may starve to death and she will need this fat for fuel." So your body may be fighting you.

Experts on obesity and dieting will tell you that if you manage to lose weight with this approach, you're going to gain it right back, because you can't starve yourself forever. They will tell you that slowly and gradually is the way to win the race. If you eat a little more, you may find you are losing weight more easily. This will happen more slowly, but more permanently. And you are looking for a permanent solution.

I would encourage you to keep exercising, because fitness is an important concept, regardless of weight. And time is a factor here. After you've had a baby, there is a change in metabolism, and it takes six months to a year for things to settle. Go back to eating between 1,000 and 1,200 calories, continue to exercise, and reestablish your eating patterns.

One piece of research that might help you over the long term has to do with portions. Eating the same portion size, or volume, of food each day is the key to feeling full, according to nutritionists at Penn State University. Their study found that both obese and lean women were able to reduce their average intake by 450 calories a day by eating a hearty helping of a low-energy meal.

While previous studies have found that fat is what satisfies us, this study found that the fat content of a meal didn't have much influence on how full a person felt after eating. The portion size, or volume, was the key to being satisfied. An example of low-energy food could be entrees that substitute vegetables and fruits for bread, pasta, or other grain products and that use low-fat versions of high-fat ingredients. This method of caloric reduction can result in losing about a pound a week.

It makes sense to me that if you consume less, like most diet plans advocate, you'll remain hungry, and it will be hard to stick to an eating routine. However, if you eat the same bulk but fewer calories by substituting low-energy food, you'll feel full and lose weight, too.

Food Allergies, Intolerances, and Interactions

Q: I have had several sinus infections and colds in the past year, but nothing serious. A vegetarian I work with has a theory about mucus-forming and non-mucus-forming foods. Whenever I come back from lunch with frozen yogurt, she tells me that I'm going to continue to have the cold if I continue to have dairy products. She says they will cause me to form more mucus, and I'll never get rid of the infection. What do you think about that?

QUIZ

Which of these foods has the most calcium in an eight-ounce portion?
A) skim milk   B) nonfat plain yogurt   C) low–fat plain yogurt
D) whole milk
(B: *nonfat plain yogurt, with 452 mg; whole milk has the least, with 291 mg.*)

A: Way back in the 1920s, Arnold Ehret wrote a book called the *Mucusless Diet Healing System*, in which he put forth the idea that dairy products make mucus and cause colds. Well, this caught on big and has not let go. One reason for the tenacity is that drinking a big, ol' glass of milk does leave a mucusy feeling in the mouth. However, there is no truth to Ehret's theory.

Mucus is produced by cells that line the nose and throat, and it has nothing to do with drinking milk fat or eating dairy products. Ear, nose, and throat doctors were asked about this so frequently that they decided to do a study to finally put it to rest. Researchers loaded people up with milk and cheese, and measured mucus flow rates. They found that a dairy diet didn't make a lick of a difference.

Q: I keep hearing the term "lactose intolerant," and I also keep seeing food products marked "no dairy." Can you explain what all this means? By the way, my sister was having some digestive problems—cramps, diarrhea—and her internist told her to stop eating dairy for five days. Is this all related?

A: Lactose intolerance is inherited and fairly common. It means you don't have a lot of the enzyme lactase, which breaks down lactose, which is a sugar commonly found in dairy products. The result can be cramping, diarrhea, and gas, but the diagnosis is often missed by doctors.

The internist gave your sister good advice, because if you stop eating dairy for a few days, and the symptoms go away, then it's either a lactose intolerance or an allergy to milk and milk products.

People who are lactose intolerant can tolerate some dairy, especially yogurt, which is partially digested. There are also products that will help your intestines digest lactose with varied success, depending on how much lactase you have in your body.

Q: What's this about grapefruit affecting medicines I take? I never thought I'd see the day that eating fruit was a problem.

A: The problem with grapefruit is that it can interfere with an enzyme in your intestines that normally breaks down drugs as they enter the bloodstream. If that happens, more drugs can enter your blood and you can wind up with a higher level than you were supposed to have. The opposite reaction is also a problem; other mechanisms have been discovered with grapefruit juice where it interferes with the absorption of certain drugs. Most commonly though, the juice raises the drug level.

This interaction is not usually of much consequence unless you are taking certain critical medications—for instance, the drug level of a heart medication should be exactly what your physician prescribed. In general, doctors are aware of this problem and will advise you to avoid grapefruit juice when they write the prescription.

Grapefruit juice is otherwise an extremely healthy beverage, and I would hate to see people stop drinking it because of this fear. When in doubt, talk to your physician or pharmacist.

Q: **My two-year-old is allergic to milk, so I give him cereal and juice with added calcium carbonate. Now I'm worried about the report about lead in calcium. What should I do?**

A: You don't need to be concerned. Natural sources of calcium, like limestone and oyster shells, are likely to have higher levels of lead than are other sources of calcium. But that's not what is added to foods like cereal and juice.

A Tufts University report estimates that Americans take in five or six micrograms of lead each day. Although no safe level of lead has ever been established, there isn't a human being on the face of this earth who isn't absorbing some lead.

It is a matter of degree. Too much of anything can kill us, and that includes toxic elements. The body is able to handle small amounts.

Q: **I grew up in the East, eating Maine lobster all of my life. I'm fifty-five now. A month ago, I went to a local California restaurant and had a Maine lobster, went to sleep, and, about twelve hours later, woke up itching. My face and eyes were swollen, too, and I was having a difficult time breathing. I took a Benadryl, and it went away in about forty-five minutes. I figured that was the end of it.**

QUIZ

Which food is most likely to aggravate an ulcer?
A) garlic   B) orange juice   C) liver   D) milk
E) chili peppers
(D: milk.)

Four days ago, I went to a sushi buffet and had a tiny piece of Maine lobster. The next morning, about twenty hours later, I had the same reaction. Can you become allergic to a food that was once no problem for you?

A: You can develop an allergy at any point in your life. But you can't develop an allergy the first time you're exposed to a food. As for your situation, you are not alone. Allergies to lobster and shellfish are among the most common of all food allergies. More importantly, you could die from this, so no more taking Benadryl and waiting to see what happens.

Also, you've got to be very careful, because you might also have a cross-reaction to other kinds of critters in this food family. It may be that you are allergic just to lobster, and it may be just species-specific, i.e. Maine lobster, but it's possible you now have allergies to shrimp and other shellfish.

See an allergist, because these things can slowly get worse, or suddenly become worse out of the blue. When you see the allergist, ask whether you should be carrying an EPI pen (a preloaded syringe of adrenaline or epinephrine). It can save your life.

As for the breathing problem, that's a sign of anaphylaxis. It would feel as if your throat is closing, and that could result in difficulty in getting your breath, as opposed to breathing more rapidly. If that happens again, head straight for an emergency room.

Q: My wife gives our kids a glass of milk to drink with their burgers or meat loaf. I don't think she should do this. I went to catering school a few years ago, and we were told that meat and milk do not go together. You should drink water with meat, right?

A: Is it possible you went to a kosher catering school? Kosher laws forbid the combination of meat and milk, and, as a religious practice, observant Jews avoid

---

QUIZ

What do chewing gum, carbonated sodas, poorly fitting dentures, and broccoli have in common?
A) bad breath   B) mild headaches   C) tension in the jaw
D) intestinal gas
(D: intestinal gas.)

that combination by keeping two sets of dishes: one set for meat and another set for dairy products.

I know of no physiological problem that occurs when you combine beef and milk. Certainly chefs put cream sauces on meat, and what about eating mashed potatoes with a steak?

These combinations are rich, and they do double your saturated fats, which isn't a healthy way to eat on a regular basis. But there's nothing wrong with drinking a glass of milk with a hamburger.

Q: I have a one-month-old son. I've been a vegetarian for about eleven years, and I'm breast-feeding him. I saw a news report that women who consume peanuts and peanut butter while breast-feeding put their children at risk for peanut allergies. Is that true?

A: Yes. What we've found is that the peanut allergin shows up in the breast milk. We are assuming that could increase the risks for peanut allergies, but we're not quite sure how all that works. In general, there has not been a lot of research on how a breast-fed baby is affected by its mother's diet.

We do know a baby can react to the effects of garlic and alcohol consumed by the mother. We've seen that some babies don't like these things, and they just nurse less often and consume less milk.

We also know that some vegetable proteins can wind up fairly intact in the breast milk, which is not exactly the way it's supposed to work, because your system is supposed to break down all protein into little amino acids, and that removes essentially the signature of the original substance. It would be like tearing down a beautiful cathedral made of bricks. Later, if you pick up a brick, you don't know where that brick came from, whether it came from a slum or a cathedral. And the same goes for amino acids; your body can't tell where they came from. But it turns out that clumps of protein in peanuts, and maybe even a lot of other substances, can get through.

They do not give out peanuts or peanut butter in nursery schools any longer, because some kids have a severe allergy to peanuts. One study cited a case where kids were playing basketball, and one had eaten a peanut butter and jelly sandwich before playing. He took the basketball and threw it to another kid, and, evidently, there was enough peanut on the basketball that the other kid who caught the basketball had a reaction. That's how little it takes.

But where do we draw the line for new moms, since there are all kinds of food allergies? Do we just ban all these foods during breast-feeding? When toddlers and infants take these substances, do they develop the allergies? We don't know.

We have plenty of indications about kids and allergies that actually work in an "opposite" way. For example, kids who grow up where there are more infections and more dirt around the house have fewer allergies than kids who grow up in a more sterile environment.

The immune system is a complex miracle, and it's very difficult to understand. It turns itself on and it turns itself off in the face of what seems to be similar kinds of insults. So, I don't have a clear-cut answer for you about peanuts. Before you make any radical changes in your diet, talk to your doctor.

Sugar and Other Sweeteners

Q: My friend is constantly nagging me about all the risks of drinking diet sodas. Every time I have one in my hand, he starts running through a litany of dangers, some of them very scary. Should I be worried?

A: To paraphrase one of my favorite Winston Churchill quotes, a lie gets halfway around the world before the truth even gets a chance to get its pants on. With the Internet today, misinformation can spread so rapidly that no one has the resources to counter it.

The scary report about aspartame is one of the most famous of a crop of scary e-mail notices that circulated around the world and continue to pop up years after they were created. The one about diet soda was completely phony—an urban myth. The names of the doctors and researchers and everything quoted in that article is untrue, yet even today there are folks who think diet sodas are going to kill us.

I'm not telling you that diet sodas are health foods, but you have nothing to worry about. If you want additional information to show your friend, check out *www.urbanlegends.com,* where you'll find a complete analysis of this hoax.

Q: I love sugar, but I feel very guilty about this pleasure. I'm thirty-five, a physically healthy person, and I'm sensible about sugar when it comes to my kids. Am I being stupid to enjoy this pleasure, usually in my coffee and in the sweets I eat?

A: Myths that sugar is fattening or causes hyperactivity in kids have led to the growing popularity of artificial sweeteners for use in everything from drinks to baked goods.

Personally, I like sugar, which only has four calories per gram, or about fourteen calories per teaspoon. (Fat, by comparison, has nine calories per gram.) And sugar certainly isn't the only reason people are fat. You put on pounds when you eat more calories than you burn, no matter what you eat. Sugar can't be blamed for this, but eating a lot of food—and drinking a lot of sugary, carbonated beverages—and being inactive can certainly cause obesity. The message is to eat less and exercise more.

Actually, using artificial sweeteners backfires for many people, because they subconsciously end up eating more "low-calorie" or "low-fat" desserts and other foods made with sugar substitutes. But those foods still have calories.

Contrary to some beliefs, you cannot become addicted to sugar, it doesn't cause hypoglycemia, it doesn't give you quick energy, and it doesn't cause heart disease or diabetes. Another myth is that sugar causes kids to become hyperactive. Most of the time people notice this at birthday parties and during holidays, when the kids are already excited; it has nothing to do with eating sweets.

And, by the way, there is no truth to the myth that some sugars are healthier than others. Brown sugar, white sugar, and honey all go into your bloodstream the same way.

DID YOU KNOW?
WHEN FREE DOESN'T MEAN FREE

According to Food and Drug Administration regulations, food packagers can use the word "free"—as in "fat-free," "sugar-free," or "calorie-free"—even when that's not exactly the case. The amounts are small, but they're there. Something labeled "calorie-free" must have less than five calories per serving. With fat and sugar, the cutoff is half of one gram—each serving must have less than a half-gram to use that label. So, if you're counting fat grams, those fat-free cookies could be a bigger problem than you think.

Sugar is implicated in tooth decay, but this doesn't come so much from white sugar as from foods and drinks that break down into sugar in the body. Fruit juices and sticky foods that are adhesive and "stick" to the teeth are the worst culprits for erosion.

There have been some health scares associated with artificial sweeteners, such as the unfounded fears generated when saccharin (Sweet'N Low) was found to cause cancer in rats in 1977. Aspartame also had a flurry of unfounded urban rumors aimed at it, but exhaustive studies have shown it to be safe and effective except in cases of a rare genetic disease called PKU or phenylketonuria.

Sugar alcohols are used in chewing gums, because they don't raise blood sugar levels and don't promote tooth decay. One of these, xylitol, which is made from the bark of birch trees, may actually prevent cavities, but there can be side effects, such as bloating and diarrhea.

Sugar's okay with me, but whether you prefer a substitute or not, moderation is the key to making sweet tastes a healthy part of your eating pleasure.

Q: I've recently eliminated refined sugar from my diet. Are there any side effects or dangers associated with stevia?

A: Stevia is an herbal sweetener. It comes from a shrub that is native to Paraguay called *stevia rebaundiana*. It tastes a little like licorice and is sweeter than sucrose. If you like the taste and don't mind the cost, I have no problem with you using it as a sweetener.

I am not aware of it causing any side effects. If you like a lot of sweet things, and if you're looking for a substitute, I think stevia would be fine. Personally, taste is a big factor when choosing what foods to eat. I don't like the taste of most artificial sweeteners, so I use real sugar, but I don't eat a lot of it.

What is surprising to many people is that dried fruits are worse for you

---

QUIZ

Which of these foods is the largest single source of sugar per serving?
A) ice cream   B) Frosted Flakes cereal   C) chocolate cake
D) candy bar   E) carbonated soda
(E: carbonated soda, with 10 to 12 teaspoons per can.)

than refined sugar when it comes to dental decay. But I think it's a mistake for people to get too obsessive about eating the "right thing," because being healthy is a lifestyle—you just need to be informed about what you are putting in your body. I would never suggest that we stop eating dried fruit.

Unfortunately some people are becoming seriously stressed about food issues, and that stress can be more dangerous for them than every little additive and every little problem they see in our food supply. Our food supply is the best in the world. Sure it can be improved, but it's our choices that louse it up.

Q: I've heard that corn syrup is not good for me—not good for my brain and not good for my liver. Should I make sure that my kids don't eat it?

A: Corn syrup (fructose) is a naturally occurring sugar in fruits. It is used by manufacturers instead of cane or beet sugar (refined sugar) because it's cheaper.

We've gone back and forth on whether fructose is better for you than regular sugar, because of questions about how the body handles large amounts of it. But it's definitely not something that should make you fearful.

What you should watch is your children's overall consumption of sugary foods. When your kids drink or eat a lot of sugary stuff, they're getting calories but nothing else—no minerals, no vitamins, no other foodstuff. So you want to make sure your kids eat more of the foods that will give them all the nutrients they need. Keep the sugar to a minimum.

Cooking Methods and Cooking Dangers

Q: I have two questions about bacterial contamination of meat. Does defrosting meat in the microwave kill bacteria like E. coli and salmonella?

QUIZ

Which sweet has more fat?
A) one chocolate-frosted doughnut   B) two chocolate truffles
C) two milk-chocolate candy bars (6 oz each)
(A: doughnut, 21 g; the candy bars have the least, 10 g.)

And does produce get contaminated when the supermarket clerk handles packages of meat and then touches your vegetables?

A: Cooking meat to the proper temperature—most pathogens die between 140 and 160 degrees—is what kills the E. coli and salmonella bacteria. If you like your steak medium-rare, you are playing Russian roulette, since that temperature is usually about 145 degrees.

Defrosting in a microwave is not unsafe, but the defrosting will not kill the bacteria. It is the temperature of the cooked meat that matters. And some microwaves do not heat evenly, which is why the food should revolve on a carousel, and should also be rotated a couple of times. Also, take the meat's temperature from a couple of different places. I know of a case of trichinosis that resulted from a cold spot in some cooked pork.

If you were to take a package of frozen contaminated meat, defrost it, and cook it until it is rare, the germs could certainly survive and be dangerous. The freezing and defrosting don't kill all germs. When frozen, a lot of critters go into a state of suspended animation, and thawing wakes them up. Germs can thrive at temperatures between 40 and 140 degrees, so this is a danger zone.

Meat packing rules require it to be wrapped so that it isn't touched and its juices stay inside the package, but we all know this isn't perfect. It is possible that meat could contaminate your produce.

Washing and separation are good rules to follow for food preparation. Fruits and vegetables, your hands, and your utensils should always be washed thoroughly—but use only water when washing the fruits and vegetables.

You are asking for trouble if the knife you use to cut chicken is the knife you use to chop lettuce, without washing it in soapy, hot water before reusing. The chicken will be safe if it's cooked to the right temperature—at least 165 degrees, but the USDA recommends 180 degrees for a whole chicken—but you're not going to cook the lettuce. For other meat temperatures, check out *www.foodsafety.gov*. And if you don't have a meat thermometer, buy one; it will help you cook your meat correctly.

Q: I like meat that is well cooked; charred if possible. In other words, I always take the end of a roast. Yet, I've heard this can be carcinogenic. Is this true? I'm confused because I also saw on public television how monkeys had used abandoned charcoal briquettes to treat their stomachaches. How does this square with the idea that anything charred is carcinogenic?

A: First, let's start with the monkeys. I had a chance to visit a chimpanzee reserve called Mahale, in Tanzania. It's the finest place in the world to see wild chimpanzees. We happened to be walking around with a guy who is the world's expert on one aspect of your question, which is primates practicing medicine. He has observed primates with stomachaches getting certain leaves and administering these leaves to cure stomach problems. We're not exactly sure how it works; it might be just an additional dose of fiber that induces the body to purge and expel the stuff, but either way, we have seen this.

Charcoal, as you probably know, is given in emergency rooms in cases of poisoning. You can buy it at health-food stores or drugstores for lots of stuff, including intestinal gas. This is known as activated charcoal, and it has the capacity to absorb toxic materials to its surface. But activated charcoal is a little different from charcoal used for cooking. Activated charcoal has a huge surface area in order to absorb the toxic materials, whereas regular charcoal isn't that absorbent. On the other hand, I don't doubt that the monkeys could be getting some benefit from regular charcoal. However, no one should even consider dipping into the grill for a quick home remedy.

Charred meat is a different subject. Charcoal is simply carbon atoms, whereas charred meat may have residues that are produced by high heat on the meat and the fat. The substance that's released, heterocyclic amine, is associated with cancers in mammals. This is why every year you hear the warnings about barbecuing. There was at least one study linking breast cancer to well-done meat. The study concluded that the more well done you like your meat, the higher your chances of possibly developing cancer. And, of course, the rarer you like it, the greater the possibility of death by salmonella or E. coli.

Yet these things are very difficult to prove in human systems. In other words, you can take the substances produced in charred meat and give high amounts of similar molecules to animals and increase the rate of cancer. However, you should keep in mind that the animals used for such research are usually genetically "preprogrammed" to be at a higher risk of developing cancer anyway.

The charcoal that remains after you thoroughly burn wood is different from the charred stuff that's a result of the heating of fat molecules and protein molecules that still retains a complex molecular structure.

But the bigger issue is this whole idea of "moral nutrition": that there are certain foods out there that will kill you, and there are certain foods that will help you live to be a hundred.

It's just not that way. Modern nutritional research is saying now that you should be able to eat anything you want as long as it's balanced and in moderation. The sum total of what you're eating is really what's important—the sum total of the calories seems to be important, not the amount of fat, protein, or carbohydrate. And that's the most recent trend that's come down in nutrition. So charred meat once in a while isn't going to kill you.

Q: I've heard that spinach, collards, and turnip greens contain a variety of beta-carotenes. I understand that this is important for the eyes. I'm sixty-four and have been trying to eat spinach every day to make up for all the years I didn't eat much of it. But then I told a neighbor that spinach needed to be cooked in order for the body to absorb and utilize the calcium in it. She exploded and said no, cooking vegetables destroys the nutrients. Who's right?

A: This is a curious and somewhat confusing topic. Your neighbor's viewpoint dates back to before World War II, when we thought that boiling vegetables removes all nutrients. Now we know that, in some cases, raw fruits and vegetables are not digested as well as after they are cooked, and cooking increases the nutrient availability of some foods. I would not make any food choice based upon whether it's raw or cooked. I eat my fruits and vegetables the way I like them.

Tomatoes are a good example. Cooked, as in spaghetti sauce and other sauces, they have more lycopene, a nutrient that, among other things, can be important for men's prostates. That doesn't mean you shouldn't eat fresh tomatoes. It's just one of those little facts that's important to know to get people to mellow out about this.

When you boil food, sometimes you lower the nutrient content and sometimes you don't. Microwaving is a good alternative for vegetables in order to preserve nutrients. And, despite all the good things we've heard about "fresh," tomatoes and pumpkins are two foods that have more value in their canned form. Incredible, isn't it?

But, overall, the differences between raw and cooked vegetables are very minor. I like fresh spinach in a salad. While I know that fresh spinach may inhibit my absorption of the calcium in the spinach, most of us are not depending on that as our sole source of calcium. Rather than splitting hairs, it makes more sense to be moderate about these things.

But you are way ahead of the class just by eating vegetables at all. That's a much more important issue than how they are cooked.

Water, Water, and More Water

Q: I have a very hard time drinking eight glasses of water a day, even though I have a water bottle near my desk most of the time. How important is this?

A: This is a more complex subject than you might think, because food provides our body with a lot of water, and many of us don't realize that.

I have never liked specific rules, such as "You must drink eight glasses of water per day to be healthy," and there's a study from Tufts University that challenges that rule. Using a small group of women, the researchers measured each drop they took in and each drop they eliminated, and found that the water, juice, and decaffeinated beverages they consumed averaged the recommended eight cups per day.

This study also found that women met almost 40 percent of their water needs just with food. And a similar study done recently at the University of Nebraska Medical Center confirmed the hydration value of both food and nonwater beverages.

Foods contain a lot of water; some are more than half water. Vegetables are about 95 percent water, sirloin steak is 60 percent water, a slice of white bread is 37 percent water.

That said, there are "exceptions," and they are important. Alcohol doesn't count when you consider water consumption, and people who exercise heavily and sweat a lot, plus anyone who is ill—especially with fever, vomiting, or diarrhea—should drink extra water. People older than seventy can be dehydrated without feeling thirsty, so they should drink a lot whether or not they feel a need.

Since most of us don't get enough fruits and vegetables, it makes sense to supplement with some extra glasses of liquid. And, for those of us concerned

---

QUIZ

Which substance has the most calories?
A) olive oil   B) canola oil   C) lard   D) butter
E) all are equal
(E: all are equal.)

about eating too much food, there's an additional incentive: Another study found that if you drink a couple of glasses of water just before you eat, you will eat less.

Q: We had a reverse-osmosis water purifier installed under our sink, because our well water has too much iron in it. The purifier connects to our refrigerator, too, so the ice cubes are made from purified water. The system works beautifully. All our guests say the water tastes wonderful. But a few months ago I heard that reverse osmosis creates lead in the water. Is that true? How can I find out?

A: Reverse osmosis is the best method of purification for getting rid of almost all minerals. It's the most effective, but it's also the most technological, it requires some equipment and energy, and it wastes water.

If there were a problem with lead in post-filtered water, the source of it would be from the pipes. If the water sits for a time in pipes that contain lead, or the pipe joints are soldered with lead, the water would pick that up. If your pipes have no lead, or if the water is flowing frequently, you're probably not getting any lead in your water.

A laboratory will test the water for you. You can find listings in the phone book, on the Internet, or by calling your local health department.

Q: I'm traveling overseas to a country that doesn't have safe water. I don't want to hassle with bottled water and lug it around. Are water filters safe?

A: In the jungles and wilderness areas, the waterborne parasite *Giardia* is a common threat, and most filters can trap it. In general, travel filters remove parasites and bacteria—and the ones with charcoal filters remove toxic chemicals, too. But in towns and urban areas, viruses are a common foe, and most travel filters won't handle those. The Centers for Disease Control recommends that travelers who carry microstrainer filters and are concerned about viruses should disinfect the water with iodine or chlorine after filtration.

Waterborne illnesses are a very real and rampant danger, so you must take all precautions. I have traveled in many parts of the world, and I always find bottled water. If you can't boil it, you just may have to bite the bullet and buy a few bottles.

Q: Frequent urination is driving me crazy. Take yesterday, for example. About an hour before I picked up my daughter from school, I was driving

around doing errands and I was drinking from my water bottle. I was at her school at three-thirty, and I desperately sought and used the bathroom. At four-thirty, I was in the same fix. Just thirty minutes later, I peed again, a lot. What's wrong?

A: That amount of urination is really not off the charts. You just told me what caused the urgency, driving around drinking a lot of water.

The more we drink, the more we eliminate. The body is very, very smart. It cues us when we need to drink, and it regulates itself. If we drink too much, we pee a lot. If we drink too little, it starts to hold onto the fluid. Our kidneys know how to do this.

The easy way to gauge if you are taking in the right amount of water is to look at the color of your urine. If it's colorless you are drinking too much. If it's a deeper yellow, you are not drinking enough.

Other common medical causes of frequent urination are diabetes, overactive bladders, bladder infection, and prostate problems. From the pattern you described, I don't think you have either disease, but anyone who urinates frequently should have a test for diabetes. A bladder infection would not produce the hearty stream that you described. It's more like squirt, squirt.

Q: My wife's health magazine says that adding ice to your water will burn calories. Is there any truth to that?

A: The work your body does to raise the temperature of the icy water will burn calories, but not enough to make any difference. This energy expenditure falls under the heading of silly little things that burn calories, like finger tapping, pencil gnawing, and general fidgeting. And, of course, coffee speeds us up a little and burns some calories there. None of this adds up to a sizable amount.

Kids and Food

Q: I have two children; one doesn't eat much of anything and the other eats a lot of not such good stuff. I try to find foods with nutritional additives, but is there any benefit to that? If they eat bread with added calcium or added iron, do they benefit in the long run?

A: We do use nutritional supplements, so to speak, in many different foods, mostly because we think we have taken out the good stuff.

White bread is often fortified, because the process used to make white breads takes out a lot of the naturally occurring vitamins, and so the manufac-turers put them back in.

Iron supplementation of many foods is fairly common, and yet we're afraid we're giving people too much iron; there are a lot of kids getting too much iron. Iron can be toxic to our bodies, and too much of it can kill children. So iron fortification is something we're questioning.

We're now adding folic acid to foods, because of the preventative effect in spina bifida and certain other birth defects. And we add fluoride to water.

Remember, getting kids to eat good foods requires persistence. I once read that you have to present a new food to a child anywhere from five to fifteen times before they accept it.

Also, you've got to be eating the same thing yourself. You can't expect to sit down to a dinner and serve yourself one thing and serve your kids something else.

When you give them something, make it count. If you're going to feed a child a piece a bread, a good piece of whole wheat bread will be better for them than the other kind, but ultimately, at the end of the day, what really matters is total daily consumption.

While food fortification can be positive, there are occasional circumstances where you want to avoid them. For example, calcium supplementation in orange juice can block the absorption of some antibiotics the way milk does. And down the line, you don't want to think that fortification will take care of everything. If you've got yourself finicky eaters, you have to deal with that straight on, because it will come back to haunt you when they get older. And if you have a child eating too much junk, you've got to get some of that out of his/her diet sooner rather than later.

Q: My grandchild is always asking for foods that we've never served in our house. I suspect that television is the culprit. Should I be worried?

A: You only need to worry when she'll *only* eat what she sees on TV. But you are right about the influence.

In a study of preschool children, researchers found that "even brief exposure to televised food commercials can influence preschool children's food preferences." It makes sense, doesn't it?

This study, according to the *Journal of the American Dietetic Association*, looked at forty-six children ages two to six in Northern California. Videos included animated shorts and commercials for "popular brands of juice, doughnuts, sandwich bread, remote-control toy cars, breakfast cereal, snack cake, fast-food chicken, and candy."

Researchers concluded that "nutritionists and health educators should advise parents to limit their preschooler's exposure to advertisements. Furthermore, advocates should raise public policy issues, given the recent epidemic of childhood obesity. . . . Children exposed to videotape with imbedded commercials were significantly more likely to choose the advertised items than children who saw the same videotape without commercials."

I watch commercials all the time. If you ask me what they were about, sometimes I can remember, and sometimes I can't. Children are much more easily influenced, and we as parents must do our part.

Q: My husband and I were both overweight as children, and we are now obese adults. I just had twins—a girl and a boy. What steps can we take to make sure our children don't become fat kids and suffer like we did?

A: Planning a healthy lifestyle for your babies in their infancy is close to a guarantee of success. Once parents find themselves with a very obese nine-year-old on their hands, they face a tremendous struggle to help that child undo many bad habits.

It is not soda or candy or any one thing that causes overweight children; it is the combination of inactivity and overeating. It simply comes down to taking in more calories than they burn.

As the father of a bunch of kids, I promise that if you feed them the right stuff from the beginning, you're set for life. You're going to have to set an example, too. If you want your kids to eat vegetables, you've got to eat them yourselves.

Remember, bad food decisions are made not in the kitchen, but at the grocery store. If you don't bring cookies into the house, you won't be burdened with keeping the kids away from them.

Keep your children active by playing with them. Running around outdoors, playing catch, bicycling, and swimming should be routine to them.

Good health is not determined by body weight alone, and body weight is not solely determined by food. Genetics play a crucial role, and be prepared to find genetic differences between your twins.

Of course, you need to love and support your children no matter what their size, but, as you know all too well, they won't be able to count on positive responses from other people if they are overweight.

See more on kids and food in chapter 5.

Food and Cholesterol

Q: **As a child, I drank a glass of orange juice every morning, and my mother was a food snob who refused to consider some of those powdered fruit drinks that other families had for breakfast. Was that just the result of a great marketing effort, or is this a particularly valuable part of our diet?**

A: The experts tell us to eat at least five servings of fruits and vegetables every day, and it seems that every day they come out with a new study that proves them right. Now they are reporting that orange juice, which is rich in vitamin C and flavonoids, actually raises HDL levels. HDL is the good cholesterol that we all want more of.

In a recent study, twenty-five people with high cholesterol gradually introduced one, two, and then three cups of orange juice into their diets. The one- and two-cup doses did not affect cholesterol, but at the maximum amount, the participants' HDL cholesterol level went up by 21 percent. In previous research on animals, LDL cholesterol—the bad kind—was reduced in animals whose drinking water was replaced with orange juice or grapefruit juice.

Q: I'm thirty-six years old, exercise moderately, and eat a high-fiber diet with very little red meat. So, I was shocked to be diagnosed with high cholesterol. It was 224. What would you do, if this was you?

A: If you are eating well and exercising correctly, I recommend that you don't worry about this. First of all, your cholesterol is not much above normal. Second, one test is inconclusive. If you are retested, you are likely to get a different result. And finally, overall health is not measured by one factor.

Hundreds, possibly thousands, of separate risk factors combine and contribute to our quality of health, and to when and how we die. Cholesterol is one important factor, but you will find people who are ninety years old living with cholesterol levels higher than yours. And you'll find a high percentage of hospitalized heart patients who have low or normal cholesterol levels.

The total cholesterol count is not as important as are the relative ratios of the LDL and HDL. Also, a family history of heart disease can predispose an individual to high-cholesterol syndromes that are independent of his/her lifestyle.

In my first book, *Eat, Drink, and Be Merry*, one of the most important messages is that we shouldn't let these isolated facts throw us off course. If you're doing what's right for your body, one test will not seal your fate.

Q: You say it's good to eat nuts, but my cholesterol is 212. I haven't had any nuts for about four months now. Can I ever eat them again?

A: You've got it backwards. For instance, we think that almond consumption is one of the reasons that people who live in the Mediterranean areas of the world have less heart disease. And a recent study published on nut consumption and heart disease concluded that the fatty acids in nuts help lower cardiovascular risk.

QUIZ

Which juice has the most iron?
A) orange   B) prune   C) carrot   D) lime
(B: prune; one cup has 30 percent RDA for men, 17 percent for premenopausal women.)

Your cholesterol is not that high, especially considering the most recent guidelines on cholesterol: 200 mg of total cholesterol is desirable, above 240 is considered high.

There is no cholesterol in nuts. Cholesterol is found in animal products, dairy, and meat.

Q: I've heard that garlic does a good job of lowering cholesterol and thinning the blood, but recently I read this isn't true. Is bad breath the only thing I'm getting from garlic?

A: Garlic certainly doesn't do any harm, but it's not lowering cholesterol as much as we once hoped. The reports on its benefits are mixed. Some tests have shown garlic thins the blood, but changes in blood factors do not automatically result in healthier human beings.

People who eat a lot of garlic may be more likely to eat a Mediterranean diet, more likely to eat tomatoes and green vegetables. So garlic eaters' reputations for good health may be due to overall healthier eating.

If I had heart disease, I wouldn't rely on garlic. The first thing to be done is to make some changes in diet and start an exercise program.

By the way, I can't see why anyone would take a garlic pill when he could eat real garlic. And it's the actual garlic that has the powerful stuff, because the garlic pills often don't have the most active components.

Q: Is olive oil so good for you that you should add it to recipes that don't call for it?

A: You mean, should you dip your pork chops in olive oil just before serving them? Or stir it into your oatmeal? No.

In some studies, olive oil—as compared to other fats—has been found to increase the "good" HDL cholesterol and lower the "bad" LDL cholesterol. It has also been suggested that an extra shot of olive oil gives an eater a satisfied feeling, thus decreasing the amount he or she eats.

The problem is that increasing oil increases calories. So, if you add the oil and don't actually decrease the amount of food you eat, then you're adding calories, which increases your weight, which increases the risk of heart disease.

I would not treat olive oil as a medicine and go out of my way to spike everything with it. Most plant oils are made of a range of fats, from the more healthy—monounsaturated and, to some extent, polyunsaturated—to the less healthy saturated fats found in butter. What's good about olive oil is that it is almost three-quarters monounsaturated fat. Canola oil and peanut oil also have more monounsaturated fat than any other type.

So you can really eat a variety of plant oils and get similar benefits.

Phony Food

Q: **Is it OK to replace meals with energy and nutrition bars? I do that a lot, because I'm always on the road, and they're really good. I'd rather eat one of those than a cheeseburger.**

A: Well, a Balance Bar or PowerBar is probably a healthier choice than a cheeseburger, but those aren't your only options. Since you're stopping at the health-food store, you'd do much better to pick up an apple and some nuts.

Nutrition/energy bars are not good meal replacements. Usually this type of product is light on fiber and heavy on fat. I think a label comparison would show that most aren't much healthier than a candy bar with nuts and raisins.

Most nutritionists bash these bars pretty heavily, but they admit that the ones with added minerals and vitamins are better than true junk food.

I can sympathize with you, because we're all very busy. I'm the same way; my solution is usually just not to eat. I figure I'm better off doing that than substituting poor nutrition, and almost all of us can do with eating a little less.

Q: **What do you think of these weight-loss plans that involve liquid meals? My mom was on one and lost quite a bit of weight, but then she gained back everything.**

A: I have not been a fan of these things, but there's one relatively small study, reported in the *Journal of the American Dietetic Association,* that shows some benefits. Seventy-five women were enrolled in this study that compared a traditional diet plan to a three-times-daily liquid meal.

Those on the liquid meal were instructed to supplement their diets with fruits and vegetables between meals. Both groups ate approximately 1,200 calories daily. Exercise for both groups was not required nor monitored by the researchers.

After one year, the meal-replacement group maintained their weight loss/fat loss. The traditional food group regained most of their initial weight loss.

I've always been opposed to the liquid diets because what do you do when you've reached your weight? Are you going to stay on this liquid for the rest of your life? Not likely.

"Good" Foods, "Bad" Foods

Q: I could eat cheese three times a day for the rest of my life. I don't do this, but I do eat some cheese almost every day. Am I asking for trouble?

A: Cheese is a nutritionally rich food that dates back to ancient times and is more popular than ever in snacks, salads, or pastas. Most of us eat twenty-eight to thirty pounds of cheese a year, six times more than the average American ate in 1910 and more than twice as much as was consumed during the 1960s.

We eat cheese because it is convenient and versatile, but did you know it is also an excellent source of calcium, phosphorus, and vitamin A? Roman emperors ate cheese for these reasons and gave it to their troops as a portable food supply.

One little known benefit of cheese is that many varieties help fight tooth decay—for reasons that I'm not quite sure of—especially cheddar, Swiss, Monterey, mozzarella, brie, and gouda.

I know many people avoid cheese because most of the calories are from fat, and cheese can contain plenty of fat. But that's no reason to cut it out of your diet completely. For one thing, having fat in your diet may reduce hunger faster, so you feel more full and eat less.

If you're worried about the amount of fat, you can still enjoy the taste by choosing flavorful cheeses and eating small portions—either grated or in thin slices—or you can choose varieties made with skim milk. For example, there's a type of mozzarella made partially with skim milk that contains five grams of fat per ounce. (See the fat content of other cheeses on page 39.)

There are a few downsides to cheese that don't affect most people. Cheese, particularly processed, contains high amounts of sodium, so, if this is a problem, you should eat less and choose low-sodium brands.

Aged cheese contains tyramine, which can interact with certain prescription drugs, especially some older antidepressants. This can cause blood pressure to rise to high levels in some people. And tyramine, which is also found in red wine, can sometimes trigger migraines.

If you're in good general health and enjoy the sensual pleasure of eating, I'd recommend cheese in moderation, as a tasty accent for almost any meal. One of my favorite salads is spinach leaves mixed with crumbled feta, red grapes, and chopped toasted walnuts, dressed with oil and vinegar. Yum.

Q: I have diverticulitis. My doctor prescribed a bland, high-grain diet, which means I can't eat raw fruits and vegetables, nuts, popcorn, caffeine, or chocolate. Must I eat like this forever?

A: Your doctor is being fairly strict. Many people with diverticulosis and diverticulitis can tolerate certain amounts, if not normal amounts, of each and every food you mentioned. Generally the afflicted are warned off fiber, which may be an irritant, but I'm surprised that chocolate and caffeine are verboten, maybe because they are favorites of mine.

Talk to your doctor about testing the restricted foods one item at a time. If you try one, and it doesn't irritate your colon, eating it shouldn't do you any harm. If you find that popcorn creates an uprising in your colon, it will have to be off limits. But if salad and chocolate cause you no pain, pass the olive oil and the Hershey bar.

Diverticulosis and diverticulitis are intestinal conditions that seem to be brought on by the lack of fiber in the typical Western diet.

When fiber is scarce, the intestines kind of squeeze down, causing little parts of the intestine to protrude from the intestinal wall between the bands of muscle. It's like squeezing a fistful of wet sand and creating globs that protrude between the fingers. Diverticulosis is the presence of these protrusions. Diverticulitis is an inflammation of the protrusions.

You can't do anything to reverse either condition, but adjusting your diet

---

QUIZ

Which food has as much vitamin C as an orange?
A) one bell pepper   B) one kiwi fruit
C) one cup of strawberries   D) one cup of broccoli
E) all of them
(E: all of them.)

DEAN'S LIST: HOW FAT IS THAT CHEESE?

I love cheese, but I know lots of folks who avoid it because of the fat content. As you can see, not all cheeses are equal in this department, but the differences are so small that you should eat the cheese you like, not the one with the best numbers. (All grams and calories are based on one-ounce portions.)

	fat grams	calories
American cheddar	9	106
Blue	8	100
Brie	8	95
Camembert	7	85
English cheddar	9.5	114
Edam	8	101
Feta	6	75
Fontina	9	110
Gorgonzola	8	100
Gouda	8	100
Gruyère	6	72
Mozzarella	6	80
Part-skim mozzarella	4.5	72
Muenster	8.5	104
Parmesan, grated	7.5	110
Roquefort	8.5	105
Stilton	9	102

will make you more comfortable and may slow down the progression of the disease.

Q: I love rice and eat it several times a week. I'm a bit confused by some health stories. Is this OK?

A: It's hard for me to believe we live in a culture where certain fad-diet gurus believe whole grains are bad for you. Rice and grains have been a staple food for millions of people over thousands of years and they have a place in a good, balanced diet.

And there is a study that indicates whole grain products may decrease the risk of diabetes mellitus, a disease that affects more than 16 million Americans. Researchers say that compared to refined-grain products, whole-grain foods reduced the risk of diabetes mellitus by about a third in a survey of 75,521 women aged thirty-eight to sixty-four without a previous diagnosis of the disease, according to a report in the *American Journal of Public Health*.

This is just another example of why we should embrace a well-balanced diet and not fall for extreme low-fat or high-protein fads. You never know what your body needs to fight off disease, but eating a variety of good foods is always a good defense mechanism.

Q: Which kind of salt is best for a person, iodized salt or non-iodized salt?

A: Iodized salt isn't necessary anymore. The practice of adding iodine to salt began in the early part of the twentieth century, when people ate locally grown food. In some parts of the world, the soil lacks iodine, and a lack of iodine in the diet put people at risk for developing goiters. Putting iodine in salt was a terrific solution, because everyone uses salt, and just a little iodine does the trick.

If you eat a varied diet, you can't miss iodine, and it's very common in fish.

I doubt there is a doctor out there who has seen an iodine-deficient goiter.

But iodine in salt doesn't seem to do any harm either. I'd pick the salt that's cheaper, or use whatever I have on hand.

Q: I'm trying to increase my milk consumption, because it's good for

---

QUIZ

Which of these foods has the lowest sodium content?
A) salted cocktail peanuts   B) doughnuts
C) buttered, salted popcorn   D) canned sardines
E) cheddar cheese
(C: buttered, salted popcorn.)

me, but I heard that there is too much phosphorus in milk. The large amount of phosphorus makes the calcium in milk unavailable for the body to use. America and Europe have the world's highest rate of dairy consumption and also the highest rate of osteoporosis. Is this correct?

A: First, you've got to consider your sources carefully. Second, you need to start with the fact that Caucasian/European people are genetically more likely to have osteoporosis.

Taking huge amounts of any one mineral can upset the balance of minerals in your body. If any source of phosphorus can affect calcium, it would be drinking too many soft drinks that contain phosphorus. Go have a glass of milk— skim milk. It's the best kind of milk you can drink.

Q: I love dried chili peppers. I eat them with every meal. I've got my best friend addicted to them, too. I fry those very hot, dark red ones in a little olive oil, shake garlic salt on them, and keep them in a big bowl. I'm having a burrito right now, and I'll probably eat five peppers with it. They don't bother me, but is it possible to overdo it?

A: Go for it. There is absolutely nothing wrong with chilies, and they even may be beneficial in relieving diseases like bronchitis. They are also high in antioxidants. However, if you have serious burning at either end of your body, change your habits.

I am glad, though, to hear that you eat other foods along with the chilies and use them as a condiment, because I don't think obsessions with one food are a good idea.

Interestingly, the capsaicin in chilies stimulates pain fibers in the mouth, rather than the taste buds. Capsaicin has been added to prescription drugs— Zostrix is one—used for nerve disorders and superficial pain syndromes.

We used to think that chilies were bad for people with ulcers, and that milk and cream were good for people with ulcers. The opposite turns out to be true. It is milk that stimulates stomach acid, not chilies. And we now know that stomach ulcers are caused by the *helicobacter pylori* bacterium.

Q: My twenty-three-year-old daughter eats tuna fish for lunch every day. Is there mercury in the tuna, and should I stop her?

A: Mercury exists in the air, on land, and in the sea, and there is no way to avoid it. But, of course, people want to avoid dangerously high levels—and mercury can be particularly dangerous for pregnant women and children.

The Edell Report
Our Love Affair with Chocolate

"Chocolate is cheaper than therapy and you don't need an appointment."

I don't know who said this, but I love it. First of all, it's true, and second, science has found that chocolate can be good for you—unless you're eating a pound a day. Being obese because of chocolate is not OK.

Most of us eat chocolate because it tastes good, but it contains ingredients that can fight bad cholesterol and help prevent heart attacks. It also has an active mood-altering chemical, but probably not enough to affect you.

Americans love chocolate—we each eat about ten pounds a year, and most of the consumption occurs between eight P.M. and midnight.

Chocolate is misunderstood, too. Eating it contributes very little to your total energy (the caffeine content is low) and calorie intake, and, contrary to popular belief, it doesn't cause acne. And not all chocolates are created equal: Dark chocolate is about twice as good for you, because it contains a higher amount of flavonoids that release cancer-fighting antioxidants in your body.

Chocolate also relaxes the inner surface of blood vessels and helps prevent high blood pressure and hardening of the arteries. It helps decrease the clumping of platelets in blood, reducing the chances of blood clots, heart attacks, and strokes.

One study involving 7,800 Harvard University alumni shows that the moderate consumption of chocolate, equivalent to about three candy bars a month, increases longevity.

The bottom line: Chocolate makes us feel good because it's good for us.

Potential danger to your daughter could depend on how much she eats in relation to her weight—but there's no across-the-board agreement on what her limits should be. The FDA has no specific guidelines for canned tuna beyond urging pregnant women to limit their consumption. But one agency, the Washington (State) Department of Health, suggests that women of child-bearing age limit their intake to one six-ounce can per week for a 135-pound person, and that children under six should also limit their consumption.

However, new research finds that the kind of mercury found in fish may not be as dangerous as once thought, and many questions remain to be answered.

Until we know more, large tuna, which is usually not canned and is sold as steaks or in sushi, should be eaten in moderation, as should shark and swordfish. All of these fish have mercury levels that are higher than those in tuna that is canned.

Considering the pathetic diet most young women have, your daughter sounds like she's trying to do the right thing. But tuna lacks several nutrients; she is eating a much more balanced diet if she's putting it on high-fiber bread, draped with a lettuce leaf and a slice of tomato. Encourage her to vary her diet a bit, and if she's skeptical about the tuna advice, suggest that she do her own research on the Internet.

Q: I've heard caffeine can leach calcium from your bones and was wondering, what level of consumption should I be concerned about?

A: It's always funny to me how we go on these witch hunts to find something wrong with only those things we really enjoy; the things we hate, no one cares about, right? Caffeine, of course, is the world's most consumed drug in the form of coffee and tea, so naturally we've been trying to find something wrong with it for years and years.

I have followed the literature very closely, and moderate amounts of coffee actually seem to be healthy. Coffee is an herb and contains all kinds of antioxidants. Can you imagine what the health-food-supplement industry would have done if coffee were discovered today? They'd be peddling it to you in capsules, because it has antioxidants and a lot of other good things. We've done research and have found that drinking coffee decreases your risk for all kinds of cancer, suicide, and depression.

Then there is a study on thinning of the bones and, yes, I have to admit that they concluded that coffee could possibly leach calcium from the bones. But it didn't seem too serious when the first study came out. There have been subsequent studies to challenge it, and I don't think it's a major factor. I think any kind of exercise is going to make up for any deficit. So, to me, right now, it's a nonissue, especially if you are taking care of yourself.

I think, nutritionally, a more important factor might be protein consumption. So all you people out there on the Atkins diet, watch out. A lot of protein seems to cause a loss of calcium in the long term.

You also need to know that taking calcium doesn't seem to reverse calcium leached from the bones, though you might be able to slow down the process and stabilize it.

Q: I'm a rare-beef lover, and I know I'm supposed to be careful with rare beef because of the germs that live in it. Does irradiation make rare beef safer?

A: Irradiation of beef can make a significant dent in the transmission of illness. It kills E. coli and renders rare beef safer. Also, chopped meat harbors many more bacteria than does a slab of meat. The more cut surfaces you have the easier it is for bacteria to grow and spread throughout the meat. So, something like steak tartare, chopped raw beef, is probably riskier than carpaccio, paper-thin slices of raw beef.

The anti-irradiation folks do make the point that rather than adding a postprocessing step to clean up after sloppy meatpacking, the slaughter and preparation of meat should be cleaner in the first place. Radiation should not mean that manufacturers can be as slovenly as they want in producing our food. It's just an added security that will save lives.

Eating a lot of meat carries health risks, whether the meat is irradiated or not. But irradiation does kill a variety of bacteria.

Q: I'm fifty-five years old and trying to stay alive as long as I can by watching my cholesterol level and fat intake. But one of my weaknesses is peanut butter. Haven't I heard you say good things about it?

A: Peanut butter provides a good lesson about using caution before turning away from foods that keep us satisfied. Peanut butter has gotten a bad rap because of its high fat content, but a recent study found that these monounsaturated fats, also found in olive oil, have a more positive cardiovascular effect than the American Heart Association's own diet.

Replacing saturated fats like beef with peanut butter or olive oil seems to be healthier than an overall restriction of fat consumption. Eating very low-fat diets, for some strange reason, seems to decrease the good cholesterol levels and increase triglycerides. We are rethinking all the recommendations on extreme low-fat eating, because some folks wind up consuming way more calories than they need, so they don't lose weight.

DID YOU KNOW?
THE BAD SIDE OF JOE

You may not be fully awake when you order your first cup of coffee every morning—but you should be. According to the Mayo Clinic Women's HealthSource, a large latte can add anywhere from 250 to 570 calories to your day. If that's too much—and for most of us it is—consider these alterations to your routine. Choose the smallest-size cup; that can save you as much as 110 calories. If you like milk, make it fat-free; that counts for 80 calories and eight grams of fat. Finally, consider artificial sweeteners instead of sugar and forget about the whipped cream, flavored syrup, or chocolate toppings.

My favorite healthy food quiz question is: Which has more calories—olive oil, lard, or butter? The answer is that they each have the same number of calories. Number nine is the nutrition number to remember: A gram of fat has nine calories whether it's a gram of canola oil, olive oil, peanut oil, butter, or lard. The difference is in the quality of the fat.

Nature designed the body to exist on all kinds of foods; we are omnivores. But having too much food forces the body to work overtime, processing, storing, and moving all that excess. The theory is that the extra work your body does to metabolize the extra food causes poor health and a shorter life.

Exercise and Fitness

Q: I have taken yoga for years, but I recently went to a new class in Bikram yoga. I registered as a beginner who had recently had surgery, to see how the teacher would work with me.

There were around thirty women and men of all ages in an extremely hot room. The instructor announced that we would feel faint, and some people would throw up, "but that's OK. This is good for you. You'll feel great. You'll sweat, and get dizzy and sick." I walked out, and many people

followed me. And later, I found out that she didn't have any credentials. Does this sound dangerous?

A: So, you pay to work out in a hot room where you can expect to faint and throw up? Sounds like a winner to me.

Seriously, rather than address this specific style of yoga, let's consider two generalizations: Exercise that makes you sick is not healthy, and beware the noncredentialed teacher.

While most people think of yoga as a bunch of fairly passive stretches, some yoga is actually vigorous, but students will not be safe if they are getting ill or have an unqualified teacher.

I'm sure people will call to say that Bikram yoga is a life-altering marvel, and I say good for them. But anyone who feels sick or endangered by exercise should absolutely walk out. Ask yourselves what you want from your exercise. Is it to feel powerful? Is it to live longer or healthier? Is it to have fun?

Q: My partner and I disagree about the best time for exercising to increase metabolism. I say that walking before breakfast gets better results than does eating and then walking, like he wants to do. Who is right?

A: Exercise before or after eating has the same effect on your metabolism, but it might make a difference in comfort, so you're both a little bit right.

For some people, walking with food on board is uncomfortable. The stomach hangs from ligaments, and the bumping and sloshing of the food while moving around could cause pain. This is one of the causes of that stitch in the side we sometimes get. Let comfort be your guide.

Q: I am the Incredible Shrinking Man. A quick history: When I was twenty years old, I was five-foot-eight and weighed 150 pounds. Today, at

---

QUIZ

How many hours of vigorous bowling—yes, bowling—would it take to work off a big turkey dinner?
A) three hours   B) six hours   C) twelve hours
D) twenty-four hours
(D: twenty-four hours.)

the age of sixty-four, I'm five-foot-five and weigh 125 pounds. **Every other day, I run 2.8 miles and do a hundred pull-ups, fifty crunches, and work with dumbbells. I eat six to seven times a day, and I can't gain weight. What's wrong?**

A: A person with unexplained weight loss and the inability to gain weight should always see a doctor, because these are signs of increased mortality.

Your case is different, because this is not a new symptom but a lifelong pattern. You have the metabolism that everyone wants. You burn a lot of calories.

In fact, you burn calories so easily that you are probably overexercising. You don't need to do all that. Twenty or thirty minutes of exercise, three or four times a week, is fine. If you do any more than that, your metabolism is going to fight you.

But it is your change of height that concerns me the most. While it is normal to lose some height as we age due to shrinkage of the discs between the vertebrae, a three-inch loss is too much. You could possibly have osteoporosis with collapsing of your vertebrae. Talk to your doctor, because thin bones can be a problem for men, too.

Q: Is swimming a good way to lose weight? Someone told me it's not, because your body doesn't heat up enough in the cool water to burn off fat. I've noticed that swimmers are very lean though.

A: As a matter of fact, swimmers are not as lean as runners. They can exercise just as much and have significantly more fat on their bodies than do runners and other athletes.

The fat on a swimmer's body gives them the advantage of riding high in the water. This is good for speed, because the deeper you are in the water, the more resistance you encounter.

Fat floats. That's why we weigh someone underwater to figure out the percentage of body fat. The muscle tissue sinks, and the fat tissue floats.

Fat also insulates. Stranded in a snowstorm, the fatter people would survive longer. Their fat would insulate them from the cold and would also provide a source of energy when food was scarce.

One fascinating study, done in the eighties at the University of California at Irvine, looked at three groups of women, averaging about 150 pounds each. Each group did a different exercise: brisk walking, stationary cycling, or swimming laps. After six months, the cyclists had lost eighteen pounds and the walkers fifteen pounds. Amazingly, the swimmers gained four pounds. What happened? We're not sure. Swimming in cold water may stimulate the appetite, so swimmers eat more, or cold may stimulate the body to produce more fat insulation.

But don't rule out swimming based on that result. We do know that swimming is a great way to exercise without stressing your joints. A swimmer is not going to wind up saddled with a cane later in life, like a lot of runners do.

Miscellaneous: Constipation, Organics, TV Dinners, and More

Q: My husband has had constipation problems for years, and we tried Metamucil, prune juice—the whole route—and nothing seemed to help. Then we came upon Dieter's Tea at the drugstore; it's not sold in grocery stores. It's made from senna leaf. I brew him a cup of that, and he's a "regular" guy. Have you heard of this treatment?

A: There was a bit of a controversy with this tea a couple of years ago, when deaths resulted from using it. The problem is that some folks use it for weight loss, and that includes young, anorexic women. I'm absolutely against that.

Laxatives do not help you lose weight, and these dieter's teas—there are a variety of them—contain a lot of powerful "herbal" laxatives, like senna. As a light laxative to get the hubby regular on occasion, it's OK, though I'm surprised the fiber didn't do it. My guess is that he just needs more in his diet.

Q: I hate to eat vegetables and fruit. Will drinking juice that has 100 percent of RDA of A, B, C, and lots of other vitamins make up for the deficiencies in my diet?

A: Pure juice that's truly extracted from fruits and vegetables, and not fiddled with, does have most vitamins and nutrients. But it lacks fiber, which is a critical part of the diet.

Beware of processed drinks that are not entirely juice and have vitamin additives. This isn't what you need, because it's missing the variety of carotenes and other nutrients found in fruits and vegetables.

A quality product from a trusted source, or juice that you make yourself, will be better for you than no fruits and vegetables at all. You've got to find a source of fiber, though. Also, you'll discover that your choice of fruits and vegetables that make tasty juices is kind of limited.

DID YOU KNOW?
FOLATE IS GOOD FOR YOU

If you want an easy way to remember this form of vitamin B, think Popeye. Folate gets its name from the Latin word for leaf (*folium*) and was first extracted from spinach in 1941. You'll find it in everything from spinach and asparagus to brewer's yeast and orange juice. Both adults—especially pregnant women—and children need folate to make red blood cells and prevent anemia and spina bifida.

Q: **What are the best foods to eat after a bad bout of the flu that includes vomiting and diarrhea? I've usually depended on dry toast, plain rice, and bananas. And am I doing anything for my body with a sports drink like Gatorade, versus just drinking water?**

A: First, to be technical, the flu never causes vomiting and diarrhea. If you have those symptoms, you don't have a classic case of influenza but possibly some gastrointestinal virus.

As you know, if you are in the middle of a stomach bug, but not quite over it, and you eat a nice, big, fatty meal, it is likely that you will see that meal again real soon. We like to gradually reintroduce solid foods. It probably doesn't matter what you eat, as long as you do it gradually. But, most important, start with fluids. And while some doctors would say Gatorade or some other sports drinks are better than plain water, because they have electrolytes that your body needs and does lose during diarrhea and vomiting, it's probably not that critical. If you were sick enough to really need the extra minerals in sports drinks, then you should probably be in the hospital getting intravenous fluids. So, plain water is fine but a little broth with salt is better. If you can hold that down, then you are on the way to a small amount of your favorite solid food.

Q: **How important is it to eat only organic fruits and vegetables? I'd like to do that, but they sure are expensive.**

A: You can decide for yourself if the extra price is worth it, but there are some myths and facts about organic foods that you should take into consideration.

A clinical nutritionist and spokesperson for the American Dietetic Association says one of the myths about organic foods is that they routinely are more nutritious than nonorganic foods. The fact is that vitamin and mineral content in organic food is usually equal to conventionally grown produce. But it might be fresher, because it is often grown close to where it is sold. Either way, small differences mean nothing to our overall health.

Another myth is that organic produce is completely free of pesticide and herbicide residues. The fact is that while organic food should be less contaminated, residues do drift from neighboring fields. This has been documented by several agencies, including the Department of Agriculture, and one sampling from a farm showed pesticide residue on 50 percent of the organic peaches. From a nonorganic farm, 93 percent of the peaches had residue. Also, regardless of how plants are grown, some (green potatoes are one example) have natural toxins that can be dangerous if consumed in excess.

Another myth I've debunked in the past is that pesticides sprayed on produce cause cancer. This just isn't true, as these bug killers mostly break down after doing their job. You may get sick from overexposure, but there's no link to cancer.

All produce is safe to eat. Wash it with water before serving or cooking it. And the best thing to do is enjoy a variety of fruits and vegetables—and not go into debt doing it.

Q: For most of my adult life I have weighed 275 pounds. The first thing a doctor says to me is that I wouldn't have X, Y, or Z problem if I wasn't so fat—like I've never heard it before. How do I get a physician to pay atten-

QUIZ

How much exposure to the midday sun do you need to get an adequate amount of vitamin D?
A) fifteen minutes/week   B) forty-five minutes/week
C) one hour/week   D) two hours/week   E) five hours/week
(B: forty-five minutes/week)

DID YOU KNOW?
FORGET THE SOAP!

Yes, you want to get rid of the pesticides on your fruits and vegetables—or just the dirt—if your produce is organic. But don't overdo it. Soap is a really bad idea, according to both the Department of Agriculture and the Environmental Protection Agency. Animal studies have shown that the residue can lead to intestinal problems.

---

tion to what's wrong with me and to realize that it may not have anything to do with my weight?

A: I have heard this complaint many times, and I agree with you that this is a problem. In my chapter on obesity in *Eat, Drink, and Be Merry* I wrote about a woman who was part of a group of very obese women who rented a public pool for weekly swims because they were tired of the taunts. She, too, told me stories of doctors who would not see past the fat.

It is no news to you that society is biased against fat people, and doctors reflect the society in which they work. Just as nonsmokers get lung cancer, all body types get heart disease, arthritis, and cancer.

One way to get your doctor to listen is to stand up for yourself. Wrap your legs around the examining table and refuse to leave until you get satisfaction. Or, for a less stressful approach, shop around until you find a doctor who respects and understands you.

One study done fairly recently found that doctors were not as biased against fat people as we have heard. This is only one piece of evidence, but maybe attitudes are changing as we learn more about the role of genetics in obesity and also that a person can be both fat and fit.

Q: My son's Japanese girlfriend told me that eating seaweed makes your hair grow thicker. True?

A: Seaweed is a healthy food, except for people on low-sodium diets, but, to my knowledge, it doesn't have any minerals or anything else that would have any effect on hair.

The ocean has almost all the trace minerals that human beings need. Boiling seawater leaves you with not only sodium chloride, but also minerals like selenium, manganese, and magnesium. Health-food stores sell pills made from mineral deposits that were mined from land that was once under water.

You have to eat a lot of seaweed to reap the benefits of those minerals, and I don't think many people eat enough to make a huge difference.

Q: I eat TV dinners for breakfast, lunch, and dinner. I read the boxes and I notice that the meals are high in sodium. Is this habit damaging my health? I know TV dinners have no nutritional value, but they fill the empty spot in a flash.

A: Plenty of people live on burgers and fries and then count those fries as vegetable servings. At least TV dinners aim at balance by packaging three little lumps of various foods, like a little lump of chicken, a little lump of potatoes, and a little lump of broccoli. They're not nutritionally empty—although, as you point out, they are heavy on sodium, and fat, too.

Processing frozen foods may diminish their vitamin value, but not always. A University of Illinois study found that some frozen vegetables had the same, or, in some cases, even more, nutrients than fresh did.

Your best bet is to supplement your TV dinners with salad and fruit. Make it easy on yourself by buying bagged salad fixings to keep on hand in the refrigerator. A meal of salad, fruit, and a TV dinner is much healthier than what many people eat.

Q: One hot night, my roommate and I had a disagreement. She said that drinking hot cocoa or eating hot soup would raise our body temperature and cool us off. My aunt, too, drinks hot coffee when she is hot and says it cools her off. I think they are nuts. Iced tea and ice cream are what cools me off. Are we all right?

A: You are all demonstrating the power of perception. Body temperature is controlled by respiration and by the amount a person sweats, so neither hot nor cold food or drink will change body temperature.

If your roommate thinks that raising the body's temperature would force it to work harder, sweat more, and therefore cool off, she is wrong. Food and drink don't change body temperature, and sweating too much can lead to dehydration, which is harmful.

As your roommate and your aunt demonstrate, perception varies, but most of us would say that drinking something cold cools us down, just like we feel warmed by a bowl of oatmeal on a winter morning. In fact, neither makes much difference to body temperature.

Someone once sent me a calculation on the number of calories the body uses to raise the temperature of a cold liquid. He asked why the calories being burned to warm the liquid wouldn't cause weight loss.

Given the mass of the body and its temperature, the bit of calories it takes to maintain a steady 98.6 degrees is like throwing an ice cube into a tub of hot water. It's not going to drop the temperature enough to matter.

A lot of this mythology comes from the notion people have that drinking hot toddies on a cold day warms them up. Alcohol dilates the blood vessels, so you feel warmer but actually you are losing body heat; the feeling that it's warming you up is an illusion.

Q: Lately my stomach has been growling more at night. This happens whether I've eaten or not. In general, what causes the stomach to growl?

A: You're talking about borborygmi. But don't worry if your life insurance has lapsed. This is the medical word for the sound that your intestines make. Your body is constantly propelling food and liquid through your intestines. This is called peristalsis.

If you take a quart of milk in a plastic container, and you shake it, and it's full, it's not very loud, because there's little air inside. But if you pour out half of the milk and shake it, it's very loud. This is because the air in the container allows the liquid to make a lot of noise. If you shake a bottle that's completely full, you don't hear any noise at all. So, if your intestines were completely full of liquid and solid matter, and the stomach and intestines were doing their jobs, you really wouldn't hear very much at all. But most of the time there's gas in the intestines.

You have long intestines, and anything you've eaten in the last twenty-four hours, or even longer, could be in those intestines. So, what you had to eat, how much air you swallowed, and when you ate, are probably the key factors. Drinking a lot of carbonated beverages or beer can also add a lot of air to your intestines. The gurgling sound comes from the interaction of that air with the food.

That does not mean that there aren't diseases that would cause this, but I think you would have a sore tummy, you'd be sick, or you'd know something was up.

The Edell Report
The Facts About Flatulence and Belching

Most of us associate flatulence with bad manners, bad jokes told mostly by men, the campfire scene from the movie Blazing Saddles, *and beans. All in all, gross stuff. But the fact is, the average healthy person passes gas between ten and twenty-two times a day. This is perfectly normal and nothing to worry about.*

Flatulence usually occurs because bowel gas builds up and needs to be expelled. This typically results from the fermentation reactions that take place when colonic bacteria break down carbohydrates that have not been completely digested by the intestines, the result being the production of carbon dioxide, methane, and hydrogen. However, not all bodies react the same way. Age and heredity can be factors, and so can your diet and the amount of air you swallow. For some of us, "problem" foods can include milk (but not yogurt), onions, beans, carrots, celery, bananas, apricots, raisins, wheat germ, prune juice, pretzels, and Brussels sprouts. Observe your own bodily patterns for the "bad guys" in your particular diet.

When excess gases are produced and passed from the body, most of them are virtually odorless, which brings us to another question: Where does the smelly gas come from?

Well, it turns out that sulfur compounds are the culprit—flatulence containing less than .001 percent of hydrogen sulfide, methanethiol, and

---

Q: I think that companies have a duty to inform consumers when they're using technologically modified foods. You always use breeding as an example of safe genetic modification that has been practiced for years. But breeding is a slower process, so, by the time a product gets on the market, its defects and hazards have been caught. We don't get that kind of chance with the speed of genetic modification. How do you feel about this?

A: Transgenic food is a tremendous agricultural breakthrough. Scientists

dimethylsufide can be very offensive—and there is very little research about how to control this problem with a change in diet. Activated charcoal is sometimes used to fight sulfur gases, but it's unreliable. One thing that may help is bismuth, which binds to sulfides and offers a solution to feces or flatus odors. Taking four tablets of Pepto Bismol a day results in eliminating the release of sulfur compounds; however, I don't recommend this on a regular basis. Remember, gas is a normal part of our bodily functions.

Another option that some researchers have suggested is the avoidance of sulfur-containing foods like cruciferous vegetables (broccoli, cauliflower, and Brussels sprouts) and beer.

Occasionally flatulence is caused by giardiasis or peptic ulcer disease, so if there is ongoing discomfort or other gastrointestinal symptoms, talk to your doctor.

While some of the air we swallow can make it to our bowels, swallowed air is the major source of gas that you belch or eructate. About 17 milliliters of nitrogen and oxygen go into the stomach every time we swallow liquid, food, or saliva. And we may swallow more air than we realize when we drink carbonated beverages or chew gum. Ill-fitting dentures, the dietetic sweeteners sorbitol and mannitol, and eating too fast or eating while stressed are other aggravating sources, and excessive fat consumption can play a part, giving you a bloated feeling. So, if belching is a problem, assess your habits.

alter the characteristics of food by splicing the desired gene of one plant or animal into the DNA of another, creating a transgenic or genetically modified food. But it's a complicated issue that has become more emotional than fact-based, and there's a lot we still don't know.

Some folks who don't even know what DNA stands for, or what genetically modified food is, are letting their views be colored by the likes of Frankenstein movies and the *Attack of the Killer Tomatoes.*

The public always meets change with fear, and the progress of genetic modification of food is being tainted by touches of mass hysteria. Such decisions should be based on science, not mob rule.

The reality is that I don't know of a single human being who has been harmed by a genetically modified food. Yes, we should be cautious. I do have a concern about how transgenic foods will alter the environment. On the other hand, we can now produce pest-resistant foods that are making us less dependent on pesticides. That's good for the environment and for us. And increasing crop yields will always be a priority as long as starvation is a reality anywhere in the world.

Right now, I have no fears about eating genetically modified foods.

Q: My husband and I are having an argument about whether a certain family member can be called "obese"—not to his face, of course. Just what qualifies as obese?

A: This is a very good question. It's kind of like blood alcohol levels and speed limits. We have to pick a number so we can begin our definitions, even though they can ultimately be inaccurate or unfair. Right now the definition is based on your Body Mass Index (BMI). This is your weight in kilograms divided by your height in meters squared. This is not simple for most people to do, so check out our chart on page 57.

Basically, a BMI of 25 is considered overweight; and over 30, you're obese. But this is not absolute. I'm sure Arnold Schwarzenegger would easily qualify as obese simply because he has a lot of weight on him—mostly muscle tissue—for his height. Also, your shape is a factor. Some people can carry a heavier BMI and look fine, depending on the shape of their body. Every human on earth is different, and it's ridiculous to think that we all have to adhere to a single mathematical formula to be considered healthy by the medical establishment. There are folks with a high BMI that will live a long life, and others with a low BMI who will die prematurely. It's not an absolute, only a guideline.

Q: Will eating spicy, hot food now burn out my taste buds when I'm older?

A: No, because it is the pain fibers on the tongue, not the taste buds, that respond to spicy food. Why we like pain on our tongues is anyone's guess.

Some people claim that capsaicin, which is the main ingredient in a lot of spicy foods, relieves everything from arthritis to migraines to psoriasis.

I think spice was originally used as a food preservative, because germs

DID YOU KNOW?
FIGURE YOUR BODY MASS INDEX

Body mass index (BMI) is used by many physicians to determine whether we are underweight or overweight. BMI uses a mathematical formula that takes into account both a person's height and weight. BMI equals a person's weight in kilograms divided by height in meters squared. (BMI = kg/m^2). For a BMI calculator, go to *www.consumer.gov/ weightloss/bmi.htm*. The chart below factors in your waist size to help assess the risk of disease.

RISK OF ASSOCIATED DISEASE ACCORDING TO BMI AND WAIST SIZE			
BMI		less than or equal to 40 in. (men) or 35 in. (women)	waist greater than 40 in. (men) or 35 in. (women)
18.5 or less	Underweight	—	N/A
18.5–24.9	Normal	—	N/A
25.0–29.9	Overweight	Increased	High
30.0–34.9	Obese	High	Very High
35.0–39.9	Obese	Very High	Very High
40 or greater	Extremely Obese	Extremely High	Extremely High
35.0–39.9	Obese	Very High	Very High
40 or greater	Extremely Obese	Extremely High	Extremely High

don't like spice. So spices were a means of keeping food bacteria-free and perhaps hiding the bad tastes of spoiled food.

Q: I'd like to know more about plastic containers. We buy gallons of milk, cooking oil, and ketchup. We even use plastic bags on our green veg-

etables. **Which containers are safe and which aren't? I know you once
warned about using plastic water bottles over and over again.**

A: When you buy food in a plastic container at the grocery store, that's OK.

The only thing I worry about is when people take those temporary containers and use them as permanent containers, and heat and reheat their food in a microwave with them. They were not meant for that, they were meant for one use only. It's not like Tupperware.

About the water bottles—that was interesting. Someone called and asked me if they could use plastic water bottles over and over, and I got some e-mails saying that a couple of times is okay, but it's not ideal. For environmental reasons, those products have been designed to break down, especially in the face of ultraviolet light. Also, water in bottles that have been reused is often contaminated with germs.

If you put water in a plastic bottle, and the water tastes like plastic, that's a sign that there is something wrong with that plastic, and it's time to throw that thing out.

The amount of outgassing from plastic is small. And if I were to list all the things in our environment that may cause problems, in terms of the air and the water and fumes from cars, etc., I'd put new plastic food containers very low on the list—but I think the way people sometimes use these things is inappropriate, and that may elevate their risks.

Q: I've heard that fasting from time to time is a cleansing process and is good for your body. On the other hand, I've heard that the lowered intake of calories may affect metabolism and the way the body stores fat. What's the truth?

A: I don't think that short fasts do any harm, but I don't think they have any major health benefits either, other than reducing overall calorie intake. The body doesn't distinguish between deliberate fasting and the nondeliberate kind—starvation. Some studies indicate that an insufficient food supply triggers the body to store what it can as fat and save it for a rainy day. So, it's possible that repeated fasting could trigger increased storage of fat.

Fasting could carry the psychological benefit that comes from feeling in control. It's similar to the appeal that running has for some people. Their jobs may be stressful, home life is chaotic, but for thirty minutes a day, it's just them and their running shoes.

So, as a mental exercise to bring discipline into your life, there's nothing wrong with a short-term fast. And, done on a regular basis, this is one way to decrease consistently the number of calories you consume. In the long-term, reducing calorie intake is probably the most powerful change most people can make in their health regimen for longevity.

Resource List

For information on every conceivable food-related subject, go to The Food and Nutrition Center at the U.S. Department of Agriculture: *www.nal.usda.gov/fnic/*

The Weight-control Information Network (WIN) is a government-sponsored national information service: *www.niddk.nih.gov/health/nutrit/win.htm*

Check out the supplements guide from the University of California, Berkeley, and Wellness Letter: *www.berkeleywellness.com/*

The National Institute of Health's Clinical Center also has excellent information on this topic: *www.cc.nih.gov/home.cgi*

Tufts University's Center on Nutrition Education provides the Nutrition Navigator, a guide to a variety of nutrition-oriented Web sites: *www.navigator.tufts.edu/index.html*

Visit the Mayo Clinic's diet and nutrition section (search for "diet pyramids") to see six variations on the classic food pyramid: *www.mayoclinic.com*

For the latest warnings and safety information on supplements from the Food and Drug Administration, go to its MedWatch site: *www.fda.gov/medwatch*

For a referral to a registered dietitian, call the Consumer Nutrition Information Line of the American Dietetic Association at 1-800-366-1655 or see the ADA Web site: *www.eatright.org.*

Check out the bean nutrient profile at *www.americanbean.org*

The Children's Nutrition Research Center at Baylor College of Medicine offers a free nutrition newsletter: ***www.bcm.tmc.edu/cnrc/index.htm***

The Dole Food Company Web site includes a fruit-and-vegetable encyclopedia: ***www.dole5aday.com***

For related questions see chapters 3, 4, 5, 6, 8, and 10.

Chapter 2

Good Sex,
Bad Sex,
No Sex

I get a lot of questions about sex on my radio show. A whole lot. Perhaps it's the anonymity of talk radio that encourages questions that folks don't feel comfortable asking their physicians—or their spouses or partners. Perhaps they just don't know where to go to get good answers. But either way, one other fact is known: Many listeners object to frank discussions about sex. And that baffles me.

Yes, I may be less embarrassed by sexual discussions because of my medical background, but every one of us owes our existence to a sexual act. (OK, sperm retrieval by needle and insemination in a test tube is an exception, but let's not get sidetracked.) Sex is a primal human instinct essential for the survival of our species, and yet we still seem to know hardly anything about it. Many married couples have a hard time even talking to each other about sex, and there is still broad disagreement about whether sex is good or bad or whether we should teach our kids about it—or keep it a secret. We have a problem here—and I refuse to stop talking about it.

I remember, when I was a kid, ordering the Charles Atlas bodybuilding kit through the mail. The cartoon in the back of the comic book said it all. If I had bulging muscles, every woman would want me. Thanks to Mr. Atlas, I would never be the skinny guy who got sand kicked in his face by the pumped-up bully. Right.

Curiously, nothing really has changed in the decades since I entertained my juvenile fantasies. Our fear of sexual inadequacy remains the most fundamental and elusive of our personal fears. More than ever, our sexual insecurities simmer as we are pummeled with messages about how thin/fat, big/small, ugly and utterly disgusting our bodies are. Our breath is fetid, our armpits rancid, and most of the time we are having a bad hair day. Our home computers flood us with e-mail spam touting penis enlargers and breast enhancers to augment our unfortunate endowments. Mix in a miasma of medieval mythologies, sprinkle with a good dose of guilt, don't forget the confusion and contradictions surrounding our political and moral attitudes, and it's no wonder we are left with a staggering amount of sexual ignorance, frustration, and unhappiness.

Unfortunately, we see the results every day, in our own homes or among those we know from work, church, or our children's schools: teen pregnancies, abortion, unwanted babies, sexually transmitted diseases, infidelities, and broken marriages. Add to this the misunderstandings and fear that still surround homosexuality, and you can see how sex has taken its toll on our society.

Doctors know—based on many studies—that there is a high rate of sexual dissatisfaction, from inhibited desire to plumbing issues to psychological disorders. Yet how often do we talk to doctors about these problems? How many marriages are lost to the divorce courts because couples struggle on their own to patch up their sex lives? Along the way, we pass on to our kids this deep-seated fear of sex because of our desire to "protect them." We teach them all the things to fear about sex, believing that will dissuade them from folly, but we don't balance the message. We seldom discuss the positives.

Sex is the most available and direct route to ecstasy that we know. It is a resource for survival, an antidote to stress, depression, and the complexities of modern life. When it works, it makes us happy. But we don't quite know the best way to communicate the fact that great sex—the real thing, not the poor substitute seen in the movies—is found within the context of a committed, loving relationship. "Good" sex in the movies almost always involves single people—or infidelities. Few young people know that the reward of understanding and managing their sexuality is a higher plane of pleasure down the road. The more common message is that great sex is found in a bar with a Budweiser in your hand—or behind the wheel of a hot car.

Amid this confusion, we fall back on a "just say no" mentality. We reinforce the message of how repulsive—how dangerous—our genitals are. We protest a one hundred-year-old statue in front of a courthouse with a breast peeking from beneath the robes. And we wonder why kids are confused.

There are countries that do a better job. In the Netherlands, sex education is routine, and they are a much more sexually open culture. While it would be shocking for the average American parent to see what kids there learn, Netherlanders have the highest rate of virginity among their teenagers, and the rates of sexually transmitted diseases and unwanted pregnancy are lower than in any other country. On the flip side, the United States has the worst statistics in the world.

How did we get to this point? Well, my profession must take some of the blame. Our training is poor—I had only one lecture on sexology—and many of us are as reluctant to discuss sexual issues as the patients are reluctant to introduce them. In many ways, the AIDS epidemic forced the door open in the medical community, but not nearly open enough. Religion and politics have also colored the discussion of sex in the United States, and we can't seem to make up our minds about how much government involvement we want to allow in our sexual lives and those of our children. That scares me.

Scientific research about sex is yet another area where we are lacking. Because of our cultural attitudes, legitimate research is difficult. First, we are dealing with human beings; there are no animal models for human sexuality. And when it gets down to real research—watching people making love, measuring orgasms, etc.—most universities are scared to death of conducting such studies. Consequently, the best quality research I see in the medical journals comes from foreign countries.

Certainly, things have changed since Dr. Alfred Kinsey's landmark reports of 1948 and 1953. But not much. We are still in our infancy in understanding this most important human instinct. While innovative Dutch researchers in 1999 used MRIs of lovemaking and masturbation to get a better picture of the basic anatomy of intercourse—what lines up with what—and the behavior of the uterus, we still have many unanswered questions about the fundamental anatomy: Is there a G spot? Do females ejaculate? Does circumcision decrease sexual sensations? Do diseases like prostatitis promote premature ejaculation? Do women have better orgasms than men?

For all the information we lack, there is research that suggests that good sexual relationships are very healthy. They can reduce the risk of heart disease and many other illnesses, and they promote longevity and mental health. One recent piece of research promotes the idea that semen has anti-depressant molecules in it. Another project found that the more sex we have, the younger we look.

What's unhealthy is our tendency to ignore or avoid the sexual parts of our body. Think how many cancers begin in our reproductive tracts: prostate, testicles, uterus, cervix, ovaries, breasts, and vulva. Almost daily, based on the calls I receive on my show, I am reminded that embarrassment still prevents some folks from getting appropriate screening tests. That jibes with a survey that found most of us would have a deep reluctance to undress quickly if ordered to do so by medical and military personnel in the face of biodisaster. Yet shedding your clothing in such circumstances is your first defense against contamination.

In this era of everything "natural," isn't it strange that something as natural and healthy as sex so confuses us?

Some public health experts now say sex is as important to health as diet and exercise, and the medical community needs to deliver that message. Sex has to become a priority in life. And there has to be an understanding that the most important sex organ is—and has always been—the brain. Communication about sex is more difficult for most people than the sex act itself, and that has to change. If husbands and wives can't talk to each other about sex comfortably and intelligently, how can they hope to talk comfortably and intelligently with their children?

Improved communication—between partners and between patients and doctors—is also essential if we are to avoid the medicalizing of sexuality. Some doctors have turned lack of desire and disinterest into a disease, perhaps because it is easier to prescribe pills for problems than to get to the root causes of our ennui. The same goes for patients who would rather have a quick fix than invest the time that good sexual relationships require. That said, new medications are giving both men and women new hope for sexual satisfaction. When Viagra spokesman and professional baseball player Rafael Palmeiro "stepped up to the plate" on prime-time television, I knew there was hope. Yes, it was just an advertisement, but we have to start somewhere. When real jocks can talk about impotence, the armchair jocks are sure to follow.

Premature Ejaculation and Impotence

Q: I have a problem with premature ejaculation. I never seem to last more than one or two minutes because I become too excited. Could you please tell me if there is anything I could do for this problem? I am in a committed relationship and have been for three years now.

A: Your problem may be easily fixed, but you should start by getting your prostate checked out by a urologist. Research has found higher incidences of chronic prostatitis among men who suffer from premature ejaculation, and you first want to rule that out.

If everything is OK, I want you to reassess your thinking on this topic; don't make it into something horrible. A minute or two is a long time, though it may be frustrating for you and your partner. In a study where women took stop-watches to bed with them, researchers found that one- to two-minutes duration is about average, so you're not starting at such a bad place. What you're asking for is the ability to control your sexual reflexes, and that's possible.

To start, men need to sit with their partners and do a couple of exercises in an open and relaxed fashion. The problem is that a lot of men with this difficulty don't have that kind of relationship. If they have an ongoing, monogamous relationship, they are already uptight about this situation and anxious and afraid to talk about it with their partner.

This issue can make both parties nervous. Your partner may be blaming herself, and you may be feeling guilty. So you must talk. And it doesn't hurt to buy a good lovemaking guide so you can become more knowledgeable about what you want and what your partner wants.

DID YOU KNOW?
YES, SEX IS GOOD FOR YOU

Is sex good for your health? Yup! One study in Wales involving about a thousand men showed that guys with the lowest frequency of orgasm had twice the risk of death from all causes, but most significantly from heart attack.

There are exercises for premature ejaculation, but before you begin them, tell your partner what's going on. If you tell her, "Honey, you excite me so much, I just can't help myself," she'll be happy to work with you.

One of the exercises is called the squeeze technique. First you stimulate yourself and bring yourself close to the edge, and then you learn to squeeze and back off, and eventually you'll recognize when you are at the point of no return.

Many men are afraid to slow down when they get to that point. But you'll find that most women are in no rush; in fact, they prefer slower lovemaking. Many men have a completely distorted view of what women like, and you are sure to benefit from reading up on foreplay, thrusting styles, rhythm, and other good stuff.

Next, get help from your partner with touching, then move gradually to insertion and withdrawal, keeping it playful and easygoing between the two of you.

People think nothing of spending hours on their golf swing, but this is the kind of thing they expect to come easily or instantly. If you don't achieve the success you want, don't get freaked out. There are a variety of medications, usually in the antidepressant classification, which are very effective. Recent studies have combined SSRIs (selective serotonin reuptake inhibitors) and Viagra to allow men to slow down and still maintain their erections. And brand-new research found that a spray-on medication combining lidocaine and prilocaine that temporarily numbs the tip of the penis extends intercourse from about one-a-half minutes to eleven minutes.

With or without medication, I promise that when you get to a point where you can relax with your partner—who knows what's going on and works with you—the two of you can have all kinds of fun.

Q: I have a theory that premature ejaculation is related to masturbation. When you don't have a partner, you tend to want to achieve gratification very quickly. I don't know if this has been tested, but do you think there's a relationship?

A: Well, that's reasonable. A lot of young men who are afraid of premature ejaculation will stimulate themselves before they go out on a date, to make themselves a little less responsive. And self-stimulation is commonly used to treat premature ejaculation. The man learns to know his response and to practice control. Later he involves his partner in the stimulation, and then they go on to intercourse.

Some current studies examine the relationships between masturbation, premature ejaculation, and circumcision. Men who are circumcised masturbate more than uncircumcised men, but both groups have a similar rate of premature ejaculation. Premature ejaculation problems seem to be a) age related, and b) experience and skill related.

Q: I was taking Viagra, and it worked for a little while, but I can't use it anymore because I get migraines from it. Is there any other legitimate medication you could recommend?

A: Because of all the publicity about Viagra, men are talking to their doctors about impotence problems like never before. This is good. But, as you pointed out, Viagra does not work for everyone, and the same goes for the next generation of impotence drugs. While Cialis (tadafil) and Levitra (vardenafil) stay active in the body for up to twenty-four hours, giving the user more flexibility with his sexual activities, both have side effects similar to those of Viagra. Another option down the road is inhaled apomorphine, which works at the brain level, not the penis level, and can be effective in eight minutes.

But don't give up hope. All this discussion about impotence is pointing us toward many other treatments that have been around for a while. Some of these treatments are even more effective than the Viagra school of drugs, although perhaps not as convenient as taking a pill.

Among the options you should talk about with your doctor are pellets you can insert into your urethra, injections, or pumps (see next question).

This brings up another point—about safety. Anyone contemplating Viagra as a cure—or just looking for the best treatment for erectile dysfunction—should see a urologist. General practitioners may not be familiar with the many other treatments available. They tell men who can't use Viagra that there is nothing else to do, and that is a disservice.

Q: I'm sixty-seven and occasionally I have some difficulty getting an erection. I've taken some Viagra and sometimes that works and other times it's not very effective. What do you think about these vacuum pumps that you read and hear about?

A: Viagra should work consistently unless there is a vascular or neurological problem. But let's make sure we understand what Viagra is good for and what it's not good for. It does not supply incentive, it does not turn you on, it does not affect libido—it simply affects a vascular response. So if it works, it should work consistently if you take the right dose at the right time, and it certainly is the easiest thing.

We consider vacuum pumps, when used appropriately, to be safe and effective. And sometimes it's beneficial for men for whom Viagra or other methods do not work, because the pump simply creates a negative vacuum around the genitalia. Blood will move slowly into your penis, and then you put a band around the base.

So, if you don't mind a little dose of technology introduced into your lovemaking, this should work well for you. I have no problem with pumps. Be careful and buy a good one. You can find these things in stores that shouldn't be selling them. They can make you black-and-blue, and there can be minor hemorrhages and coloration changes. Obviously you want to remove the elastic band when you're done, because if you leave that on, you can get yourself in real trouble.

Also, do not use just any elastic band you find around the house. The specialty bands are designed to exert a pressure that is enough to allow venous flow to be blocked back to your heart but not to block arterial flow coming in. If you make the band a little too tight, and it blocks the blood flow coming in, you'll get gangrene.

Q: I called an 800 number that I heard on the radio and was able to order Viagra over the telephone after answering questions about my age, height, weight, drug allergies, and the medications I'm taking.

The salesman said that if my information cleared with the medical staff, they would get Viagra to me within three days. I asked how they could prescribe a drug without me seeing a doctor, and he told me there are two types of prescription drugs, controlled and noncontrolled.

QUIZ

Between the ages of forty and eighty, which gender has higher statistics for sexual dysfunction?
(Men, by a long shot. A study of almost 28,000 adults from thirty countries showed that women become sexually dysfunctional at about half the rate of men.)

Viagra is supposedly noncontrolled, because it has minimal side effects. Is that true?

A: Doctors are supposed to see patients face to face before prescribing any kind of drugs, although they do prescribe to their own patients over the telephone if they know a patient's case and history.

Your story is a perfect example of the dangers of violating that rule. A recent urologists' study reported that 15 percent of the men at one clinic who asked for Viagra for erectile failure had cancer of the bladder, prostate, or some part of their reproductive systems. In a different study, 14 percent of the men had diabetes and didn't know it. A number of men also had undiagnosed heart disease.

Imagine these men skipping medical exams and getting Viagra while their cancers, diabetes, and heart disease go undiagnosed and untreated. Treating impotence without finding the root of the symptom, and without knowing the whole body of a patient, is the same as playing roulette.

Q: My husband was diagnosed with Peyronie's disease about two years ago. He has tried all the traditional treatments, including taking vitamin E, but he has gotten progressively worse. Will Viagra help him?

A: Peyronie's disease—a curvature in the penis during erection—can be painful. A prolonged erection induced by Viagra could mean more unrelenting pain. That won't help anyone's sex life, and I don't recommend it.

Peyronie's has been known to go away on its own, but I am concerned that your husband's condition is worsening. He needs to get aggressive in looking for solutions. The drug verapamil is showing some promise. Also, although I'm sure he wants to avoid it, surgery is sometimes a solution. As for vitamin E, there is no evidence that it helps at all.

Q: The newspaper recently had an article claiming that men suffer depression as a result of male menopause. It also claimed that male menopause causes decreased sexual function. I certainly notice this problem with my friends. Do you think zinc and saw palmetto can help a man's ailments?

A: Many people do not believe there is such a thing as male menopause. It depends on how you define it. For a woman, menopause is a sudden change. Her ovaries stop producing estrogen, she doesn't ovulate anymore, and her periods stop. She knows, uh-oh, it's here. This can bring on rumination and depression. We do not think that decreased estrogen causes the psychological upset that plagues some women during menopause, because many women go through menopause with no trouble.

There is no sudden change in men. With aging, the testosterone levels decrease gradually. But men also ruminate on and respond psychologically to getting older, and that can lead to stress and depression, which can also play a part in sexual function. If a man's testosterone is low, a testosterone patch should fix things.

Saw palmetto may be effective for an enlarged prostate, but unless a man is zinc deficient, zinc isn't going to do anything for him. As a matter of fact, too much zinc can be toxic. Zinc is overhyped by health food advocates.

One last thought on this topic: Most people report that sex improves as life goes on. It may not be as frequent, but it can be better.

Q: I don't care about sex, because I'm seventy years old, but I'm wondering if my impotence will hurt me. I took the "postage stamp" test four nights running and nothing happened. I'm single, so it's not a big deal. But do I need to do something about this?

A: C'mon guy! Seventy is too young to throw in the towel. There are good women your age out there, so don't give up on your erections. Even if you never have sex again, I want you to see a doctor because aside from causing erectile failure, impotence is a symptom of several ailments, including diabetes, vascular disease, and neurological disorders.

Impotence has a cause, and it responds to medication, Viagra being only one option. So, see a doctor for a checkup, so you aren't relying on just the "postage stamp" results.

However, this is a cheap (depending on the cost of the stamp), do-it-yourself test for erections during sleep, which is one way of knowing if your erectile failure is physical or psychological. (To do the test, you make a ring of postage stamps and lick the ends together. Licking the stamps after they are in place is not a good idea unless you are a contortionist. Put the stamps around your flaccid penis just before you go to sleep. Broken perforations in the morning mean that you probably had an erection during sleep, and your dysfunction is more likely to be psychological.) Of course, your doctor has more accurate testing methods, and I highly recommend those.

Q: I recently read an article in the newspaper about bicycling and male

impotence. I was planning to take up the sport; now I'm not so sure. Is this a legitimate report?

A: Impotence is a bit of a disincentive, isn't it? In fact, this may be a real problem. With frequent riding, both male and female cyclists suffer pain and numbness in the groin, and some male cyclists become impotent. I should emphasize that these symptoms were seen in serious bicyclists, not the occasional rider.

In his research at Stanford University Medical Center, urologist Robert Kessler found that a specially designed bicycle seat relieved symptoms and "reversed erectile dysfunction." The seat, manufactured by Specialized Bikes, is called the Body Geometry Seat. I recommend it. You may as well have everything working to your advantage.

The Web address, for those wanting more information about this seat, is *www.specialized.com*.

Good Orgasms, No Orgasms

Q: Can you recommend something to help with female orgasms? I want them, but I'm not getting them, and my husband knows it.

A: If you are heading for menopause—or already there—that can change your ability to achieve orgasm. If that's the case, talk to your doctor; this can be remedied.

If menopause isn't the cause, you can fix this problem yourself, but your husband must be an active participant in the remedy.

You have two choices: Work with a sexual counselor or therapist—someone you are comfortable with, who has appropriate credentials (see the Resource List on page 105 for referral organizations). Or, if you are uncomfortable with that, there are books with exercises that the two of you can do together.

Most of the time the inability to have an orgasm is not a physical thing. It may be a matter of just relaxing, or feeling you are being cared for—two things you and your husband should work on together. It is important to look at the roles you and your husband might be playing within your relationship. Sometimes it just comes down to teaching your husband what to do. Many men learned sex as a formula and they think they know the principles of female sexuality. Often, they don't. Usually, the best place to begin is with masturbation, with the gradual participation of your husband.

Q: Whenever I have an orgasm with my husband, I start crying. Can you explain this? I'm not in pain. The orgasm feels good, but I actually cry, tears and all.

A: I don't think there is any medical literature that exists on this, but, personally, I've seen this before, and it wasn't in a pathology laboratory. And I am going to assume that this is a good sign, that you're overwhelmed by your orgasms, which is the way it ought to be.

Crying is a wonderful, positive emotion. It is something we do when we're very sad, obviously, but it also is something we do when we're ecstatic and happy. When you're overwhelmed by an experience, almost any kind of an experience, you cry. Why shouldn't that be the case with sexual experiences?

Q: When my wife and I have sex, everything is fine, but when I climax, she says it burns like a hot poker. What's wrong?

A: Strange as it sounds, a woman can develop an allergy to her husband's semen. It's not an unknown phenomenon, and that is one of the manifestations—often a burning, an itching, or redness. One way to test this theory, just to make sure we know what's wrong, is to have sex with a condom and to see if there is the same burning. If there isn't, you've pinpointed the source of the problem.

This is not a very well understood or well known ailment, and the treatments can be tricky. Some doctors use desensitizing shots derived from semen to build up tolerance.

In rare cases, the man may be taking a medication or drug that shows up in all bodily fluids—and the partner is very sensitive to that. This is not purely an allergy to the husband's fluid, but to what's in the fluid. If that's the case, do some more detective work—as long as it's medically OK to stop taking the medicine—and see if she still gets that burning reaction.

Viruses, Infections, and Diseases

Q: My boyfriend took an HIV test, and he is negative. He's my first sexual partner, but I'm not his first, and before we met he had a bisexual lifestyle. Is that one negative test enough for me to be sure he's truly negative?

A: Bisexuality is a major way HIV winds up entering the heterosexual female population. No, one negative HIV test doesn't guarantee security. If he tests negative again six months down the road, and if you are certain you were his only sexual contact for those six months, you can then rely on the test results.

Over the next six months, the only way you can keep yourself absolutely safe from HIV is not to have sex with him or to always use condoms. Beyond the six months, it comes down to trust. You may decide never to have unprotected sex with him. If you trust him, and he lies to you, that lie can cost you your life.

Q: My wife recently had an outbreak of genital herpes for the first time. What precautions do I need to take and be aware of? I have herpes in my mouth. Could I have transmitted it to her during oral sex?

A: Herpes is much more common than most people realize. In fact, among affluent suburbanites in the United States, more than 25 percent tested positive, though only four percent knew they had it. That should tell you why it spreads so easily. But overall, herpes is poorly studied, and you raise a lot of issues, some of which are seriously misunderstood.

First, you could have transmitted it to her during oral sex, but your wife may have had herpes previously and not known it. However, there is a blood test for herpes, and a lot of people find out that they have it, though the majority don't remember ever having a lesion.

It's easy for women not to remember a lesion, because they have a lot of inside parts. For guys, it's almost impossible to ignore. But let's talk about your

---

DID YOU KNOW?
FIVE SYMPTOMS YOU SHOULDN'T IGNORE

If you or your sexual partner experiences anything on this list, make an appointment with your doctor.

1. Sores or rashes anywhere on the genitalia
2. Chronic pain before, during, or after intercourse
3. Total lack of interest in sex
4. Bleeding from the genital area
5. Unusual discharges

---

case. Because we now know that the virus that causes cold sores is contagious and can take up residence in the nether regions, your suspicion about passing it along during oral sex is appropriate.

However, I've seen relationships break up over the issue of herpes, even when there's no proof of infidelity. People will call their lawyers before they think to call their doctor to get this straightened out. This virus can hang on for a while, then, with a little stress and irritation, pop out. You think it's the first attack, but you've actually had it for a long time. Add to this one more frustrating fact—you can spread the virus without active lesions, though it is more common for it to spread with active lesions—and you can see why it's hard to protect yourself and others.

Are you doomed to barrier methods of birth control for the rest of your life? A lot of folks would disagree with me on this, but I believe that when you're married, you need to figure that you're going to share your microbes, and that if your partner has something, you're probably also going to get it. If they have a cold, you're likely to get a cold, too.

In terms of precautions, while she has lesions, the reasonable thing would be to protect yourself, because if you don't have it, you don't need it. As far as oral sex goes, that is a no-man's-land. How common is it for genital herpes to transmit to the mouth? I think that is still an unknown.

One way to look at your situation is as an opportunity to explore new habits of intimacy. You might try something you wouldn't normally do, and it can often add something to the relationship. So, if layers of latex sound unappealing during a breakout, have fun experimenting. If you need help with ideas, there are plenty of books available on that front.

Q: I used to think that oral sex was pretty harmless. But a friend insists that there's a risk of cancer and infections. Does he know what he's talking about? Is there any way to protect my girlfriend and myself?

A: I think oral sex is a very pleasurable part of lovemaking, and some researchers believe it can contribute to a healthy pregnancy (see page 161 in Chapter 4). But there are risks; you need to be informed, and prophylactics are an option to consider.

The *Journal of the National Cancer Institute* did report that the virus found in certain oral cancers is also a sexually transmitted virus. But nothing is simple about this finding, because it's difficult to prove how the transmission occurs. Researchers cannot put people in cages, make them do certain things,

DID YOU KNOW?
THE DARKEST SIDE OF RELATIONSHIPS

Nearly one-third of American women (31 percent) report being physically or sexually abused by a husband or boyfriend at some point in their lives, according to a 1998 Commonwealth Fund survey. And another study shows that intimate partner violence is primarily a crime against women. In 1999, women accounted for 85 percent of the victims of intimate partner violence (671,110 total) and men accounted for 15 percent of the victims (120,100 total).

and wait a year. It was very difficult to prove or disprove how HIV could be transmitted, and there is still disagreement about how easily HIV can be transmitted orally.

I would say that since herpes crosses both ways—between the mouth and the hinterlands—it is reasonable to believe that a virus in oral cancer could be sexually transmitted. All we have now is the fear, but we don't have enough evidence.

As for other infections, researchers have found that oral sex increases the transmission of streptococcus. Perhaps the most common germ passed to women by oral sex is yeast.

So, it makes sense to consider both condoms and dental dams—a sheet of latex that acts as a barrier between the vagina or anus and the mouth—if there is any concern about spreading infection.

Q: My boyfriend wants us to try anal sex, and it sounds gross to me, but I don't want to be a sexual prude. Is there any medical reason not to try this—at least once?

A: Anal sex is the most dangerous sex act because of the ease of spreading HIV. To decrease the risk of spreading disease, we have advised people to use condoms. However, it turns out that may be incomplete advice. Based on research involving condoms with Nonoxynol-9 added to the lubricant, your best bet may be unlubricated condoms plus a nonpetroleum-based lubricant.

The spermicide Nonoxynol-9 has been known to peel epithelial cells when tested in mice. This is serious, since the cells form a layer of protective membrane lining the rectum.

To test Nonoxynol-9's effect on the epithelial cells, lubricants with and without this spermicide were applied to four individuals. The rectal canal was then washed out. Hundreds of epithelial cells were found among the Nonoxynol-9 users. No epithelial cells were found from using the other type of lubricant—carrageenan and methylcellulose.

The Population Council in New York City, which conducted the research, subsequently issued a warning about Nonoxynol-9: "It is reasonable to assume that the loss of the protective epithelium would render a person more at risk for infection by HIV and other sexually transmitted pathogens. We therefore caution against the use of N-9."

Separate of the condoms issue, one other study on anal sex found that people who indulge in this practice frequently have looser sphincters and higher rates of incontinence.

Some people enjoy anal sex, but not everyone does. If you are uncomfortable with it, it's OK to say no.

Q: My girlfriend and I are committed to each other, and we want to spend the rest of our lives together. The doctor told me that I have genital warts. My girlfriend is getting tested. Can we keep this disease under control with proper medical treatment and by using condoms?

A: The warts need to be treated. When they go away, you can consider having unprotected, monogamous sex, but until then, keep the protection, especially if you haven't gotten a clear diagnosis from the doctors yet. The family of viruses that causes warts—HPV—also causes cervical cancer, so it's worth keeping under control.

For more information on HPV, see page 79.

QUIZ

At all ages, which group is more likely to contract gonorrhea, chlamydia, or genital herpes—men or women?
(Women)

Q: I'm forty-four and have had chronic vaginal yeast infections since I was seventeen. My doctor has prescribed Diflucan, which I use once a month, but I don't like to use it all the time because I heard it's bad for my liver. I eat yogurt and use Monistat, and I've tried a candida destroyer, but I only have relief until my next sexual relations with my husband. I also get it from oral sex. And he's been treated, too. What can I do?

A: Recurrent yeast infections in a woman are not unusual, and the best chances for wiping them out depend on the special care of a gynecologist who is willing to consider all of the alternatives. When using medications, the best way to treat a yeast infection is to use the medication directly where the infection is. Since your infections go away when you use medication, we know we can cure them.

When it comes back, it's coming from someplace. We used to think that certain types of tight clothing, the acid-based balance inside a woman's body, or diabetes could be possible causes. But oral sex is probably the most common, underreported cause.

Yeast can come from the colon, and it can come from the mouth. To stop the cycle, your husband can get a prescription for an oral rinse. He can also use a dental dam, or you can even stop oral sex for a while, to see if time helps you get it under control. Finally, instead of just eating the yogurt, try using live yogurt as a douche.

Q: My friend has been married nine years and is pregnant with her second child. Recently the doctor told her she has chlamydia. The only way she could have gotten it is if her husband had sex with someone else, but she believes they have both been monogamous. Does this make sense?

A: First, she's lucky she got pregnant. Chlamydia is one of the most com-

---

QUIZ

Which is the most common sexually transmitted disease (STD) in the United States?

A) HIV   B) gonorrhea   C) HPV   D) hepatitis B
E) herpes

(E: herpes; about 45 million people in the United States are infected.)

The Edell Report
How Serious Is HPV?

Just a couple of years ago, many of us had never heard the term human papillomavirus (HPV). Yet now it is the second most-prevalent sexually transmitted disease (herpes is No. 1) in the United States, and it's a killer for women, so no one can afford to be in the dark about it.

According to one of the latest studies, published in winter 2002 in the New England Journal of Medicine, *there are eighteen strains—yes, eighteen—that are high risk, and one of the most serious dangers is cervical cancer. Other types of HPV also may have links to cancer of the cervix, vulva, vagina, anus, and penis, so this is nothing to fool with.*

Who's most likely to be exposed to HPV? According to one report, the lifetime incidence of genital HPV infection is estimated at as high as 70 to 80 percent of the sexually active population. While the virus can be dangerous, it does not affect all people the same way; for many carriers, the virus clears out on its own, and no cancer develops.

In total, there are about a hundred types of HPV, and, rarely, it includes a symptom of genital warts in both men and women. The good news is clinicians have an array of therapeutic weapons available to diagnose and treat genital warts, so if you have them, see a physician.

But a great many people have been infected with HPV and don't even know it, because the condition is latent and in most cases there are no symptoms. And condoms don't eliminate the risk of virus transmission, since HPV can also be spread during foreplay and other sexual contact. It even has been found under fingernails.

According to the study reported in the New England Journal of Medicine, *the virus usually causes cancer in women when they have carried it in their system for years. Scientists are working on screening tests that can be incorporated into Pap smears, and a vaccine for HPV-16—which is most frequently linked to cervical cancer—has shown good results in a controlled trial.*

mon causes of infertility. It is a bacterium that can cause pelvic inflammatory disease (PID), which can be chronic.

Second, I can understand why you are suspicious, and I would be, too—more so than I would be if we were talking about herpes or even genital warts, which could lay dormant from a time before she even met her husband.

But your girlfriend is far from alone in her response to her diagnosis. A recent study of three hundred heterosexual couples by researchers at the State University of New York found that both men and women have less information about their partner's sexual experience than they think they do. Both genders underestimated the number of sexual partners that the other person in the relationship had had. And eighty-two men and sixty-three women in this study said they had had sex with another person—not their current partner—within the past six months, though most couples had been together at least six months.

Your friend needs to have a frank discussion with her gynecologist and her husband.

The Penis, Prostate, and Testicles

Q: I read an article about penis-reduction surgery. I'm a twenty-five-year-old newlywed, and I guess I have an abnormally large penis. We are having trouble with our lovemaking. What's my next step?

A: I've talked to newlyweds with this problem, and when we get down to numbers, we find out that the man's penis is entirely normal or even on the small side. Discomfort and pain can occur regardless of the size of the penis if your positions or technique are wrong.

When a doctor examines a woman's vagina, he uses a steel speculum, which is larger in girth than the penis of even a very well-endowed man. So the width of your penis should not be an issue.

A penis can be uncomfortably long for a woman's canal. Lubrication, position, and a man's sensitivity to his partner's needs almost always resolve this. Communicate with her about which moves and positions hurt. And give her what she needs to get turned on, to get her juices flowing.

I would never recommend surgery. Such a drastic solution is unnecessary and just not done. Reducing the length would require detaching the penis from the pubic bone, which is also what we do to increase the length. It's a very unreliable procedure.

Q: I have a friend who wants to have foreskin reconstruction, because he thinks that will allow him more pleasure from his sexual relationships. Is he right?

A: Isn't it curious that our society accepts women enlarging their breasts with surgery, but when a guy wants to restore a foreskin that was removed when he was a young child—his normal body structure was altered before he was old enough to have a say—people don't really get it.

There is no doubt that circumcision alters sensitivity. The tip of an intact man's penis is mucous membrane that's only one-cell-layer thick, while that of circumcised men is ten to fifteen cell layers of thicker, drier skin. Men who were circumcised as adults and men who had their foreskins restored talk about definite decreases or increases in sensitivity. In fact, I remember one fellow, circumcised as an adult, who said that sex after the surgery was like living in black-and-white, where once he had known color.

There are urologists who will do foreskin restoration. And many men do it themselves by stretching the skin as far as it will go with tape and weights (see next question), then getting surgery to finish the job, if necessary.

There is a good book about this subject, called *The Joy of Uncircumcising*. And the organization NOCIRC has a Web site, *www.nocirc.org*, if your friend wants more information.

Q: I think my boyfriend needs a penis extender. What can you tell me about these?

A: First, don't tell your boyfriend you asked this question. Second, these products are a total and complete scam. Instead of focusing on the size of your boyfriend's penis, try initiating a healthy conversation with him about what *both* of you would like to experience in your sexual relationship.

If that advice doesn't satisfy you, here are a few facts on penis length: An Italian study conducted with 3,300 men ages seventeen to nineteen years old determined that the average flaccid penis, stretched taut, measures 12.5 centimeters or about 4.9 inches. And a study at the University of California that measured men with erect penises found an average length of 5.1 inches.

One interesting thing to note: The Italian researchers found a correlation between penis size and height and weight. And Greek researchers found a relationship between the length of the index finger and the penis.

Q: Every time my husband and I have intercourse, his left testicle both-

ers him. It's not swollen or anything. He wants to push it down and in. Is this a good idea?

A: This is a real guy thing. Many men's testicles disappear into the inguinal canal after or during sex. The testicle either gets pushed up, simply by the act of intercourse, or the muscles pull them up.

It can be uncomfortable. A man has to reach up to the outer quadrant—I assume most men know this—and push on it to kind of pop it out. However, if a man complains of pain in this area after intercourse, there's an outside chance there is something going on in the prostate, and he should see a urologist. This would be "referred pain," so named because if you hit a man in the testicles, he will first grab his stomach, because that's where he feels it. That's because the nerve to the testicles comes from the stomach area, and the pain is "referred" there.

Q: I'm fifty-eight and in excellent condition. I feel great and I'm never tired. However, I've noticed that I have less and less semen when I ejaculate. Is this a problem?

A: A decrease in volume is natural as you get older, but no semen is not natural. If that's the situation, see a urologist. You could have retrograde ejaculation, where semen goes backwards into the bladder.

Q: I have a sixteen-year-old son who has an undescended testicle on the right side. He had an ultrasound, and it shows the testicle in the inguinal canal. The urologist has given us the following options, and I don't know which direction to take. One is to do nothing, which he advises against because of the cancer and fertility risks. The other is to have surgery, but he's uncertain—given that my son is well past puberty—that he will be able to bring down the testicle into the scrotum. He said the testicle might have to be removed, but he won't know that until he does the surgery. Can you help us make a decision?

A: We had to go through this with one of my sons, but he was just a few months old. Usually when boys are very young, there is a better chance of bringing it down.

This is a very difficult situation. Since it's in the canal, the doctors have a better chance of pulling it down. When it's up in the abdominal cavity, it's a little more challenging. If the doctors go in and cannot pull the testicle down, you're in a tough spot.

Doing nothing is not a good idea, because an undescended testicle has a much higher rate of developing cancer than a descended testicle. Also, this situation may have an impact on his fertility, although it's highly unlikely that the testicle will be fertile at this point.

It is possible to put in a prosthetic, so that whatever happens in surgery, when your son comes out he'll have two testicles—though one will be real and one may not be. He's reaching the age where this might be a factor, so the two of you should talk to the urologist about that.

Bottom line: I don't think you have a choice; you've got to go for it.

Q: It's been recommended that I have my testicles removed because of chronic pain. The pain is in the actual testicles themselves. Are there any long-term side effects?

A: There are several things to consider about removing your testicles. First, the nerves from the testicles come from the abdomen. You need to be absolutely sure the pain you are experiencing is from the testicles and not from your stomach; in other words, if you haven't gotten a second opinion, you should. And the specialist should be a urologist.

Second, it would be much easier just to snip the nerve to your testicles, and then you could keep them. Are you going to get a prosthesis? Do you care? Also, you must weigh the testosterone question: You are removing your source of testosterone. Aesthetics aside, would you be willing to take hormones for a period of time?

Testicular cancer does not always begin with pain, but a shriveled, painful testicle should be removed because the index of suspicion is high. Just make sure your doctor has taken the things I mentioned into consideration.

Q: When my husband and I have intercourse, there are lots of brown and black spots in his semen. Is it from an infection?

A: This is a common question. Usually brown and black spots in semen are from old blood. With all the pressures involved in the ejaculatory reflex, it's not surprising that blood shows up every once in a while. And as upsetting a symptom as this can be, I have rarely seen it due to anything serious.

Just to be sure, though, you should have your husband see a urologist and take the opportunity to get his prostate checked out.

Q: About fifteen minutes after intercourse, I get a sharp pain and

burning in my rectum that goes away within another fifteen minutes. It happens very infrequently. I sometimes have the same symptoms when riding my bicycle. Is that a spasm of the rectum or prostate?

A: The prostate is surrounded by muscles that can contract, reducing the flow of blood and possibly causing cramping and pain, though this has never been proven. And, of course, pain in the prostate can easily be felt in the rectum, because the prostate and the rectum are next to each other.

It's impossible for me to know the exact source, but the pain during bike riding is a helpful clue. Bike seats can irritate the nerves in the region (see the Premature Ejaculation and Impotence section in this chapter, too).

Many men report this kind of elusive discomfort or pain. Spasm in the rectal area is also a very real phenomenon.

Q: I'm a fifty-year-old guy who's been diagnosed with chronic infectious prostatitis. The antibiotics aren't working too well anymore. I tried to massage my prostate myself, but my arms aren't long enough, so I ordered a prostate massager on the Internet. It came in the mail the other day, but I haven't had the nerve to try it yet. It's shaped like a forefinger with a little attachment. Do you know if these things work or if they can do any damage?

A: Maybe I lead a sheltered life, but I'm not familiar with a nonhuman prostate massager, and if you were my patient, I'd write you a prescription for orgasm. What do you have to lose?

Nothing I know of empties the prostate as effectively as an orgasm does. If a man were to feel his prostate before and after an orgasm, he would be amazed at how much it shrinks. The prostate is surrounded by a muscular capsule, and during orgasm that muscle contracts and then empties the gland pretty thoroughly. In fact, one recent study from Australia comparing men with and without prostate cancer found that the more men ejaculate between the ages of 20 and 50 the less likely they were to develop prostate cancer.

But you're talking about an infection, not cancer, and we're not exactly sure about all of this, because this topic isn't the type that attracts major research funds. However, based on what we know about glandular infections elsewhere in the body, shedding the infectious material can be assumed to be helpful.

For example, if a breast-feeding woman has mastitis—an infection in her breasts—we encourage her to express her milk as much as possible. Getting rid of the infectious material makes the job that much easier for the antibiotics.

Fortunately for you, infectious prostatitis can be easier to treat than the noninfectious kind. For the latter, you just have to hang in there until you hit the right antibiotic. Ask your doctor about doing a culture to further identify the infection.

The delivery system for the antibiotic, namely swallowing it, is another potential obstacle to knocking out this infection. The medicine goes into your stomach, then to your bloodstream, which carries it to the prostate with the objective of making a direct hit in the area where the infection is percolating. Sometimes it works, sometimes it doesn't.

Q: On the side of the head of my penis, I have an area that looks like the skin is slightly raised, like a scratch. Every three or four days it flakes off and then comes back again. I've had this for a couple of months. Should I be worried?

A: When the skin flakes off and then returns and flakes off again, it suggests something could be growing, such as a basal cell carcinoma. Most often, growths are benign, but because there is such a thing as cancer of the penis, you need to see a urologist.

I'm not suggesting that you have cancer, but you want to know for sure. You would not want the consequences of its spreading. Both men and women can make the sad mistake of letting treatable, genital cancers grow because they are too embarrassed to see a doctor. Urologists and gynecologists are not going to be surprised by anything "down there." They've seen it all many times. Of course, almost every dermatological disease can affect the genitals, so there are lots of possibilities here.

Q: Three months ago, I had prolonged intercourse and oral sex with a female partner. Afterwards, my penis was sore to the touch; even my clothes irritated it. I've had friction sores before, but this was different. The pain lasted for about two months, and then it went away. Last month, I had sex with the same partner, and again I developed the same problem. The pain is mostly at the tip of my penis. What's going on?

A: I want you to see a doctor, because you could have urethritis. The sensation you are having could be caused by an infection of your urethra or by a sexually transmitted disease in your urethra.

Simple physical irritation is not unusual, particularly if lubrication is insufficient. Some men find dryness to be more stimulating, but it can also cause irritation. In your case, the irritation has been going on way too long.

Vasectomies

Q: Forty years ago, shortly after I had my vasectomy, I heard a rumor that vasectomies cause hardening of the arteries. Is there any truth to that?

A: There seems to be some truth to that rumor for monkeys, but not for men. Around the time you had your vasectomy, researchers studied two groups of primates that were fed a higher fat and cholesterol diet than normal. One group of animals was given vasectomies. This group had a higher rate of arteriosclerosis than did the other group.

When we got those results on primates, we began to watch for similar patterns with men. Five years went by with no such problems developing, but five years isn't enough time to observe. But twenty years later, there were still no increased levels of arteriosclerosis in evidence. And that's where things stand.

We have an expectation that results that turn up with lab monkeys will turn up with humans, but that's not always true. If a vasectomy does have any effect on hardening of the arteries, it is a tiny one compared to the known risks of poor diet, lack of exercise, and hereditary predisposition.

Q: My wife is bugging me to get a vasectomy. I have a question. Where do the sperm go?

A: They don't go anywhere. They hang out, die, and get absorbed. But, obviously, if you have your vasectomy reversed, that restores the flow of sperm through the vas deferens. However, what many people don't know is that there are several microsurgical procedures for extracting sperm directly from the testicle, in cases where a vasectomy reversal doesn't work. Pregnancy rates vary according to the procedure.

Libido: Too Much and Too Little

Q: I know this sounds strange, but is there a drug, herb, or something else that could help to lower my libido? I'm not married.

A: I'm going to guess that having a strong libido all the time can be a nuisance; it's like you're sitting there and you want to watch a ball game, and there you are with all this libido stuff.

Well, in the most serious cases, with sex offenders, there are drugs to turn off their ability to have sex. And sometimes their testicles are removed. But I'm sure you don't want to consider either of those options. When it comes to mythology, there is saltpeter—but it doesn't work.

Probably the largest group of medications that lower libido are antidepressants. The selective serotonin reuptake inhibitors (SSRIs) represent most of the antidepressant market. But these drugs are meant for something else. So, if you were serious about it, you and your doctor would try to find a medication that is the most benign for what its primary usage is, and then see if the side effect helps you.

I'm giving you this information, but I'm not recommending it. I think there are easier solutions that relate to your own personal life, including masturbation, exercise, and/or meditation. Once you find a partner, you can address this with him or her, directly and honestly, and see if the problem persists.

Q: My partner wants sex every single day. It has to be every twelve hours, or every day, three times a day. We're in our forties and fifties and it's always been this way. Is there a medical condition that could cause this? I'm exhausted, and this is becoming a big problem for me.

A: In my first book, *Eat, Drink, and Be Merry*, I cited what I consider the most important consensus statement from sexual medicine doctors on the definition of sexual health. It is a fairly broad and encompassing definition that covers a range of individual tastes. It defines sexual health as the enjoyment of sexual activity of one's choice without causing or suffering physical or mental harm.

Every couple has their own definition of the "right" amount of sex, but problems arise when one partner changes the definition or grows tired of something that was once tolerable but no longer is. On a pure numbers level, many of my listeners consider once a day the ideal, while others would consider that to be very intrusive. And one earth-shaker a month satisfies some. As for three times a day, I think most folks would find that extreme. But there is no right answer; it really depends on what we look to sex to be.

As far as medical conditions go, they are very rare in this situation. People do get tumors in some parts of the brain that will increase the sex drive, and

DID YOU KNOW?
ENJOY SEX, DRINK WATER . . .

I think we all realize that sex is a form of exercise, so it doesn't surprise me that people could become dehydrated after a flurry of lovemaking. The answer to this is to drink lots of water, which is also the conclusion of a study done at Aberdeen University in Scotland on behalf of a bottled-water company. Researchers point out that a half hour of making love can be as strenuous as a three-mile run, but I don't think many couples have intercourse for that long—a few minutes is more like it, according to studies I've seen. Nor is postcoital dehydration filling up emergency rooms. Of course your heart rate increases, and you can work up a sweat during sex, and some people later have headaches or become lethargic, but this varies from person to person.

there are hormone abnormalities, too. It's also possible your partner is using testosterone. But I think it's more about you and your partner—what sex means to you and what it means to him or her. Resentments have built up, and if you continue to let a dissatisfying situation go on without talking about it, your relationship could be damaged or destroyed. But do not try to solve this problem in one day. I urge you both to seek a good counselor. Sit down for a few hours and discuss this in front of an objective third party, possibly someone who specializes in sexual medicine. Often it has nothing to do with sex, and there is something else going on. There are many creative solutions here, but until you start talking, you can't know how to fix things.

Q: I'm forty-one and I'm just not interested in sex like I used to be, and I'm wondering if birth control pills could affect my sex drive?

A: I saw one study that showed some brands of the pill improve sex drive while others dampen it. So that's a possibility, and you should discuss this with your gynecologist. A pill switch might change everything.

However, you need to begin with the basics. Look at the possibility that depression, stress, or difficulties with a relationship might be the cause. One of these is most often the case, and folks just don't want to acknowledge that.

Q: What can you tell me about a new pill that may allow men to have multiple orgasms in a short period of time? My best friend said he heard something about it on the radio, but he was short on the details.

The Edell Report
Who Gets the Headache?

Are men more likely to suffer from sex-related headaches than women? Apparently, the old joke, "Not tonight, honey, I have a headache," isn't very accurate, according to the findings of German neurologists.

Men can get sexually related headaches that are described as "a thunderclap," coming on suddenly and with great intensity. They frequently appear at the base of the skull, at or near the moment of orgasm, transforming pleasure to pain in seconds. The pain can last anywhere from ten to fifteen minutes.

Although they are sometimes referred to as "coital headaches," this term is not exactly accurate, since it can occur during moments of self-pleasure.

Most people flush just as they get turned on. This is caused by vasodilation—the blood vessels dilate. This may be the cause of these headaches.

What is the cure for this problem? The first step—you're going to hate this prescription—is a brief period of abstinence, a couple of weeks.

Other cures include varying sexual positions to cut down on sexual exertion, losing weight, and lowering blood pressure.

If you think you need treatment, it's important to see a neurologist or a physician that specializes in headaches and ask about antimigraine medications.

A: Well, if preliminary research proves accurate, we will all soon know a lot more about a drug called cabergoline. As strange as it sounds, this drug is normally used in the treatment of Parkinson's disease, but during medical trials it was found to enable men to have multiple orgasms in rapid succession. The drug had no side effects on men during the tests, according to an article about the findings, and further trials were planned to see if the drug would have the same impact on women.

The downside, for me, is how this plays into the old numbers game, where we seem to measure sexual performance in quantity rather than by the pleasure quality. One good orgasm in a man would seem to be the way it was designed, although many women may differ. There are men who seem jealous of women's common capacity to have multiple orgasms, and while this drug is not routinely prescribed for this use yet, I am sure once the word gets out, some drug company will turn this into a best-seller.

Q: Can anything be done when a woman's physical and mental interest in sex is totally destroyed by a hysterectomy? My lack of interest is hurting my marriage.

A: A woman's uterus is involved in her physical sexual response, so it makes sense that its removal could reduce her interest in sex. If a woman's ovaries are removed along with her uterus, her libido is even more likely to plummet.

For some women, the uterus is an emotionally powerful representation of their womanhood, so losing it can make them sad and depressed, and that alone is enough to quash the sex drive.

The good news is that there are solutions. First, you should find out if depression is a part of the problem, and your gynecologist should be the first person you talk to about that. Second, you should talk to your doctor about taking testosterone, particularly if your ovaries were removed along with your uterus. Testosterone acts as an aphrodisiac, increasing a woman's libido. It's available as a pill, a patch, or an under-the-tongue tablet.

Some research suggests that a hysterectomy actually improves a woman's sex life. After all, a woman who has had a lot of bleeding or a tumor may feel much better when her uterus is removed and her health improves. However, a recent study says that many women do feel their sexual response changed after a hysterectomy.

Q: I'm a fifty-five-year-old man, and I have been taking Depo-Testosterone for a low libido and low testosterone. I heard a doctor on TV say that taking testosterone can shrink a man's penis. Is that true?

A: A man with normal testosterone levels in his blood who begins taking testosterone is one thing, but taking testosterone because your levels are low is something entirely different.

I don't think shrinkage should concern you, because you're trying to get your level back up to normal. I have no knowledge of testosterone causing a man's penis to shrink in that situation.

The doctor may have been warning men with already normal levels of testosterone who are taking even more. When that is the case, testicles can become smaller, and other things can happen, too.

This is why I'm so opposed to DHEA supplements and androstenedione (see page 128 in chapter 3 for more about this). When a man with already normal levels of testosterone takes these hormones, his testicles will say, "Hey, there is a lot of testosterone in the bloodstream already, so I better turn off any further androgen production."

As a result, his testicles can turn off because of the additional testosterone from the pills in his system. This can, indeed, cause some genital shrinking— but this is not your situation.

Q: I'm a happy, healthy, forty-one-year-old guy, and I've been in a monogamous relationship for a number of years. For the last two years, I've had no libido. I was discussing this with a friend, who happens to be a physician, and based on answers I gave him to his questions, he said it sounded like my problem was physical. He suggested that I get an extensive blood test to find out if it may be caused by diabetes. Do you know of any connection between diabetes and libido?

A: Loss of libido is the No. 1 sexual complaint that people go to their doctors for. So you're not alone.

Usually, diabetes is associated with erectile failure rather than libido. But certainly there's the possibility that you might not be enthusiastic about sex if you thought you were facing erectile failure. When you hear hoofbeats, you think of horses and not zebras, and in medicine we're trained to look for the most likely explanation for a patient's symptom and then move down the list.

That said, if you walked into my office, I would first go down the common list of things that can explain this, and we would certainly look at physical things and hormonal illnesses and low testosterone. But the primary cause is stress, fatigue, depression, or anxiety; low libido at your age usually relates to your life, your wife, your relationship, etc.

Men, especially, place a lot of pressure on themselves and think they're supposed to feel turned on all the time, like the guys in beer commercials. Sex is an extraordinarily complicated subject and not a simple reflex. I find that when you approach a problem like this, you've got to keep an open mind and consider all of the possibilities.

Diabetes wouldn't be the first thing on my list, because you haven't mentioned other symptoms—fatigue and frequent urination come to mind. But certainly, get everything checked out. You need a physical at your age if you haven't already had one.

Q: How do you view the relationship between marijuana and sex? I am a woman who had an active sex life up to age thirty-five. From thirty-five to forty-seven, I smoked a lot of marijuana and had a wonderful sex life. Now I'm fifty-nine and have had no sexual desire since I stopped smoking marijuana twelve years ago.

A: I would have expected the opposite reaction, but this is a confusing subject. Very early on, we found that a lot of people believed marijuana to be an aphrodisiac. And I received many notes sharing details about wonderful sex.

Then research began to show that chronic abuse of marijuana had the opposite effect—it depresses libido. I also believe that chronic abuse of marijuana can cause depression, and one of the prime symptoms of depression is a loss of libido. But most side effects of marijuana use go away once you quit, so I don't think it's related. Perhaps the marijuana was covering up an underlying depression. Talk to your gynecologist about your options. You're too young to be missing out on sexual enjoyment.

Q: I'm a widow, age sixty-six, and I'm not on estrogen. Last fall, I met a gentleman and had a sexual experience, just once. After that I developed very strong sexual feelings, and they got a little bit out of hand. In a two-month time frame, I was up in the middle of the night putting on CDs and dancing around the kitchen; I didn't need much sleep.

Then suddenly, I got up one day and that feeling was gone. I thought that was the last of this craziness, until two weeks ago, when the sexual

feelings became so intense that I went to my doctor. My blood work indicated that I have an abnormally high testosterone level, and now I'm taking Synthroid (hypothyroid medication). The doctor checked my estrogen levels, and they were fine, but physically or vaginal-wise, I'm like I was when I was young. What do you think is going on?

A: You should ask your doctor to refer you to an endocrinologist. When you see the endocrinologist, you should ask to have the blood work repeated; one has to be very careful in measuring hormone levels in a woman.

Increased sexual desire could be caused by your pituitary gland; sexual hyperactivity can be a part of bipolar disorder (manic depression), and there are rare disorders of persistent sexual arousal.

Start by getting an explanation for your high testosterone levels, and I think an endocrinologist will help you get the answers you need.

The Questions Kids Ask and Don't Ask

Q: My seventeen-year-old son wants his girlfriend, who is also seventeen, to stay overnight one night per weekend. He's a great kid in every way, and we like his girlfriend, too. But we are really torn up about this and have had several arguments with him. Oh, by the way, his sixteen-year-old brother lives in the house, too. What would you do?

A: This is never an easy subject, and I don't feel one answer fits all situations. But here are some questions to consider.

First, do her parents know about this request? If so, have you talked to them about it? Don't get your information on this point from your son or the girl; talk to the parents directly. If the parents are opposed, your decision is easy: There should not be any overnights.

Second, if the girl's parents are comfortable with the idea in general, what other issues have been discussed? Would they ever sleep at her house? Would they share in joint family activities—such as dinner or a movie—when they are at your house? Or are they going to act like no one else exists in the house? Have there been frank discussions about birth control?

Other things to consider: Is the younger son comfortable around the girlfriend? Does he have an opinion on this? Is he already sexually active himself? If you let one son have this living situation, when will the other son be "eligible" to have girlfriends stay overnight in his room?

Finally, if you decide that weekend overnighters are the best way to ensure a safe environment for your sexually active child, insist on a face-to-face meeting with both sets of parents and the teenagers to outline expectations, so there are no surprises or misunderstandings later on. Overall, though, I think most parents would object to this.

Q: I feel that the best sex education for my sixteen-year-old daughter should follow the abstinence-'til-marriage line of thinking, and this is what my church supports, too. My older sister, who also has teenagers and goes to our church, thinks I'm being unrealistic in this approach. Who do you agree with?

A: I have no objection to the goal of abstinence-'til-marriage, but the practicality of that and how you get there is the problem. The "Just Say No" antidrug program gave us evidence that abstinence programs, at least in their current incarnation, don't work. And as with the antidrug program D.A.R.E., there is a possibility the current abstinence programs could backfire and increase an interest in the behaviors they seek to discourage.

Like you, I feel the best sex can be had in the context of monogamy, but it may be hard to convince a sixteen-year-old. And you have to ask yourself,

---

DID YOU KNOW?
WHO KNOWS WHAT?

According to a study by the Sexuality Information and Education Council of the United States, more than four in ten (43 percent) parents of nine- and ten-year-olds have not discussed the basic facts about reproduction with their child. Even those with teenagers have not tackled some vital topics. Two in ten (20 percent) parents with thirteen- and fourteen-year-olds and one in ten (11 percent) parents of kids age fifteen to eighteen admit they have not discussed relationship and sexual-activity issues with their child.

do you want your daughter rushing into a bad marriage just so she can experience sex?

The best evidence we have from other countries is that the most effective way to get teens to abstain from sex is to provide comprehensive sex education programs that teach young people all aspects of sexuality, including how to use birth control to prevent unintended pregnancy and how to protect against sexually transmitted diseases. Add to this your own personal discussions with your daughter, and you are more likely to get the results you want.

By the way, I do think it's important to be honest about sex when talking to kids. We find it easy to tell them of the fears and pitfalls and scary negative things that can happen to them, but we seem to have difficulties discussing the joys of sex and why it is such a draw. I assume that your goal is for your daughter to have an ecstatic and loving sex life for the rest of her life. Tell her that's why you want her to wait.

Q: I suspect that my fifteen-year-old daughter—who's my oldest—is either sexually active or on the brink of it. We try to be good parents, but I'm constantly battling with her about everything, and I am not sure what to assume on the sex question. Can you help?

A: Don't assume anything. And don't go into this looking for a fight. If your primary goal is that your teenage daughter remain virginal, communication at home is what is most likely to get you to that goal.

If you don't know this intuitively, which I hope you do, consider this data from a ten-year study of two hundred Wisconsin girls that looked at their school activities and grades, drug and alcohol use, sexual behavior, and relationships with their siblings and parents.

Over the course of the ten years, some of the virginal girls became sexually active. But the girls who ranked highest in communication with their parents

---

QUIZ

What percentage of STDs occur in people age twenty-five or younger?
A) 45 percent   B) 52 percent   C) 75 percent
D) 66 percent   E) 38 percent
(D: 66 percent; one out of four new infections occurs in teenagers.)

DID YOU KNOW?
TEENAGERS AND CHLAMYDIA

Two and a half million teenagers in the United States contracted chlamydia in 2002, making it the most common sexually transmitted disease among teens. And new research shows the majority of teen girls get chlamydia from boys their own age. Chlamydia can lead to pelvic inflammatory disease (PID), infertility, and an increased risk of contracting HIV. A simple cervical swab or urinalysis can diagnose it.

delayed the onset of sexual intercourse. "Even after correcting for age, communication with the mother was significantly better in patients who maintained their virginal status."

If, through your conversations, you determine that your daughter is already sexually active, tell her that the only thing you will insist on is that she see a gynecologist about the best method of birth control, then ask her if there's a particular doctor she would like to see. If she doesn't have a doctor in mind, ask her if she'd like to see your doctor or someone who doesn't know you.

This sounds tough, doesn't it? But it could be a lot tougher if you don't talk with her frankly and openly. Also, encourage her to talk about any problems with you at any time. If she doesn't want to talk to you, tell her about Go Ask Alice, a great Web site produced by Columbia University (details on page 105).

Q: Should we keep the medicine cabinet in our son's bathroom stocked with a supply of condoms? He's seventeen, and we know he's sexually active. My husband says our guy should take the initiative and make the purchases himself. I figure the more we do to encourage safe sex, the better.

A: Instead of talking to each other about this, you and your husband should be talking to your son. Just stocking his medicine cabinet and walking away is not a complete solution to the perceived problem. If you know he's sexually active, you first need to ask him if he's protecting himself. And while it's nice to think that he's not embarrassed to walk into a store to purchase a condom, it sounds like you're not sure if he's protecting himself right now. If he's not, you need to know that and have a discussion. Encouraging safe sex requires more than just putting condoms in the medicine cabinet.

Q: I am only sixteen, and I just lost my virginity. I've now had sex a few times. I know that some girls bleed a little the first time they have sex, but I seem to bleed every time. It scares me, and I haven't gone to a doctor because I don't want my mom to ask a lot of questions. Did I catch a disease?

A: First of all, you've got to talk to your mom. Even if she's angry or frustrated with you at first, she's the one person who can make sense of this for you.

From a medical point of view, you should not be bleeding every time. In fact, most women do not bleed the first time they have sex. So you should see a doctor to find out why you are. It sounds like sex is causing you a lot of worry and not very much fun, so why don't you consider putting it off for a while?

Miscellaneous: IUDs, Vibrators, and More

Q: I have an unusual problem. When my girlfriend and I talk about having sex, I sneeze. Not so much while we're having sex, but if there is some suggestive sexual talk prior to the act, I will sneeze. A long time ago, a woman told me I have honeymoon nose. Have you ever heard of this?

QUIZ

In their first experience with intercourse, how many teenagers use condoms?

A) less than half   B) more than half   C) more than two-thirds

D) almost all

(*C: more than two-thirds.*)

A: Honeymoon nose is a new one to me. I'd be interested in knowing the origin of that, because what you're describing may be real, and it's very interesting that it happens before the act. I have had many questions over the years about people develop sneezing attacks *during* intercourse.

Some allergists will say it's because your face is buried in the pillow, and you're stirring up the feathers and you're allergic to them. That's not the most likely explanation. The nose can react in strange way to body reflexes. For instance, the photic-sneeze reflex is a condition where you come out of darkness—out of a movie theater, for example—and into the light, and you start to sneeze.

What we think is going on is that the nose has tissue in it that's very similar to erectile tissue. And when many people have sexual thoughts, they can feel a flush go through their face and their body. In fact, we have observed the swelling of turbinates, which are these ribbed structures inside your nose. That can certainly induce a sneeze.

Unless this becomes obtrusive to your lovemaking, I don't see any reason to treat it. You could try an antihistamine, but you don't really need it.

Q: My wife has an IUD, and every time we have sex I bump into it. She fears that it could get infected. I can feel the end of it, and it's a real drag. Can this be fixed?

A: This isn't unusual. She should tell her gynecologist to snip the tail of the IUD (intrauterine device). That will take care of it.

There was once a bad model of IUD, the Dalkon Shield, which had a multi-

---

DID YOU KNOW?
WHEN CLEAN ISN'T A GOOD THING

Don't douche! I've said it again and again, but if you don't believe me, here's hard proof: A 2002 study shows women who insist on being "clean" are 40 percent more likely to have mild bacterial vaginal infections than those women who don't douche at all.

The Edell Report
A "Heat" Period for Women?

Sexologists have always wondered if human females have a heat period within their menstrual cycle similar to that found in other mammals. But despite many attempts to prove that women are more likely to initiate sexual activity while they are ovulating, there have been no conclusive results. And studies on sexual arousability, masturbation, desire, and intercourse frequency during women's cycles have yet to be fruitful.

The newest thinking is that so many external, environmental events determine how often a person makes love that subtle internal drives and cycles would not cause a noticeable shift in something as broad as how many times a month a woman has sex. However, studies that look at more subtle aspects of sexuality have found that during ovulation women do exhibit increases in sexual expression other than coital frequency.

For instance, women will judge normally unattractive, sweaty odors of men as more pleasant during ovulation. They seem to prefer a different look in a man's face during ovulation. Using morph programs on a computer, women seem to prefer a more masculine face during ovulation compared to other times in their cycle, when they seem to prefer a more feminine look in a man. In addition, men seem to find the scent of women more attractive during ovulation than during the phases of the cycle before and after ovulation.

As fascinating as this is, these changes are so subtle that psychological and emotional factors, I'm sure, would overwhelm any physiological increases in sexuality. Human beings are among the only animals that make love for recreation as well as procreation, and it seems to work well for us.

filament tail that could carry infection into the uterus. So now IUDs have a single-filament tail. It can feel sharp against the tip of a man's penis.

Because of past problems with the Dalkon Shield, American women have shied away from using IUDs. That's too bad, because they are a great method of birth control and are widely used elsewhere in the world. They have the highest satisfaction rate of any method of birth control.

Q: I have a bet with my friend. He claims he can make his girlfriend ejaculate. I say he's nuts. Who's right?

A: It's amazing, the amount of spirited debate that surrounds this issue. There is no secret organ hidden within the female pelvis that has eluded anatomists for thousands of years that could possibly contain the amount of fluid that people claim to emerge during orgasm.

I attribute any fluids to a condition that urologists are very familiar with, called orgasmic incontinence. During the moment of orgasm, your sphincters are atwitter, and the loss of urine is totally compatible with what is described

---

DID YOU KNOW?
A CONDOM IN A PANTY?

I think this is a cool idea, and I hope it flies. The Zebra Woman Panty Condom—disposable bikini-style underwear fitted with a lubricated latex pouch that is inserted in the vagina just before foreplay—is being tested by the Zebra Foundation, a U.S.-based nonprofit organization working internationally since 1996 to support research and development of new HIV/STD prevention tools. For more information, check out *www.zebrafoundation.org*. However, I can't recommend a similar condom made in Colombia and being sold on the Internet, which does not use latex. Right now, there is only one condom for women, the Female Condom, but some women find it awkward to use, visually unappealing, and it can make squeaky noises. (For more information on contraceptives see page 178 in chapter 4.)

---

as female orgasm. While many people are embarrassed about it, and think this is a negative, I see it as one example of achieving peak sexual ecstasy. It's simply a sign of how excited the woman has become. However, if you don't want this particular display of excitement to occur, urinating before intercourse is one way to prevent this. And we advise women to urinate after intercourse to prevent bladder infections.

Q: I heard on your program that you do not recommend genital shaving "for obvious reasons." Could you elaborate? It's not obvious to me.

A: Pubic hair removal has become fashionable among women, especially teenagers, and this is one fad that can lead to the doctor's office.

Pediatric dermatologists are seeing cases of vulvar folliculitis, which is an inflammation or infection of the hair follicles. This often requires antibiotics and cortisone to cure.

Other factors to consider: Once a woman starts, she has to commit herself to regular shaving or waxing, because the stubble is very irritating. And one of the functions of pubic hair is to help decrease friction during intercourse. Pubic hair also helps keep you lubricated. So, if you remove the hair, you may regret it most during vigorous lovemaking.

Fads come and go, and I have no objection to this one, but I'd consider the comfort issue as well as the nuisance factor. This is not a low-maintenance trend, either.

Q: Periodically, usually after some new uproar over gay rights, my brother and I get into an argument about homosexuality. He feels that people choose to be gay. I feel there is too much research that says this is genetic. Am I right or wrong?

A: Parents of gay men often will tell you that they noticed differences in their child's personality and play patterns when they were toddlers. Others will tell no such story. Both experiences fit with genetic evidence we have today.

If you look at twins that were separated at birth and raised by different parents and never knew each other, you have a very unique laboratory. When one of those twins turned out to be gay, there was a 50 percent chance the other would be gay also. Not 100 percent, but 50 percent. Considering that in the average population there would be a 3–10 percent chance (depending on what rate you accept for the percentage of gay people in our population), you can see the role of genetics. There have been studies on brain structure, on whether gay folks are more likely to be left-handed or to hold different kinds of jobs, and yet they all dance around the fact that with one individual you just can't know the answer to the nature-versus-nurture question.

For some people, there may just be attraction to same-sex attributes with no genetics playing a role, and for others there never was a question. And when it comes to attitudes about homosexuality, there is one study that is sure to stimulate conversation. Men with the most homophobic views are the most likely to be suppressing their own bisexual feelings. When shown gay porn and wired to machines that measure blood flow to the penis, the most homophobic men had the most blood flow. Draw your own conclusions.

Q: I have been on and off methadone for several years to treat pain related to back surgery. I think it's one of the best painkillers, and it has a lower potential for abuse than a lot of the prescription drugs. When I am on methadone, though, during orgasms my urethra burns a little. It makes sex somewhat unpleasant. When I'm off methadone, my orgasms are fun. What's going on?

A: I don't have a specific answer, beyond the possibility of a touch of urethritis. But we know that any opiate or opiatelike drug will interfere with the body's natural endorphin system, which is linked to sensations of pleasure.

Even drug-free orgasms are often described as a sensation that's close to

---

DID YOU KNOW?
WHILE YOU WERE SLEEPING . . .

Researchers at Stanford University's Sleep Disorders Center found that it's possible for people to be involved in unconscious, sexually aggressive activities, from violent masturbation to sexual assault while in deep sleep. Several patients involved in this study were diagnosed with psychiatric disorders, including depression and obsessive-compulsive disorder, and some had a history of sexual abuse. In most cases, once the patients were treated for their core disorders, their nocturnal sexual activities stopped.

---

pain. And often, a person has a pained expression during orgasm. It is easy to imagine that a pharmacological manipulation that blocks endorphins could tilt an orgasm to the pain side.

People mistakenly consider drugs to be aphrodisiacs. With prolonged use, both marijuana and heroin will depress libido, as any addict will tell you.

Since I haven't seen any literature listing painful orgasm as a side effect of methadone, my general answer is that it is altering your body's normal chemistry, which is what drugs do. As for a bigger issue, I would love to see you find a nonpharmacological solution for your back problems.

Q: What does it say about my lovemaking with my husband if we need to use lubricants? I always thought that if there was enough foreplay, you shouldn't need them. But my girlfriends say that's silly.

A: Walking through the aisles of drugstores should tell you that lubricants are a popular commodity. Personal lubricants now occupy many shelves, and for good reason. Human lubrication not only differs from person to person but will differ with the time of the month during which you are making love—not to mention stages of life. In menopause, women notoriously have a condition called atrophic vaginitis. It is one of the most common symptoms of menopause.

Several years ago, the *Journal of the American Medical Association* reported that the more you make love the less likely you are to have this dryness problem, but it plagues many women. Natural lubrication is a sign of being sexually stimulated and turned on, but it is so inconsistent that you shouldn't rely upon it. In other words, women should not get upset if they don't lubricate, and men certainly should not think that they are doing something wrong if a woman feels drier than he thinks she should be.

Lubricants can also introduce creativity to your lovemaking in the form of new styles of stimulation. That can be very positive.

Q: What's your opinion of sex toys? My girlfriend has a vibrator that she bought before I met her, and she asks me to help her with it occasionally. What does that say about our lovemaking?

A: This is usually a question I get from men, because many guys feel threatened if a woman wants to use sexual aids. I think the message your girlfriend is sending you is that she is sexually open and may become a more creative, interesting sexual partner. The fact that she is able to communicate her needs to you is also a big plus. One of the most fundamental problems in lovemaking is that people don't express what they want or enjoy, out of fear of hurting their partner's feelings. So, I think this is a positive, and I'm told that most customers in stores that sell marital aids are women.

The basic tenets of lovemaking are: Don't hurt your partner or force him or her to do something against their will. Once that's understood, there's a whole world of fun and enjoyment out there.

DEAN'S LIST: GET INTIMATE WITH INTIMACY
Books are a *great* resource when it comes to sex. Who can't benefit from good illustrations and fresh ideas?

Passionate Marriage: Love, Sex, and Intimacy in Emotionally Committed Relationships, by David Schnarch, Ph.D.
The Complete Idiot's Guide to Amazing Sex, by Sari Locker
Doing It: Real People Having Really Good Sex, by Isadora Alman
The New Male Sexuality, by Bernie Zilbergeld, Ph.D.
The New Joy of Sex and More Joy of Sex, by Alex Comfort, M.D., D.S.C.
Sex Matters for Women, by Sallie Foley, MSW; Sally A. Kope, MSW; Dennis P. Sugrue, Ph.D.
Secrets of Better Sex, by Joel D. Block, Ph.D.
The Tao of Sexual Massage, by Stephen Russell and Jürgen Kolb

Resource List

Having a hard time talking to your seventeen-year-old? Send him/her to Columbia University's Go Ask Alice site: *www.goaskalice.columbia.edu* or Sex, Etc., the Web site from the Network for Family Life Education at Rutgers University. It was created by teens for teens: *www.sxetc.org*

At the National Institute of Aging, type "sex" in the Search box and look for "Sexuality in Later Life" health information: *www.nia.nih.gov*

Check out the results of an AARP sexuality survey: *www.research.aarp.org/health/mmsexsurvey_1.html*

Find frequently asked questions on a multitude of sexuality-related topics at The Kinsey Institute: *www.kinseyinstitute.org/resources/FAQ.html*

To find a licensed sexual therapist or counselor, check out the American Board of Sexology at *www.sexologist.org* or the American Association of Sex Educators, Counselors, and Therapists: *www.aasect.org*

For a variety of information, including publications to help you communicate with your children, visit the Sexuality Information and Education Council of the United States: *www.siecus.org*

At the Planned Parenthood Web site, click on Health Info for information in both English and Spanish on birth control, emergency contraception, and sexually transmitted diseases, as well as a list of their centers: *www.ppfa.org*

For comprehensive information on sexually transmitted diseases, check out the American Social Health Association: *www.ashastd.org*

For more information about impotence, go to the National Institute for Diabetes & Digestive & Kidney Diseases Web site, type in the words "erectile dysfunction," and hit the Search button: *www.niddk.nih.gov*

For related questions see chapters 4, 6, 8, 9, 10, and 11.

Chapter 3

The Good, the Bad, and the Ugly: Alternative Medicine

Many of you already know my feelings on this subject, but I'll say it one more time: There's no such thing as alternative medicine. Unproven medicine, yes. But a viable alternative? No.

So why devote a whole chapter to it? Because many folks want to believe that "alternative medicine" is better medicine. They want to believe in something "natural," in something new, in anything that "guarantees" a cure. Often, they are looking for the quick fix after years of paying too little attention to their health. And, for many, it is also an issue of alienation and fear: They no longer trust the traditional medical community.

But what's the option? Why are we willing to trust people who sell their wares through cheesy magazine ads or infomercials, providing very little or no research to back up often outrageous claims of success? Many alternative medicine marketers and practitioners have no qualms about tapping into our most base fears, and millions of us are letting them do just that—which scares the hell out of me.

When folks first hear me bash a bogus supplement, herb, or therapy, they often turn a deaf ear, especially if they are among the true believers. They don't know that I was once one of them.

Thirty years ago I was in the thick of the alternative medicine movement, though we called it holistic medicine then. I read all the books and got involved in all the movements. As I look back now, I know this was a result of my disaffection with mainstream medicine, which I saw as cold, scientific, and unyielding—and sometimes ineffective.

I was an iconoclast and, yes, I wanted to see the day when all the romantic and magical healing traditions of primitive people took over the world. But I had no idea that it would get as big as it has—and that I would come to believe that there is no such thing as "alternative medicine."

This is not an extreme view but a statement of fact. The course of scientific medicine is such that as healing approaches are tested and proven to be effective, they are incorporated into the practices of the modern physician. In other words, honest medicine is the constant pursuit of the best possible ways of healing, no matter what the roots of that approach—and you will find in this chapter some treatments that have proven results. Do I refer to these treatments as "alternative medicine"? No, because massage, for example, is not an "alternative" as far as I'm concerned. It's a practical treatment that works for certain ailments. But it is in this chapter because that is how it is known among many medical practitioners today.

Some segments of the medical community like to use the term "complementary medicine." If a neurologist who encourages yoga as an option for reducing the frequency of headaches calls that "complementary medicine," that's fine with me. But why tag it as anything other than part of a program of traditional medical treatment, if a doctor thinks it will work for his or her patient? What scares me is when someone with frequent headaches doesn't see a neurologist first but instead pursues a self-treatment program with an acupuncturist or yoga instructor. That's just plain crazy. That headache could be caused by a serious disease.

And, of course, there are "natural" roots in a lot of traditional medicine. Today, a huge number of the medications that doctors write prescriptions for are derived from herbs. The difference is that these are herbs that have been tested, investigated, extracted, retested and finally marketed with a proven efficacy. But in our overzealousness for a simpler time—and cures for everything—we seem to want to believe that all herbs are effective just because they have been used by some exotic culture for thousands of years.

Though I wish herbs were a medical miracle, research has been extremely disappointing. Nothing is simpler than putting an herb through double-blind testing to see if it does what its backers claim, and some of our favorites have just simply failed, or performed modestly. Echinacea has not been found to cure the common cold. St. John's Wort has not been found to be a highly effective antidepressant—it is not as good as current medications on the market. Saw palmetto seems to show some results as a treatment for enlarged prostates, but maybe not more so than the medications currently used by doctors.

My stance on alternative medicine doesn't mean I oppose exploring any creative ideas for curing human beings, because that's the only way we will find out if they work, and science is the only standard we have for evaluating those ideas. It got us where we are and will continue to move us into the future.

Every herb has hundreds or thousands of chemicals in it, and if we find out what the active ingredient is, we can make even more effective medications. If we can prove that acupressure on a woman's forearms helps her with nausea during pregnancy, hallelujah. But how do we justify the death of someone who used an "alternative medicine" that's known to be dangerous yet remains on drugstore shelves for anyone to buy, even your teenager?

Don't be naïve—or reckless. Many people continue to be harmed by the injudicious use of these products, some of them simply because they want to lose ten or twenty pounds or reduce their high blood pressure. If you insist on taking herbs, tell your physician, because interactions with other medications can be critical, and I'm not talking just about prescription pills. We're seeing brain hemorrhages in people who take aspirin and ginkgo biloba, which is also a blood thinner.

Occasionally, an alternative medicine advocate will invoke the "Galileo principle." Galileo was mocked for his views about motion of the stars and other planets, but he turned out to be right. What they don't mention was that science proved him right. Cases do exist in the history of medicine where people were laughed at by the establishment, only to be proven right. But the vast majority of those who are scorned turn out to be wrong.

This is your health; insist on standards. First, make sure that what you do doesn't harm you. Second, try to learn as much as you can to make sure you are helping yourself.

Does your doctor have all the answers? Of course not. Are there medications that were tested, approved, and prescribed, which later proved to be bad for us? Yes. But just imagine what can happen without testing. Modern medicine is not perfect and never will be. We have to educate ourselves every step of the way—asking questions, reading the fine print, listening to our doctors and our bodies. If we each don't take responsibility for our bodies, who will?

Many folks, when arguing with me about alternative medicine, come armed with anecdotes from family, friends, and coworkers. These stories can be very convincing—an end to headaches, the elimination of allergies—but step back and ask yourself: Do they feel better because the treatment worked or because they wanted the treatment to work? The placebo effect is a real thing, proven in many studies. If you believe you're going to get better—or that someone else is going to make you better—it's very likely you will improve. The power of the mind in this regard is not a bad thing, but in the process many people are duped, while a few get rich.

One other reason alternative medicine has thrived is that there are almost no regulations concerning its use. Supplements, for instance, do not have to meet any standards for efficacy, safety, or quality of manufacturing. This is a huge loophole created by Congress through which many quacks pass. But most of these folks are savvy marketers, and they know how to appear as if they have science on their side. If ninety-nine studies find a particular herb worthless, yet there is one that found it helpful, that's what you hear about from practitioners. Remember, if something sounds too good to be true, that's probably the case. When you get on an airplane, you expect standards for the mechanics and the pilots. When you are assessing healing experts and techniques, see what standards they apply.

If I can't convince you to be a skeptic, read some of these questions. There's a lot of crazy stuff out there, and people are buying it.

Herbs, Plants, and Oils: User Beware

Q: I'm taking ephedra to boost my metabolism. I'm getting results, but it's hard to ignore the newspaper headlines about it. Is it really that dangerous?

A: Ephedra is not a "natural" weight-loss and energy-boosting supplement—it could be a killer. Yet, because of the ridiculous way the laws are written protecting "natural supplements," the Food and Drug Administration (FDA) can only ban drugs in extraordinary cases. I don't know how many more people have to die before the FDA feels they have enough evidence to get it off the shelves. This situation has become absurd, and warning labels are not enough.

According to the *New England Journal of Medicine*, two physicians reviewed 140 cases of adverse reactions to ephedra that have been reported to the FDA.

The reactions involved the cardiovascular system—including heart attacks and high blood pressure—and the central nervous system. They included 13 permanent disabilities and 10 deaths.

"Because of the severity of the adverse effects that we reviewed and, in particular, the occurrence of events that caused permanent disability and death, we conclude that dietary supplements that contain ephedra alkaloids pose a serious health threat to some persons," their report said.

The deaths of at least two professional athletes also have been linked to ephedra, and the National Football League, the National Collegiate Athletic Association, and the International Olympic Committee were among the first sporting groups to ban it.

When something goes wrong with a prescription drug, and inevitably mistakes do happen, we are quick to blame the pharmaceutical company that has spent millions of dollars testing the safety and efficacy of the product before it was allowed on the market.

Supplement manufacturers, on the other hand, face no such expense or scrutiny before they sell their "natural" products. And when "nature's cure" goes wrong, the government—ultimately, that means you and I—has to pay for the mistakes, in dollars and with our health. Chinese herbalists have great respect for, and show great restraint with, ephedra. You should, too.

Q: I read somewhere that the herb St. John's Wort can promote the growth of cataracts. I'm taking it for depression, and I do feel better, but this has me worried. What do you know about that?

A: The popularity of St. John's Wort puzzles me. Here is an herb, with a host of side effects that we don't have much data on, that may or may not provide mild relief from depression, and it is one of the top-selling herbs in America.

Why are we so interested in this? Because it doesn't require a doctor's exam and a diagnosis? Because it's "natural"? Because it's cheap and available over the counter? Is that it?

Depression should be treated by professionals; studies indicate a high rate of success in treating it with medication and talk therapy.

As for your question, there is some concern that St. John's Wort can damage protein in the eyes when they are exposed to bright sunlight. This can lead to cataracts.

And other possible side effects of St. John's Wort keep popping up—and researchers have found that it can impact the effectiveness of certain HIV and

The Edell Report
Kids and Alternative Medicine: Don't Do It!

While you have the right to do anything to your body that's legal, no matter how stupid it may be, you have a responsibility to make sure your kids aren't victims of the latest health fad.

Their young bodies are very sensitive, and you shouldn't meddle in their development. Some supplements, like soy and DHEA, contain hormones. And some vitamins have too much iron for kids. In extreme cases, where parents have applied their personal health and healing beliefs to a child to that child's detriment, the parents have faced prosecution for child abuse.

Less extreme are the parents who put their kids on low-fat or low-calorie diets, thinking they will improve their health. Unfortunately, a condition called "failure to thrive" sometimes results, because children (including infants) have not received adequate nutrition to gain weight and grow. Since a baby's brain growth is critical in the first year of life, poor nutrition early on can have a permanent effect.

Rule No. 1 for kids: Restrictive, extreme diets are not healthier diets.

Please, please, please check with your pediatrician before risking your child's health.

---

cancer drugs as well as birth control pills. So, anyone taking other medications should talk to his or her doctor before trying this supplement. Is that too much to ask?

Q: I know you don't like herbs, but how can you be against echinacea and goldenseal? Hasn't it been proven that they prevent colds?

A: In Europe, echinacea is widely used in the belief that it prevents and treats colds, and I once thought there was something to this thinking as well. But ever since I read about the results of a 1998 German study, I have had serious doubts. The herb totally flunked a high-quality, double-blind study of three hundred people.

DID YOU KNOW?
HOT FLASHES AND HISTORY

If you are over forty-five and you're a woman, you're the target of black cohosh supplement marketers. But that's nothing new. This native North American plant belongs to the buttercup family and it was used in Native American medicine for gynecological disorders, among others. In the late 1800s, the Lydia E. Pinkham Medicine Company made it a key ingredient of Mrs. Pinkham's legendary "vegetable compound" for women's ailments. However, the most notorious ingredient in her "medicine" was alcohol—about 20 percent. In 2001, black cohosh went mainstream again when the American College of Obstetricians and Gynecologists stated that the herb may be beneficial in the short term (six months or less) for some menopausal symptoms. The key words here are "may be." A variety of studies have produced mixed results on the effectiveness of this herb, and further studies are under way.

Some people got a phony pill, and some people got the real echinacea, and there was no difference between the groups in terms of how long they went without colds or how many colds they got. The researchers concluded that no difference existed between the group that took placebos and the group that took echinacea. Researchers at the University of Wisconsin got similar results with a smaller study in 2002.

Now that you know that echinacea has failed these tests, you've got to ask yourself if you want to keep spending your money on it. The best way to prevent colds is to prevent people from sneezing in your face.

Echinacea is also supposed to boost the immune system. People get a glow on their faces when they talk about boosting the immune system. Well, that is not a good thing. Rheumatoid arthritis is what's called an autoimmune disease; it is the result of an immune system in high gear.

One other issue is liver damage. People who take echinacea every day can do damage to their liver in as little as two months.

Goldenseal, *hydrastis canadensis,* does seem to relieve some topical skin rashes and wounds. While I have seen many poorly done European studies on goldenseal, which would not pass research standards in America, I have not seen any high-quality research showing it to be effective when taken internally.

As for my not liking herbs, that's a simplistic assessment. Many prescription drugs are based on herbs—from digitalis for heart disease to opiates for pain. So science is very interested in herbs. When scientists examine an herb to discover the source of its effectiveness, and then make a pill out of it, it becomes a pharmaceutical and is no longer considered herbal or alternative medicine.

Over-the-counter herbs, though, fall under the Dietary Supplement Health and Education Act, which means manufacturers can make almost any proclamations about them that they want, without any proof. But once herbs are modified and become pharmaceutical drugs, the FDA requires that those drugs pass rigorous tests. This is the greatest consumer loophole in the history of consumer law, because herbs share many properties with drugs, and yet herb distributors can claim their products will improve sleep or melt fat or cure colds, without any proof of effectiveness, or, even worse, of safety. So, keep asking questions.

Q: I am very confused about essential oils. Do you eat them or do you rub them on your body? And someone told me they fight bacteria. Which ones do that?

A: My first introduction to essential oils was on a safari, when we had to board a small plane that was filled with the awful smell of a water buffalo head (it was part of the cargo of a previous group of travelers). Our guide whipped out some fresh handkerchiefs, put a few drops of lavender oil on each one, hung them up in the plane, and that was all we needed to make the flight bearable.

The basic concept is simple: Essential oils are essences of plants (from herbs to nuts to vegetables), created by extraction processes that vary somewhat from brand to brand. They have become very popular in the alternative-medicine community, particularly for aromatherapy, and they are very big in the beauty business, too. You can find them in bath soaks, moisturizers, and massage lotions.

Some folks do add a drop or two of certain types of essential oils to certain foods as they cook, but don't do it unless you know what you are doing.

As for killing germs, if you put an essential oil on top of a germ, it will probably kill it. But so would vodka. That doesn't mean vodka is good for your skin.

I don't know that many people have a problem with germs on their skin. Also, you could make a case that if you put essential oils directly on your skin to kill germs, it could upset the natural balance of good germs and bad germs on the skin.

One study, conducted by the University of Munich, found that water has the same effect as all those expensive aromatherapy oils, as long as a patient believes they're given the real thing. Volunteers wore surgical masks, and one group was sprayed with essential oils that are supposed to make people feel more alert: peppermint, jasmine, and ylang-ylang. The other group was sprayed with plain water.

They found there was no difference in reaction times between people who were given aromatherapy oil and those given water. The results imply that aromatherapy causes a placebo effect where patients actually become healthier when they believe it.

Still, good smells make you feel good. The researchers plan to look at the effectiveness of massaging the oils into the skin to see if there is any effect when they are absorbed rather than inhaled.

Q: Is it true that saw palmetto helps restore hair and, if so, is it safe? What about Rogaine?

A: Saw palmetto is a safe herb; and its pharmacological properties indicate it could regrow hair, but I have not yet seen any scientific evidence that it does.

More significantly, lots of men are taking saw palmetto because of its benefits in treating enlarged prostate glands. I expect we would hear a roar if it were also growing hair.

The problem is, hair growth can be erratic. Sometimes just massaging the scalp and increasing the blood flow can result in a little more fuzz, and that will fool you.

Here is a good example: When researchers studied Rogaine—the only real pharmaceutical that can help you grow hair, and it's not great, really—some men were given the real thing and others just used a thick cream that looked like Rogaine. An amazing number of men using the placebo reported hair growth because they were so sure it worked.

Q: Have you ever heard of cod liver oil being used to treat arthritis? I know my father was given lots of it as a boy, but I have no idea why it was considered valuable back then.

A: You are right, cod liver oil is an old-time remedy. There are all kinds of jokes and cartoons about the horrors of a daily dose of cod liver oil. There are also many unsubstantiated claims about its health effects.

But cod liver oil and fish oils in general have been found to be anti-inflammatory, which means they may relieve the pain of arthritis, but probably no more than a powerful ibuprofen or aspirin-type drug can. Unlike drugs though, fish oils won't do damage to your stomach.

There is a concern, however, that the vitamin A in cod liver oil can cause bones to thin. This is a problem among the Northern Europeans, whose diets are unusually high in fish. So, don't overdo it. Nature has given us nutrients in balance. Yes, we need vitamin A, just like we need the sun, but too much of any good thing can turn dangerous.

You can get your fish oil just by eating cold-water fish, and salmon is one of my personal favorites. It's a lot more pleasurable than pills.

Q: I have been taking chromium and ephedra and other herbs for a few years now, because this combo gives me a lot of energy for my workouts. When I got pregnant almost eight months ago, I reduced my dosage and told my doctors, my herbalist, and my midwife what I was doing, but no one had much advice about this. Now I'm having second thoughts about what I've done. What are the chances my baby will have birth defects?

A: So, let me get this straight: You were willing to put your baby at risk so you could get a better workout? What are your priorities?

First, let's address your question. The answer won't make you feel very good: Nobody knows what risks your baby faces, because this is such a difficult area to research.

Second, let me be clear on this topic, and if I don't sound very sympathetic, too bad: DON'T mix supplements and herbs with pregnancy, unless your obstetrician is calling the shots. No one gave you direct answers about the impact on your baby because the effects of these substances on a developing baby are big unknowns. We don't experiment on pregnant women to see what kind of birth defects result when they gobble the supplements du jour. Medicine is extremely conservative when it comes to babies' lives, as everyone should be.

However, women who take supplements while they are pregnant must talk to their doctor. While there are screening tests for some abnormalities, there's a lot we still can't detect.

Chromium is a toxic metal in large amounts, but I doubt that you've been taking large amounts. There is evidence that, in tiny amounts, it can negatively affect cell growth. Chromium is also worthless in terms of affecting your workout.

Unless sound medical research concludes that a substance is safe, don't listen to anyone who tells you otherwise. Do not fall for someone telling you that it's an ancient practice so it must be OK. Bloodletting is an ancient practice, too.

Natural is popular, but nothing is more natural than leaving your baby alone while it is in your womb. Unnatural is running to the health food store to buy a bunch of chemically extracted nonsense over which there is no regulation.

Q: I've read so much about how soy helps women in menopause. But what does it do for men? The reason I ask: My son drinks a lot of soy milk.

A: Right now soy is a very confusing substance in both its food and supplement forms. And that applies to both genders.

Eating the food may not be a problem for menopausal women or your son, but no studies have been conclusive, and more research is needed. However, the soy isoflavone supplements are a different story, and I am very opposed to people taking them right now. In the supplements, the natural plant-based

QUIZ

Which of these substances are dangerous if taken at the same time as kava?
A) sedatives and sleeping pills   B) antipsychotic drugs
C) alcohol   D) drugs used to treat anxiety or Parkinson's disease
E) all of these
(E: all of these. Kava can be trouble on its own—it has been linked to severe liver damage—and when it's mixed with any of these other substances it can lead to deep sedation and, in some cases, even coma. It is banned in several countries.)

estrogen found in soy is present in such an unnaturally high concentration that it is suspected of possibly accelerating the growth of breast cancer, among other problems.

Natural soy has estrogen-like (possibly cancer-causing) effects as well as estrogen-blocking (possibly cancer-blocking) effects. It's the balance of these two reactions that determines what happens in your body, and that's not consistent.

We run into trouble whenever we expect health to come in the form of a magic food. There's no such thing. I want more research before I can be comfortable with high-dose soy supplementation.

Q: Can you tell me everything you know about kava, please? My friend is taking it, and I'm not sure she did any research before she started using it.

A: Your friend is playing with fire. To drive home the point that herbs are powerful drugs, please tell her about a man who, after taking kava for two months, ended up with a damaged liver. Then you can mention that it's been banned in several countries, including Canada, Great Britain, and Switzerland. If that doesn't catch her attention, nothing will.

Forms of the kava plant, which has long been brewed into a narcotic-like drink in the South Pacific Islands, have gained popularity as a sedative, and extracts from kava are made into drugs to treat anxiety. But the bad far outweighs the good.

The *British Medical Journal* reported that a man who had taken three or four capsules of kava per day for two months was admitted to the hospital with symptoms of dark urine, jaundice, and fatigue. Within four days he had deteriorated so seriously that he needed, and received, a liver transplant. This man did not drink alcohol or take any other drugs. That's scary stuff.

Consumers need to realize that "over the counter" does not equal "safe." Before you put any supplement in your mouth, ask your pharmacist or doctor—not the clerk at the health food store—about its safety. And when your doctor asks if you're taking any drugs, don't omit the vitamins, herbs, and supplements in your daily regimen.

Q: My husband has cancer, and it has metastasized in his lungs, so he started chemotherapy four days ago. Someone told me about a tea that has burdock root, slippery elm, and rhubarb root. I did some research on these herbs and found they were a good blood purifier with vitamins and other

things. So I started him on that. It seems to be helping the side effects. Could I be hurting him without knowing it?

A: This is a tough question, especially since chemo can be so debilitating.

First, there really is no such thing as a blood purifier. That's a nineteenth-century term that has no meaning today, so I don't know what a blood purifier would do.

Second, talk to your husband's doctor about what you are doing, because herb-medicine interactions can be dangerous.

Third, we have found some shocking things about several vitamins and supplements on the market, and some may actually accelerate the growth of cancer. The reason for this is that cancer is simply a rapidly growing cell, and when you feed it supplements, you may be nourishing it.

While you are simply trying to help your husband with the symptoms that occur with chemotherapy, and not cure his cancer, you are still in a no-man's land. I have no reason to doubt that some of these herbs might work. After all, marijuana is an herb, too, and it's very effective with chemotherapy symptoms. Yet I don't know of any objective evidence that other herbs help. In fact, most of the studies on herbs and cancer have been dismally disappointing so far. I wish it were different.

Vitamin, Fiber, Mineral, and Food Supplements

Q: Is there really much difference between taking a cranberry supplement and drinking cranberry juice? I want to avoid any more bladder infections, but I forgot to ask my doctor if either approach would have the same impact.

A: I will never understand why someone would rather pop a pill than drink a nice glass of cranberry juice or eat a nice piece of fish or enjoy a bowl of strawberries. Food is pleasure, folks, and we need as many moments of pleasure in our lives as possible.

OK, enough of my rant. Here are the facts, and it reminds us that too much of anything is seldom a good thing.

Cranberry juice is popular among women because of its ability to prevent bladder infections. This is because a substance in the juice discourages bacteria from adhering to the wall of the bladder. However, cranberries also have a high concentration of oxalate, which contributes to forming kidney stones.

According to a report in *Urology,* a patient came to Stanford Medical Center with terrible kidney stones and reported that she had been taking cranberry pills that she had bought at a "nutrition store," prompting her doctors to measure the effects of cranberry pills on a small group of volunteers.

The researchers measured the oxalate levels in the urine of five healthy women, who then took cranberry pills for seven days per instructions on the label. On the seventh day, their urine was measured again. The oxalate level had increased by an average of 43 percent. That's a big increase in a short time!

In addition, University of Alabama researchers found cranberry pills were not effective in fighting bladder infections.

I've said it before and I'll say it again: Eat fish, eat garlic, drink cranberry juice, eat soy. But don't take your food as pills. If nature had meant for us to consume concentrates, cranberry pills would grow in the bogs, fish oil pills would swim through the ocean, and garlic pills would grow in the ground.

DID YOU KNOW?
THE REAL THING VERSUS THE SUPPLEMENT

Here it is, folks, even more evidence that foods that are good for you have no substitute.

If you're looking for the beta-carotene that comes naturally in carrots, spinach, broccoli, and other foods, don't expect to get the same impact from a pill. In fact, beta-carotene supplements can be dangerous. Two studies confirmed that beta-carotene supplements increased the risk of lung cancer for smokers. And another long-term study of 22,000 doctors who took a beta-carotene pill every other day for twelve years showed that they did not reduce their risk of cancer or heart disease.

Don't waste your money *and* risk your health. Take a few extra minutes every day to eat right. Consider it the best long-term investment you'll ever make.

Q: My friend gives a small dose of melatonin to her three-year-old son at night to help him sleep. What do you think of this?

A: Melatonin is a hormone, and kids should not be given hormones without a doctor's recommendation. Aside from regulating sleep cycles, melatonin plays a role in growth patterns, so I would not give it—or any other supplement—to a child.

Not only could your friend be hurting her child, but in this particular case, the treatment doesn't work. Melatonin seems to have no effect on children's sleep, because their bodies produce enough of it. If supplemental melatonin helps anyone get a good night's sleep, it would be an older person, but even in that population the evidence is weak.

Melatonin supplements were designed to relieve jet lag, and it was a miserable failure in a test of its efficacy there.

Your friend can teach her child to sleep better. Establishing healthy habits—a practice known as sleep hygiene—will pay off for a lifetime. We are a pill-popping society, and many of us lack the patience to solve a problem with effort and time. Encourage her to talk to her pediatrician about what steps to take to improve the situation without hormones.

Q: My girlfriend is selling some supplements that have iron in them. I have heard about a book that is totally against iron. Is iron safe to take? And how much do I need? I'm a twenty-eight-year-old woman in good health.

A: First of all, before you buy anything, read the labels on any packaged food you eat over the next week or so—and check out the label on your multivitamin, if you take one. You may be surprised at how much iron you are already getting. Iron is now added to breakfast cereals and breads, and it is combined with many supplements.

This is not necessarily a good thing. Evidence is showing that we may be pushing too much iron on people in general, and women in particular. Because women have less iron in their blood than men, we encourage them to take supplements, but a better approach might be to just accept that this is how women are made and it's not a disaster.

Iron has a very narrow therapeutic range. This means that the difference between too little and too much is small, and we don't have much wiggle room for finding the amount that is just right.

A little extra iron may increase the risk for heart disease. Too much iron can be very toxic and is associated with specific diseases like hemochromatosis and polycythemia. It is also the No. 1 over-the-counter pill that children accidentally poison themselves with. It can be very toxic.

Now, most people are not getting too much iron, but research is arriving at the conclusion that people should have their iron level tested and then take iron based on the need.

In general, I would not take an iron supplement, unless a doctor specifically told me that I had significant iron-deficiency anemia. So, bottom line: Find another way to be supportive of your friend.

Q: I have seen ads for a health bar that has arginine in it. The ads say that the arginine will improve the blood flow to the heart and reduce painful symptoms of heart disease, such as angina and leg pain. Is this true?

A: An arginine "health bar" is a funny idea. Arginine is an amino acid contained in most proteins, and it would be hard to avoid eating it even if you tried. Many hormones and neurotransmitters are made of amino acids, and research indicates that taking large amounts of certain amino acids can increase levels of those hormones. But the effect is very minimal.

Eating a bunch of arginine is not going to resolve someone's heart disease. To my knowledge, there have been no clinically relevant studies regarding amino acid supplements and heart disease. In fact, it's dangerous for a person

---

QUIZ

Deficiency in vitamin A possibly can lead to which ailment?
A) scurvy   B) osteoporosis   C) kidney stones
D) tennis elbow
(*C: kidney stones. A vitamin A deficiency is fairly common and can also lead to night blindness, eye disease, and dry skin. Many breakfast cereals, dairy products, and other foods are fortified with vitamin A. And many fruits and vegetables also contain beta-carotene, which the body can turn into vitamin A. However, too much "pre-formed" vitamin A such as that found in vitamin pills can lead to blurred vision and liver toxicity.*)

with heart symptoms to think that eating a "health bar" can be a substitute for medical treatment, a healthy diet, and exercise.

Someone with angina or leg pain needs to be tested by a doctor, and they may be told they have impaired blood flow. They may be told to exercise and eat a low-fat diet. I know most people would rather eat what is essentially a candy bar than do hard work, but no candy bar will turn heart disease around.

Q: I read in an article in *Newsweek* magazine that Americans lack essential fatty acids in their diets. One of them, DHA, promotes brain growth, especially in the fetus. So I took a DHA supplement. Later I became pregnant and had a miscarriage. Is there any link? I know miscarriages are very common, and everything can't cause them, but I'm curious.

A: You're very smart to have this figured out about miscarriages. Even a cigarette smoker who gets lung cancer cannot blame the lung cancer on the cigarettes, because people who have never smoked get lung cancer. Each individual case has to be evaluated on its own.

DHA is docosahexanoic acid, one of the essential fatty acids. Essential fatty acids are more than just a food and do have a lot of complex metabolic roles. And a substance that seems innocent can surprise us. But miscarriages are very common, as you said, and the odds are DHA had nothing to do with yours.

As with most nutrients, you should get your essential fatty acids from eating a balanced diet. Taking just DHA as a magic pill means you are getting a disproportionate dose of that fatty acid compared to the others. That's out of balance.

You are very likely to become pregnant and have a normal, healthy baby without taking any of this stuff. Next time you're pregnant, don't take anything before you talk to your doctor.

Q: My girlfriend's eighty-year-old grandmother has osteoporosis. She read that DHEA might help. Is this a good idea or a bad idea? My girlfriend and I have already been on the Internet and have read a lot of articles on DHEA, but we didn't find anything about its effect on older women.

A: Your grandmother is lucky to have such caring folks around her. Now, let's clarify a few things. First, there's the matter of osteoporosis in an eighty-year-old woman. Most of the success in battling osteoporosis lies in stopping its progression. There are newer, nonestrogen drugs on the market, but their effect on an eighty-year-old is unknown. Taking calcium and vitamin D and being active are also important, but not a cure.

DHEA (dehydroepiandrosterone) is confusing at this point. It may indeed have medical uses, but I would like to see it banned from the over-the-counter, health-food-store market. Once ingested, DHEA triggers powerful hormones. It is sold as a food supplement and promoted as a testosterone booster, but it actually seems to boost estrogen in men. If it's a food supplement, then show me the "food" that has male and female hormones in it.

It may be a safer, gentler way of giving people steroids, but endocrinologists—not health-store clerks and sports figures like Mark McGwire—should be calling the shots on that.

Until DHEA is approved by someone other than its manufacturers, I'm dead-set against giving it to your friend's grandmother or anyone else. I think it could be dangerous, and whether or not it would relieve osteoporosis is unclear.

Q: I just read an article about the benefits of phytochemicals. Do you have any opinion on this?

A: Phytonutrients (*phyto* means "plant") are a very important subject these days, but first, here's a little background. When you take a multiple vitamin pill, for instance, it likely includes beta-carotene. This is a vitamin A phytonutrient that is contained in carrots and easy to manufacture.

Once upon a time it was thought that beta-carotene was the most active vitamin A phytonutrient. But, unfortunately, a lot of studies done on the effects of beta-carotene supplements have found that it doesn't do much good. In fact, it seems to increase the risk of cancer in some people, especially those who smoke and drink alcohol.

Then scientists found out that there is more than just beta-carotene in a carrot—alpha and gamma carotene, zeaxanthin, and lutein are just a few of the other carotenes—and some of these elements may be more effective in preventing disease. In fact, they may be most effective when working together naturally. So the supplement manufacturers said, "Maybe we should pack in some of those other ones that scientists are discovering now."

Well, in a living fruit or vegetable, there are so many of these things that scientists will never find them all. Furthermore, it's crazy to trust the primitive science that is used as the basis for manufacturing these kinds of supplements.

So, instead of taking the supplements that are supposed to contain the phytonutrients in fruits and vegetables, I would just eat real fruits and vegetables. This way, you're sure to get any phytonutrients that scientists have yet to discover or understand.

I don't think we have any proof that phytonutrient supplements will do you any good, because when you take one, it creates an imbalance in your system. You will notice that manufacturers don't tell you the ratios. Unfortunately, there are no manufacturing standards that are law right now.

The only way these people make money is by convincing you your health is bad, because if we perceive ourselves to be healthy, they won't have customers.

Q: My physical therapist suggests that I take an eighth of a teaspoon of sea salt every morning and night to relieve muscle pain and help with hydration. What do you think of this treatment?

A: This is a BAD idea. Sea salt is still salt—it's 99 percent sodium chloride—and doctors are trying to get people to cut down on it. This is particularly true for someone with high blood pressure.

The recommended daily maximum amount of salt for a typical healthy person is 2,400 milligrams. A quarter of a teaspoon is almost 600 milligrams, so this dose of salt would be one quarter of your daily intake.

Sea salt has no magical ingredients that ease muscle pain. It is a source of trace minerals, but those are also available in most foods. Huge deficiencies of calcium and magnesium can cause muscle dysfunction, but you would be noticeably ill in that case, and sea salt would not be your cure.

I have come to believe that the human body may need microscopic amounts of most elements on the face of the earth. We need all these strange-sounding metals—vanadium, boron, molybdenum, etc.—in tiny amounts, because they hook up with certain enzyme systems.

So, if anything, I'd rather see you take a mineral supplement, without the salt. You can buy these in the health food store.

Q: What's the big deal with antioxidants? It seems like every time I go to the grocery store, I see this word somewhere. Why should I want these as part of my diet? Or is this just a lot of sensational packaging?

A: Yes, there has been a lot of hype on this subject. But, for once, there is some truth here; they seem to be a key to our good health, even though a lot is still unknown. And while antioxidants are a darling of the "alternative medicine" movement, there's absolutely nothing "alternative" about them, as far as I'm concerned.

In short, antioxidants help protect the body's healthy cells from damage caused by "free radicals," which are out-of-control, oxygen-based molecules in our bodies that cause what's called oxidative stress and have been linked to dozens of diseases and ailments, from cancer and hardening of the arteries to macular degeneration.

Your body has many built-in antioxidation systems, so you don't need any supplements to get antioxidants. There are hundreds of different ones, and they are almost everywhere, especially in foods rich in vitamins C or E. What are some of the best sources? Try fresh berries, all kinds of citrus, grapes, sunflower seeds, walnuts, peanut butter, wheat germ, kale, sweet peppers, cabbage and spinach, to name just a few. But don't overdo it, especially if your diet is heavy on foods with lots of vitamin C. In excess (more than about 1,000 milligrams per day), vitamin C can lead to nausea, stomach cramps, diarrhea, and even kidney stones.

As valuable as they may be, antioxidants aren't a cure-all, and one of the most popular "alternative" claims has been that vitamin C and other antioxidants prevent the common cold. Well, that sounds great, but the most rigorous studies have been very disappointing. So, don't grab something just because it has antioxidants, hoping for the quick fix. It ain't going to happen.

Q: Why do I pay a lot of money for a potassium supplement and get only two percent of the recommended daily requirement in a pill?

A: The main reason is because potassium can be very dangerous. It can stop your heart cold. I would discourage you from going near it. Instead, put your money in the bank or invest in bananas, physically and fiscally.

Potassium is a very important nutrient that's in almost everything we eat, and the 2 percent of the daily requirement in a pill is a sign that most of us are getting the other 98 percent anyway.

The only exception that comes to mind is if your doctor has you on water pills or diuretics, or you have kidney disease; then he might recommend upping your potassium intake. But the rest of us can get all the potassium we need from fresh fruits and vegetables. Bananas, in particular, have lots of potassium.

Q: I have had a fuzzy, white tongue for about a month. At my doctor's suggestion, I've been taking zinc lozenges for three weeks, but my tongue is still white. What do you suggest?

A: I'd keep my tongue in my mouth and take up bird-watching instead.

Once upon a time, before we knew better, doctors thought that a coated tongue meant something. And my mother and traditional Chinese medical practitioners still think so.

But now doctors know that if the tiny filiform papilla that pave the surface of the tongue are not abraded by food, they can grow a little bit long, like grass on a lawn. This can result in a visible white coating. Rougher foods like apples and granola bars mow the "grass," so to speak.

Antibiotics that kill good germs and allow the bad germs to grow and make pigment can turn a tongue black. Of course, a tongue can get infected, and a sick tongue can be a symptom of disease, but white fuzz isn't anything to worry about.

Besides, zinc lozenges taste bad. Don't bother.

Q: I take calcium pills, but now I'm wondering if I should change to coral calcium. Can you explain how it's different from "regular" calcium pills?

A: Don't waste your money! Coral calcium is simply calcium carbonate—think Tums with a tiny sprinkle of minerals—that you could get from food or your regular vitamin pill. The claims for this are preposterous and have been condemned by many reputable scientists.

If I had ten dollars for every supplement scam I've discussed on my shows in the last twenty years . . . oh, you know the cliché.

Historically, calcium supplements haven't always been safe: Years ago calcium carbonate from bone meal or oyster shells, for instance, was used in some supplements—but was later found to contain high levels of lead. Since then the government and manufacturers took action to reduce lead levels in existing calcium supplements. But new supplements can go untested.

There are, however, plenty of reliable calcium pills. Generic calcium carbon-

---

QUIZ

Which vitamins are most likely to harm you if taken in excessive amounts?
A) A   B) B   C) C   D) D   E) K
(Vitamins A, D, and K. Fat-soluble vitamins are always more dangerous, because they cling to existing body fats and more easily reach toxic levels.)

ate pills can cost as little as five cents a day, compared to as much as a dollar a day for coral calcium.

Q: My eighteen-year-old, mountain-biker son wants to take glucosamine and chondroitin because he's heard they are good for the joints. Are they safe for someone so young?

A: Glucosamine and chondroitin sulphate are two things that people often buy at the same time or in combination in one pill. They're substances derived from cartilage, and there have been studies that suggest there might be something beneficial about them—but I'm waiting for better research. And I don't see any reason for a young person to take these supplements.

If he is having problems with his joints at his age, he should see a doctor. If he's talking about prevention, I'm not aware of any studies on the benefits of young people using these supplements preventively. To my knowledge, cyclists don't have anywhere near the joint problems that runners and soccer players do.

So, tell him that since he is a biker, his joints should not give him problems, and that being in good shape and training properly will take care of him. I hope he'll listen to you, but if he doesn't, this isn't big enough to worry about or to turn into a family fight.

See more about glucosamine on page 536 in chapter 12.

Chiropractors and Osteopaths: Yes, No, Maybe?

Q: What can chiropractors do and not do for bulging discs? I have a bulging disc in my cervical spine. The chiropractor says he can fix it with adjustments and traction. The surgeon says surgery is the only way. What would you do?

A: I number chiropractors among both my friends and my enemies. I have enemies because some chiropractors step beyond the bounds of their field and hurt people in the process.

Here is THE question to ask to determine if a chiropractor is on the up and up. "Doctor, is it true that pinched nerves can cause diseases like asthma or appendicitis?" You should run from the chiropractor who replies "but of course" and shows you the chart of the spinal column with all the little pinched nerves going to all the organs. This is thirteenth-century anatomy.

The Edell Report

The Facts About "Andro"

The fact that androstenedione ("andro" to all you sports enthusiasts) is still on the market tells you just how screwed up our laws are when it comes to supplements.

Baseball's home-run star Mark McGwire made this supplement headline news in 1998, when he admitted taking it to improve performance. McGwire subsequently stopped taking the hormone. Andro's side effects have been well documented, but I wonder how many folks who buy it have read the fine print.

If you have any reason to think this supplement is OK for you or a family member, read on. These facts come from the Endocrine Society, the American College of Sports Medicine, and scientific studies published in the Journal of the American Medical Association.

- Androstenedione is a hormone made by the body in the testes, ovary, and adrenal cortex that is naturally converted to the male sex steroid testosterone. However, there is no evidence that taking over-the-counter supplements of andro will generate increased testosterone levels, as claimed by some advocates.

You also want to beware of a chiropractor who is an M.D. wanna-be. The telltale signs are that he wants to treat diseases, he won't give referrals to physicians when appropriate, and he won't consult with your M.D.

A patient with a neckache caused by meningitis may be dead in three hours if he or she first seeks treatment from a chiropractor who believes that pinched nerves are the source of all neckaches. A backache may be caused by metastatic breast cancer, kidney stones, or something else. So you need a diagnosis first.

Diagnosis is one area where Western medicine has no peers. So, after you are diagnosed by a medical doctor, I have no objection to you seeing a chiropractor about a diagnosis that is within the scope of his field. A chiropractor

- Taking andro supplements does increase levels of estrogen—a female sex steroid, which could result in adverse side effects.
- Elevated estrogens in males may cause a drop in "good cholesterol" and put athletes at greater risk of heart attacks and strokes.
- There may also be these side effects of anabolic (muscle-building) steroids in men: acne, enlarged breasts (gynecomastia), premature balding, irritability, aggressiveness, kidney and liver dysfunctions, testicular shrinkage, and decreased sperm count.
- Women may experience these side effects: acne, decreased breast size, clitoral hyperatrophy, deepened voice, unwanted hair growth, irritability, aggressiveness, kidney and liver dysfunctions, and menstrual irregularities.
- In adolescents, the use of andro or other steroids is known to stunt growth.
- Andro is banned in Olympic competition, by the National Collegiate Athletic Association and the National Football League, but not by major league baseball.
- Because andro is unregulated, its purity and dosage may vary.

So, be smart. Don't pay the price that comes with using this supplement.

can deal with some back and neck problems and some musculoskeletal injuries.

Now, about your bulging disc. Some of them go away with exercise, physical therapy, or no treatment at all. So you have a good chance of avoiding surgery. But this depends, of course, on the specifics of your injury. If I were you, I'd get another opinion from a medical doctor.

A tiny piece of broken disc pushing on a nerve can cause permanent damage. So, you can't take a wait-and-see attitude with something like this.

If an M.D. tells you that you aren't in imminent danger, and if you have a diagnosis that's appropriate for chiropractic care, you can give it a try.

Finally, avoid any chiropractor who follows the practice of MUA—manipulation under anesthesia—unless he is working with an M.D. who is an orthopedic specialist. I find this treatment particularly curious since chiropractic medicine is consistently described by its practitioners as "drugless, natural medicine."

Q: My daughter had her first child six weeks ago, and I'm very concerned. She's going to be taking her daughter to an osteopath for manipulative treatment. As far as I can tell, the doctor is going to squish the child's head in order to "restore the function of surrounding tissue." Is this a common thing? Is there any benefit?

A: This is a century-old superstition and has no foundation in fact. Any practitioner who insists that a healthy child needs "adjustments" to stay healthy is just preying on the gullible. This practice has been condemned by all pediatricians that I know of, and it makes no sense based on human anatomy.

While I have just described manipulation of the neck, there is another therapy called craniosacral therapy, which sounds more like what is being done to your grandchild. This is also worthless and has been condemned by mainstream osteopathic organizations.

Osteopaths are physicians—often in primary care—who are licensed to prescribe medications and perform surgery in all fifty states, and they have a D.O. after their names. They practice a more "hands-on" approach to medicine, with an emphasis on whole-body treatment that can include massage and various manipulations of your musculoskeletal systems. Many states, including California, offer the D.O. a choice of having D.O. or M.D. after their name. Just as with M.D.s, there are good osteopaths and bad ones.

In this case, I would encourage your daughter to get a second opinion about her baby's health needs.

Q: I recently went to a chiropractor for bad spasms in my back and now, after the adjustment, I feel much worse. I know my muscles are tighter; they feel inflamed. It's spread around my back and my neck. I don't want to go back, but I still feel out of alignment. What's my next step?

A: Here is where I'll make some chiropractors angry, and others will agree with me: There really is no such thing as your spine being out of alignment.

We've taken spines out of dead people, put them on drill presses, and tried to misalign vertebrae, and you really can't. It's a hundred-year-old theory that diseases are caused by subluxations—mythical misaligned vertebrae. There is no such thing as a subluxation causing disease. If you have a chiropractor who is telling you that you have diseases based on pinched nerves and subluxations, I would say, "Prove it."

Some believe that chiropractic adjustments can stretch the fibrous capsules that surround joints in your spinal column. As a back is worked on, you may hear a popping sound, which is actually gas. When you pop your knuckles, you make little gas bubbles in your knuckles and the same may go on in these little joints—when the capsules are stretched, it may make things feel better.

Well, not all backaches are caused by the same thing, and for a chiropractor to say—not that your chiropractor would say this, but some would—that all backaches are caused by the same thing and can be cured by an adjustment is ridiculous. You can get a backache from kidney problems, bone problems, arthritis and inflammation, muscle spasms, and tendons and ligaments that are torn and pulled. So how can adjustments be good for all backaches?

In fact, a recent study of five years' worth of stroke cases found that spinal manipulation significantly increased the risk of stroke because of artery tears during the chiropractic therapy. Two of those strokes occurred within seconds after the spinal treatment.

Your next step should be a visit to an orthopedist who specializes in backs and who will make sure you don't have some of the things I mentioned, from slipped discs to other kinds of problems, which would be made worse, I think, by an adjustment—or at least not helped.

As for the feeling of being out of alignment, that would be very unusual, unless you had terrible osteoporosis and your vertebrae collapsed, or you had something broken back there. An orthopedist should shed light on what's going on.

Q: My doctor wants to operate to relieve my chronic sinus condition, but I'm diabetic and I'm not too keen on surgery. Someone suggested I go to a chiropractor. What do you think?

A: First, you need to ask yourself a basic question: How could tweaking your back or neck change something inside your head?

I may be able to help you find alternatives to surgery, but chiropractic treatment isn't one of them. Chiropractors have no business treating sinus problems.

A sinus problem is basically caused by a swelling that clogs the opening, prohibits draining, and fosters infection, because of trapped germs. I have known people to avoid surgery just by getting the sinus to drain. The simplest solutions are often overlooked.

Good decongestant nose drops, properly used, can sometimes do the trick. Doctors often recommend oral decongestants, but you'll have a better chance of success spritzing directly to the sinus openings with drops. After you spritz, if you are vertical, the drops will be useless. I advise you to get on all fours, drop your head down to your chest and hold it there a bit to let the drops seep in. If you get them right to the sinus openings, you may prevent future problems.

If you have allergies, be scrupulous about following the plan your allergist has given you for fighting them, because allergies are another source of clogged sinuses.

The position you sleep in also can affect your sinuses. Propping yourself up with a few pillows, or even tilting your entire bed by putting blocks under the headboard, can eliminate the edema—swelling and puffiness—that naturally occurs from the pull of gravity when we lie flat.

Finally, if you haven't discussed this already with your doctor, ask about simple saline irrigation. This has its roots in yogic nasal-flushing treatments dating back three thousand years. But now you can buy inexpensive spritz bottles of saline (salt water) at the drugstore.

Depending on how rip-roaringly bad the sinusitis is, you may need surgery anyway. But first try these tricks, because the results of surgery are inconsistent.

The Worst of the Worst: Iridology, Chelation, and Other Bad Ideas

Q: My girlfriend swears by iridology. Is it a trustworthy indicator of general health and well-being?

A: Iridology is totally bogus, but you'll never convince the true believers, of course. This practice is based on the belief that the iris of the eye represents all the organs and systems of the body. One spot is the stomach, another the uterus, and yet another the feet—you get the picture. Colors, shapes, and spots on the iris supposedly give information on the health of the corresponding organ.

The ludicrous premise that the body would be organized in such a way, that the iris would be the window to disease, was put to the test a few times and failed miserably. For instance, a bunch of patients dying from kidney disease were presented to several iridologists, and their accurate-assessment rates were no higher than the odds for accuracy based on an outright guess.

A Hungarian physician is believed to have invented iridology in the nineteenth century; health-food guru Bernard Jensen popularized it in America in the twentieth century; and, to my amazement, the superstition has lasted into the twenty-first century. The believers tell me they won't allow numbers and facts to trample their belief systems.

It's like psychics. I get chills up my spine when I'm watching a quality health program on cable TV that is interrupted by an ad for a psychic. I know the stations have to survive, but those ads undermine my faith in them.

As adults, we have the opportunity to choose whatever treatment we want to try. However, I will always have a problem with people who prey on the less fortunate or the emotionally desperate in our society.

Q: My friends want to involve me in something called a "colonic detoxifying program." The program says that junk is left in our colons for years—one friend told me one speck of black pepper can last nine years—and the treatments will get rid of it. My friends say it's agony when they're going through it, and I'm not eager to share the pain. What's your opinion?

A: Colonics, or colon hydrotherapy, is total bunk. Your friends are having herbal mixtures flushed into their rectums, based on the idea that rotting matter in our colons is poisoning us—a belief that dates all the way back to the time of Hippocrates. The standard "treatment" is to flush the colon with twenty-five or thirty quarts of liquid. Infections and, very rarely, ruptured colons are two of the dangers of colonics.

A doctor named John Kellogg popularized this process early in the last century, before we had colonoscopies. Now that science has invented a flashlight and a tube that lets us look into the colon, we can see that it is pink and fresh like the inside of the mouth. You don't need a "professional" to flush out your colon. Nature does an incredibly fantastic job.

Mostly, I'd consider this harmless, but it does damage the name of good health and good sense.

Q: How accurate is hair analysis in determining proper nutritional balance? I would really like to improve my eating habits, and this seemed like a good place to start.

A: If your diet is out of balance, the healthiest, cheapest thing you can do is read the advice in the rest of this chapter and start making food decisions based on what you learn here.

Hair analysis is one of the most popular scams going, and it's absolutely worthless. The Federal Trade Commission, the FDA, and every medical association I know of has condemned it. The usual scheme goes like this: You send in your hair and, in return, the company sends you an analysis with promotional material for various vitamins and supplements that they sell. The only times hair analysis is used in medicine is to look for levels of certain toxic heavy metals, such as arsenic, mercury, and lead. That test should be administered by your doctor. Of course, hair also can be used to determine a person's DNA.

Q: I'm forty-one years old and I enjoyed good health until about three years ago. I started experiencing a lot of angina, and now I have diabetes and hypertension and I have ballooned to three hundred pounds. I don't eat red meat or drink alcohol.

I've seen a cardiovascular surgeon who says I might need a quintuple heart bypass. Nowadays I run into so many people who have had bypass surgery that it almost seems routine. But I'm deathly afraid. I don't want to have my chest cut open, and I don't want to have a scar on my leg from vein harvesting. A friend suggested I look into chelation, but I haven't done much research yet. Would you consider this a reasonable option to surgery?

A: You're very, very young for this kind of a problem, which leads me to believe that it is linked to your family history. Even a person who eats roast beef three times a day would not have angina at the age of forty-one.

Our genes are largely responsible for our health. Some of us are tall and some are short. Some of us have soft arteries, and some of us develop hard arteries. So, don't blame yourself.

I understand your fear because I hardly ever go to doctors myself, but I know intellectually that this can be a very bad attitude. Now is the time to make good decisions about your health. Thankfully, we live in a time when we have the ability to go in and replace those arteries. This is an incredible achievement that was not brought about by hanging crystals around our necks and waiting for a cure.

I've been challenging chelation (pronounced "key-lation") since my first day on the radio back in 1978, when there was less evidence supporting my point of view.

Chelating agents were developed after World War I to fight nerve-gas damage. The chelating agent grabs poisons like arsenic or lead and takes them out of the body. It also takes good minerals, like calcium. So, in the early fifties, the idea became popular that chelating agents could root out the calcium from hardened arteries. A huge industry was born.

Then along came angiography, which allows us to look directly at the arteries, and we saw that chelation did nothing. The industry that was already in place started hollering, and the fight has been going on ever since.

We have done double-blind studies where one half of the group was injected with the chelating agent and the other with plain salt water, and it made no difference. There is no evidence that chelation does anything except take your money.

However, there is one legitimate option to surgery. Dr. Dean Ornish's program might well be able to spare you this particular operation by getting you on a zero- to ten-percent-fat diet while turning you on to meditation and exercise. Only a huge commitment from you gives this a chance for success, and you would need to see if your profile meets his criteria. His book is titled *Dr. Dean Ornish's Program for Reversing Heart Disease*.

If the Ornish program is not an option, and I were in your situation, I'd lay my chest down on the table. That's saying a lot, because I was once opposed to this surgery. However, bypass now has a huge success rate, and careful documentation shows this is a highly effective treatment.

Q: I have trouble digesting food; I get intestinal inflammation and all sorts of gas. My doctor says that I have food sensitivity or food allergies, and he wants me to do a NAET program, which is a combination of kinesiology, acupressure, and chiropractic techniques. He is an M.D. Have you heard of NAET?

A: In this case, M.D. stands for "miserable doctor." Kinesiology is as close to witchcraft as medicine can get. Run while your wallet is still intact.

My concern is finding something to help you. You could have colitis and ileitis, which are intestinal inflammatory diseases that are not triggered by food at all. Irritable bowel syndrome or lactose intolerance are other possibilities. Or you may simply be eating too many gas-producing foods.

"Diagnosis first" is my basic rule. Find out what's wrong and then go after a treatment. If you haven't yet seen a gastroenterologist, start there, and ask for a full evaluation. Tell the doctor you're only leaving the office when you have a diagnosis in hand.

As for kinesiology, it was really big in the seventies and eighties, and I still remember how some health food–store clerks would provide an "assessment" of food allergies. The prospective "patient" was asked to stand with his arms out and to resist when the clerk pushed against them.

Then, the seller put the offending food in a glass vial and held it above the patient's head or put it on his tongue. The seller pushed down on the customer's arm again and—wham—it slammed right down to his side, because it had been weakened already.

Time and again, the Skeptics Society has demonstrated this as a parlor trick.

Q: What are your thoughts on body wrapping? How does it "melt away inches" and eliminate toxins?

A: Isn't "melt" a wonderful word? The FDA guidelines on questionable medical practices with regard to weight loss always warn about the word "melt." You melt butter in a frying pan, but, of course, there is no way to melt fat off the human body, though many of us wish it were that easy.

Then there is the word "toxin." Ask proponents of toxin elimination to name just one of the actual toxins, and they fall silent. If their service or product eliminates these awful things, why can't they tell you a little about the evils they are so anxious to flush from your system?

I have no objection to anyone going to a spa and wallowing in mud or getting wrapped for fun and relaxation, but when these establishments claim to cure you or to "melt" fat, they are breaking the law.

Of course, you sweat when you're wrapped, and the loss of water will show up as a weight loss if you get on the scale right away. As soon as you drink some water and eat something, your weight will go back up.

You won't lose any inches, and an objective measurement is impossible to attain. For example, the abdomen is constantly changing in rhythm with respiration, so hip and waist measurements will frequently vary. And the measuring tape's tautness varies from measure to measure.

These promoters should wrap their mouths shut.

Q: I've seen ads for hyperbaric tanks, and they claim to give you pure oxygen that will heal fractures and soft-tissue injuries. How does that work?

A: This is an example of the misuse of a substance that has a legitimate medical application. Hyperbaric oxygen, which requires a doctor's prescription, aids in wound healing, especially in people with vascular insufficiency.

But it is certainly not a cure-all. The hopes we had that it could be used to treat multiple sclerosis and to prevent heart attacks have not been fulfilled.

Oxygen—like heat, water, and food—is necessary for life, but too much or too little can kill you. More is not better. With oxygen, as with temperature, the body regulates its systems very closely. Just as body temperature doesn't waver from 98.6 degrees, whether it's 10 degrees or 100 degrees outside, other systems protect the lungs and tissue from too much oxygen by slowing respiration. So, pumping in extra oxygen will backfire, because your body will fight the invasion.

For a time, hyperbaric oxygen was a fad among the Hollywood set and some famous rock 'n' rollers who thought it would keep them forever young. As you can tell by looking at most of our aging rock musicians, that's bull.

Q: I'm familiar with your opinion that magnets don't have special healing powers, but I read an article on a magnetic device for healing fractures. The research is pretty convincing. Is there something new going on here?

A: You are confusing different types of magnets, a common misconception. In contrast to the refrigerator magnets that men are told to strap on their testicles to make them more potent, or the magnets that people wrap around their neck for neckaches and things like that, the power of electromagnetic fields to diagnose and to heal has been used by medicine for many years now.

If a broken bone isn't healing well or in a timely manner, we apply electricity to the limb to promote healing. And at least one study is testing the effect of alternating magnetic currents on a certain part of a schizophrenic's brain to reduce hallucinations.

Of course, the magnets on the mass market are mostly junk, and range from cheap trinkets to expensive magnetic mattresses that miserably flunk tests to measure their healing powers. Yet the industry goes unfettered in selling promises they cannot deliver.

Acupuncture and Acupressure

Q: A friend has urged me to see an acupuncturist about my sore muscles. I'm not crazy about needles, but I'm curious, too. Will I get results?

A: Maybe, maybe not. If you exercise when you're out of shape, and your muscles tense up and become sore, you don't need an acupuncturist for relief.

A carefully designed study has found that acupuncture was not very effective at reducing pain or tenderness caused by delayed-onset muscle soreness, according to a report in *Clinical Physiology*.

Researchers used a standardized exercise regime to induce elbow soreness and then divided forty-eight volunteers into four groups. One group got twenty minutes of rest, the second group got a placebo treatment of minimal needling at nonacupuncture points, the third got needles at classic acupuncture points, and the fourth got acupuncture at "tender" points.

Elbow range of movement, tenderness, and pain were assessed before and after the treatments, and researchers found no significant interactive effects from acupuncture after all the measurements and comparisons were made.

While acupuncture, especially with electricity, may have some benefit for mild pain syndromes by distracting you from the discomfort, it cures no illness—and it's apparent from this study that it won't relieve muscle soreness due to exercising.

More acupuncture studies are in the works, looking at its impact on everything from osteoarthritis to heart disease, but don't get your hopes up. The highest-quality studies done on acupuncture to date have shown the most disappointing results.

Q: I'm in the early stages of pregnancy, and the nausea is killing me. A friend says she used some kind of wristband to help her when she was pregnant. What is she talking about?

A: One area of Chinese medicine that's becoming more popular is acupressure, which simply involves putting external pressure on different parts of the body. No needles are involved.

Several studies have claimed that placing pressure on the P6 "acupoint" above the wrist on the inside of your forearm will reduce nausea and vomiting for pregnant women. You can use your fingers, but wristbands are sold just for

---

DID YOU KNOW?
MASSAGE VERSUS ACUPUNCTURE: NO CONTEST

If you have ever dealt with back pain, read this. A study compared acupuncture, therapeutic massage, and self-care education for treatment of persistent back pain. Researchers looked at 262 patients between the ages of twenty and seventy, and participants were randomly placed into one of the three treatments.

Ten acupuncture and massage sessions were allowed over ten weeks.

The bottom line: Massage beat acupuncture hands down.

Once you have a diagnosis for your back pain, and the doctor thinks massage might help, make sure you have a certified massage therapist, and try a few different people to see whose style best suits you. Then lie down and enjoy.

---

this purpose, too. Ask your doctor if he or she has any objections. I can't see how it can hurt, although I believe most of the effect is due to placebo, and a recent University of Pennsylvania study concurred. But so what, if it helps.

Homeopathy: The Good, the Bad, the Useless

Q: I'm worried about the two homeopathic medicines that my sister-in-law gives her eight-year-old child. One of them is belladonna, and the other has arsenic in it. How can I talk her out of this?

A: I have good news for you, with one little caveat. Homeopathic compounds contain such tiny, tiny amounts of a particular substance that ingesting it is comparable to one molecule in many, many swimming pools of liquid.

So, are belladonna and arsenic poisons? Yes. But the child isn't ingesting enough to make a difference. In other words, homeopathy compounds are safe, but they are useless, too. Save your energy for a bigger battle.

Q: I'm going to Italy next month, and when I was in my local pharmacy, I saw a product called No Jet Lag, which is made in New Zealand. I bought it just for the heck of it, because it was cheap. The active ingredients are mostly herbs: leopard's bane, daisy, chamomile, and ipecac. Do you think this product will help reduce jet lag? Is it safe?

A: Somewhere on the label there probably is a hint that this is a homeopathic remedy. Homeopaths believe that if you give someone a few molecules of ipecac, which in normal amounts makes you throw up, that it can cure nausea. It's a nineteenth-century idea that was invented by a guy named Samuel Hahnemann. It's amazing that this idea is still very much alive today.

Homeopathic practitioners believe that if a substance causes a certain state in an individual, then exposing the person to a little bit of that substance will actually prevent or cure that state. For instance, if a person is vomiting, give the person something that makes them throw up, but in such a low dosage that there is nothing really there.

A lot of people believe this stuff. And it's fine to believe it and to use it. Taking these pills won't harm you. But I think the best thing to do, if you really have to be alert when you land, is take a short-acting sleeping medication that will put you down for three or four hours on the plane. This will allow you to get some sleep, even though it's out of phase with the sleep routine you had when you departed. It also helps if you don't drink alcohol, and you should try to get some sunlight once you arrive, before you go to bed for the night at your destination.

Another way to deal with jet lag is by slowly synchronizing your body. When my family plans to travel overseas, we try to go to bed an hour earlier or an hour later every night for three to four days, so that our bodies won't notice such a dramatic time difference. For example, if we're flying from San Francisco

QUIZ

Acupuncture has been proven helpful in controlling:
A) smoking   B) weight   C) depression   D) drug abuse
E) none of the above
(E: none of the above.)

to Paris, since Paris is nine hours ahead of us, we would try to reduce the impact of the time-zone change by going to bed an hour later every night for three to four days. So, if we normally go to bed at ten, four days before the trip we would go to bed at eleven, then twelve, then one A.M., and finally two A.M. Obviously, you can't adjust your clock entirely, but I promise you will notice the benefits once you arrive at your destination.

Q: For about a year I've been having periodic hearing loss and dizziness. Then I got a severe bout of vertigo when my family practitioner was out of the country, so I went to an ear, nose, and throat specialist whom I found in the phone book. He looked in my ear and then said that I probably had Ménière's disease. He gave me a prescription that only one special pharmacy could fill. It turned out to be a homeopathic medication for vertigo.

This doctor is a licensed M.D. I wrote him a letter saying that a minuscule amount of deadly hawthorn is not a cure for vertigo, and that he shouldn't be a doctor. I sent a copy to the county medical society. Is there anything else I should have done?

A: One important issue that medical consumers should remember—and that this experience proves: M.D.s can be quacks, too.

I'm not saying that all M.D.s who practice homeopathy are quacks, but at best they are poorly trained physicians who don't understand scientific evidence and how to evaluate the medical literature.

If homeopathy worked, if the equivalent of one molecule diluted in fifteen swimming pools of a substance were a cure, it would be one of the grandest discoveries in the history of science and biology. Homeopathy requires the same proof for its claims that traditional medicine does—many carefully controlled studies conducted on hundreds or thousands of patients. Well, the field of homeopathy has done no such thing.

Behind closed doors, the M.D.s I know who practice homeopathy tell me they do it for lots of reasons: Patients pay cash. The doctors don't have to work for HMOs, and they don't have to deal with blood and death. Also, patients really want this stuff, and they are better off getting it from M.D.s, who can properly diagnose them. The M.D. will know when a patient's stomachache is actually appendicitis and will not send him out the door with a potion or a referral for acupuncture.

The doctor who believes in what he's doing, however wrong he may be, is different from the one who deliberately sets out to rip people off. Whereas the first guy is stupid, the second one is a creep.

As for the original question, what else would I have done? I would have asked my friends if anyone could recommend a new ear, nose, and throat doctor. Dizziness and hearing loss are no small issues.

The Good News: Massage, Tai Chi, Biofeedback, and More Cool Stuff

Q: My sister has a weekly massage, and she says it's the best thing she's ever experienced for relieving the stress that comes at the end of a hard week at work. Would you say she feels better because she wants to, or are the effects of massage legitimate? And is there any chance of being injured by having a massage?

A: In general, I am positive about massage, and studies have shown it can be very effective in reducing stress, which, of course, relates to lots of different illnesses. And a good facial massage may bring at least temporary relief for those who deal with chronic sinusitis.

However, there are so many different types of massage in the market these days that it's difficult to keep track of them. Also, practitioners can vary dramatically in their abilities, so I always look for someone with certification from a recognized organization.

It is possible to do physical damage with inappropriate massage. There are people, for instance, who have back pain due to various diseases, from osteoporosis to metastatic bone cancer, who have had serious consequences with overvigorous types of manipulation.

However, for musculoskeletal problems from aching backs and necks, massage is now taking its place within hospitals as a less expensive and more effective therapy than pills, shots, and surgeries. As for the medicinal effects of massage, I would be very skeptical of any massage therapist who says he or she can cure or ameliorate a disease.

Finally, don't try to save money by having your partner or spouse give you a massage. Only a pro knows where to work in those fingers for real results. (See page 139 for results of a comparison between massage and acupuncture.)

Q: Is there any ailment that is effectively treated by hypnosis? I know

that hypnosis as a stage act is totally phony. But I want to quit smoking, and I wonder if this works.

A: Hypnosis does have practical and therapeutic uses, but in some studies it has not proven to be better than or even as good as other standard means of helping people to stop overeating or smoking. However, you have to consider that people who are attracted to using hypnosis to quit bad habits may be people who don't want to do it the hard way. They may be a special group that is more likely to fail because they aren't up for a big struggle.

Certain people can be hypnotized more easily than others, and judging by how a person's eyes respond to movement, some hypnotherapists can tell how easily they'll be able to put someone under.

We don't have much understanding of how hypnosis works. One reason is that setting up controls for experiments is tough. I mean, how do you do a placebo on hypnotherapy? By saying, "I'm going to fake swinging a watch before your eyes"? You can't do that.

Hypnosis has a checkered past and a checkered present. Always ask about the provider's training and experience, and realize that there are no seals of approval or guarantees on things like this.

Q: My husband has Parkinson's, and his doctor suggested he try tai chi. Does this sound crazy to you?

A: No. If your husband's Parkinson's has not gone too far, and he's capable of doing tai chi, I would recommend it.

It's a great beginning exercise for those who are still sitting on the sofa wondering what they can do for themselves. Tai chi has been described as "meditation in motion" and it involves a series of slow body movements performed while standing. It seems to help a lot with balance and muscle tone in elderly people. It's not an aerobic activity, but any activity is a positive for people who otherwise get none.

Q: I have carpal tunnel syndrome, and my New Age neighbors said that yoga may give me some relief. My job depends on me getting to the root of this problem. In your opinion, is this worth exploring?

A: I think you are getting good advice. First, for those of you who've been living in a cave for the past ten years, carpal tunnel can occur in the wrist area because of repetitive activities. The most well-known culprit is probably work at a computer that involves a mouse and a keyboard. This ailment can be painful and debilitating, and treatment can include everything from simple splints to surgery.

A small study conducted by doctors at the University of Pennsylvania School of Medicine involved twice-weekly treatments for eight weeks. It found that those treated with yoga (participants practiced eleven different postures that worked on strengthening, stretching, and balancing of the upper torso, as well as relaxation) showed significant improvement in grip strength and pain reduction.

However, this was just a preliminary study, and I want to see a lot more research on yoga's benefits. But, in the short-term, I can't see any harm in pursuing this type of treatment for carpal tunnel, and it is certainly less intrusive than shots or surgery—or changing your career.

Fortunately, therapeutic yoga—not to be confused with some of the aggressive yoga methods you'll find at a lot of health clubs—is the subject of several studies, and in the near future we should know a lot more about how well it works on a variety of ailments.

Q: I suffer from severe blushing. I get hot, turn very red, and beads of sweat form on my forehead. I've tried everything, including breathing exercises and special foods, but nothing works. Can you help me?

A: Biofeedback helps teach people to alter their blood pressure and other body functions, so it might give you a technique to control blushing. A sensor that catches your blush impulse at a very early stage will send you an audio or visual cue. You learn to respond to the cue to stop the blush.

Do make sure you don't have early signs of rosacea. (For more on this subject, see page 323 in chapter 7). Also, lasers can help some blushers.

Q: My brother suffers from chronic constipation, and now his doctor has him using biofeedback as part of his treatment. Is this legit?

A: Constipation is mostly due to a lack of fiber in the diet. Fiber attracts fluids, which keep things kind of loose and allows you to evacuate properly. I always advise people to increase fiber in their diet or to use one of the many fiber supplements now in the market. Laxatives can be a downward spiral to nowhere and should only be used on the advice of a physician.

Biofeedback can be effective, according to the most recent studies, in helping people learn how to recognize certain cues, and it is definitely worth a try. The problem is that many biofeedback practitioners are not equipped with the proper technology, but the method is legitimate.

Q: My girlfriend swears by daily meditation to control her headaches and overall mood. This sounds suspect to me, but I want to be supportive. Does this work because she believes it will work, or is there something more here?

A: While meditation can be part of some unusual spiritual practices, in and of itself it has the endorsement of most physicians. We call it the "relaxation response," and certainly most humans can use an extra dose of relaxation. It seems that when one's mind is focused on a simple repetitive phrase or on one's breathing, the brain's electrical activity duplicates a state of relaxation.

There is argument, though, among neurophysiologists about whether meditation is more effective than doing something as simple as sitting down with a glass of wine and listening to your favorite music. Nevertheless, part of the attraction of meditation is that you purposely set aside time for this break in your life on a very regular schedule.

Focusing your mind on anything you enjoy distracts you from the daily issues that may cause stress, and stress can lead to mood swings and headaches. So, appreciate the fact that your girlfriend has aggressively tackled the stress issue, but she should make sure that her headaches are stress related and not the result of some illness.

Interactions with Prescription Drugs

Q: My dad is taking Coumadin and would like to continue taking a dietary supplement that contains omega 3, 6, and 9, gamma-linolenic acid, organic flax seed oil, ginkgo biloba, borage seed oil, water, and glycerin. Do you have any concern about him combining this drug and supplement? When he asked his doctor, the doctor said, "I don't know."

A: You are right to be concerned. Coumadin is a powerful blood thinner prescribed for patients at risk of stroke or blood clot. I assume there is a very important reason your dad is taking it, and his life could depend on it. He must take exactly the right amount, or his blood gets too thick or too thin, either of which can have devastating consequences.

The interaction of pharmaceutical drugs with supplements and herbs is a no-man's-land. People gobble these nostrums at the drop of a hat, and it takes science years to catch up and figure out which combinations are dangerous.

In your dad's case, I can't help but wonder what he told his doctor. And I would question what benefits he is even getting from the supplements. While fish oil may be beneficial, fish itself is probably a better way to go. The other oils are considered healthy oils, but there are no long-term studies to show that popping pill-sized amounts is a good thing. Ginkgo, while popular, has no real benefits and can thin the blood too much in combination with the blood-thinning drugs; there is a risk that hemorrhaging can occur.

So, encourage your dad to at least consider dropping the supplements while he's on the medication. At the very least, ask him to discuss this one more time with his doctor.

Q: My daughter-in-law says I could give up Zocor and substitute soy and flax seed. Have you ever heard of that? And how does it work?

A: While soy, flax seed, and many other vegetable oils may favorably alter

---

DEAN'S LIST: WORDS TO BE WISE TO

The next time you spot an advertisement for a supplement, herb, vitamin, or any treatment, see how many of the following words or phrases pop up. Any one of these should make you nervous. More than one and you know this product could be trouble. If you want to do more checking about a product, check out *www.quackwatch.org*. This Web site, operated by Dr. Stephen Barrett, is devoted to spotting bad stuff—and it does a great job of it.

Guaranteed	Holistic
Revolutionary	Neutralize
Natural	Essential minerals/vitamins
Toxins	Cures cancer
Clinically Proven	Organic
Nontoxic	Melts fat
Wellness & Healing	Revitalize
Ancient remedies/practices	Detoxify
Top-selling	Rejuvenate
Boosts immune system	Alternative
Cleansing	

cholesterol profiles, there have never been studies to show that heart attacks and death rates drop as a result of such changes. But there are studies to show that Zocor can dramatically reduce heart attack rates. Now which would you choose? Take a chance on your life based on what your daughter-in-law says or go with your doctor's recommended treatment? The answer is an easy one.

Resource List

For consumer advisories and general health information and research, explore The National Center for Complementary and Alternative Medicine at the National Institutes of Health: *www.nccam.nih.gov/*

The Office of Cancer Complementary and Alternative Medicine at the National Cancer Institute has information on clinical trials as well as a list of frequently asked questions: *www.cancer.gov/occam/*

A Herbal Medicine directory can be found at MedLine Plus, which is provided by the U.S. National Library of Medicine and the National Institutes of Health: *www.nlm.nih.gov/medlineplus/herbalmedicine.html*

For extensive information on herb and drug interactions and other herb-related topics, see the Food & Nutrition Center at the Mayo Clinic Web site, then click on "herbs": *www.mayoclinic.com*

The Dietary Supplements section of the Food & Drug Administration Web site includes warnings and safety information and a Frequently Asked Questions page: *www.cfsan.fda.gov/~dms/supplmnt.html*

Here's everything you should know about herbal use and anesthesia, from the American Society of Anesthesiologists' Web site: *www.asahq.org/patientEducation/insideherb.htm*

For a directory of herbs and supplements—with information broken down by evidence, unproven uses, potential dangers, interactions and dosing—click on the Healthy Lifestyle box at Intelihealth.com, then go to the Complementary and Alternative Medicine section: *www.intelihealth.com*

Find a certified massage therapist at the American Massage Therapy Association Web site: *www.amtamassage.org*

For related questions see chapters 1, 2, 6, 8, 10, 11, and 12.

Chapter 4

The Women's Room, from Fertility to Fibroids

I will never forget the moment. It was 1972 and the home-birth movement was in its heyday. Parents were told to seek out everything "natural." Mothers-to-be were made to feel guilty if they took pain
medications to ease the delivery, or had a cesarean.

Hadn't we medicalized something that should be left to Mother Nature?
And what better place to be born than at home? My wife and I took the
bait. After all, I was a doctor, even if babies weren't my specialty.

What fools we were. There I was, the very uneasy spectator as my wife
squatted on the floor in our bedroom. The Harvest Gold shag carpeting was
soaked with blood and amniotic fluid. My wife was dilated and pushing and
I had no business being there. Luckily, I had a doctor friend standing by, just
in case. He bailed me out; Caleb is now in his thirties; and it makes for great
party conversation.

It was then that I first fully appreciated the female reproductive system:
So much more complex than the male equivalent, so much more to go
wrong, yet when one realizes it exists solely for the purpose of conceiving,
carrying, and delivering a baby, it becomes more understandable.

The subject of gynecology still confounds and confuses many physicians,
and medical schools are to blame. I earned my degree without ever hearing
a lecture on breast-feeding or menstruation, and I had only one lecture on
sex. I didn't know how to advise a woman about lactation or menopause.

I still remember one of my first days as a student at a gynecology clinic. We could all see each other, a long row of mostly male medical students perform-ing—and witnessing—our first pelvic exams. The looks on the faces of my cohorts—the sweat, the pallor, the concentration, and, of course, the fear—told it all. We barely knew how to put on rubber gloves, much less be gentle with a female patient whose most private parts we were about to examine.

It was clear to me, even as a novice, that this field of medicine was des-perately in need of a fix. It had become almost reckless in its physical assault on women's bodies, from hysterectomies to cesarean sections, and was deeply tinged with sexism, paternalism and misogynistic practices. Some gynecologists of that era were known to hide a husband's affair-born gonor-rhea or herpes from the wife, treating her with antibiotics under the guise of vaginitis. Childbirth was seen as an illness—and a painful one, at that. Sex-ually inappropriate conduct between doctor and patient wasn't unheard of, and a general ignorance about women's bodies prevailed.

As late as 1980, a respected gynecologist made headlines when he advised women not to jog because they risked having their uterus fall from their pelvis.

Amazing to think that just two decades later, women are playing profes-sional basketball without leaving body parts on the court, the scientific advancements surrounding fertility have made women more knowledgeable about and in control of their bodies than ever before, and the complexities of breast cancer have empowered women to challenge doctors about their medical care.

Fortunately, today the male domination of the OB/GYN field is fading fast, and while some bad habits and bad practices have been passed on to female gynecologists, the new generation of women doctors is likely to spend more time with their patients and to talk more about preventive and social issues, inspiring a new vision of what this specialty should be. They know firsthand what women are experiencing, so how could they not be as good or better at what they do than most male doctors?

But we in medicine, both genders of doctors, have fallen into the habit of routinely medicalizing natural body functions. Nowhere is this more acutely felt than in obstetrics/gynecology, where pharmaceutical companies have seized on any opportunity for a new market, while some doctors have been willing to medicate even the smallest complaints of their patients.

Unfortunately, many of these practices often backfire. Douching is one of the most blatant. It has been promoted for years as an aid to "cleanliness," capitalizing in part on the fact that some women aren't comfortable with the natural smell of their bodies. Yet studies have shown that douching increases the rate of fertility-threatening infections.

The shelves of douching products in the drugstore tell me that women aren't talking to their doctors about this issue and are just doing it on their own, or the doctors are encouraging it. Either way, this is a bad health-care habit.

The medicalization of birth isn't as bad as it once was, but it remains a problem. We still have too many C-sections in this country, and induced labor is overused. Are we really improving maternal and fetal health with most of these operations?

The episiotomy is equally invasive, and it refuses to die. The surgical cutting of the vaginal opening just before the baby's head pops out is supposed to open up the birth canal and speed up delivery. As if Mother Nature needs this much help. The fact is, it can increase, not decrease, birth trauma, and what woman really wants to deal with the urinary and fecal incontinence that frequently results from this procedure? Yet the percentage of mothers undergoing episiotomy is still much higher than it should be.

Are the menstrual period and menopause in need of the constant medical attention we give them, or have doctors just responded to a market full of "remedies"? The estrogen fiasco is perhaps the most embarrassing chapter in modern gynecology. I'm no medical psychic, but twenty years ago I first started questioning the evidence—or lack of it—that estrogens were helpful. It was not a view shared by most gynecologists.

But the treatment of menstruation and menopause is also a response by the medical community to women who want to suppress or ignore a physiological chapter of their lives. I know I'm on difficult ground here, especially because I have no idea what it feels like to have constant hot flashes or crippling cramps. Yet society has told women over and over again about the horrible symptoms they are supposed to have, and that alone can induce symptoms in many individuals. It's called "the nocebo effect."

In cultures where women aren't bombarded by books, magazine articles, and news reports about the horrors of the menstrual cycle and menopause, the women have fewer symptoms and seem to suffer less. Of course, other factors could play into these findings. And I absolutely believe there are menopause-related problems that require medical attention and further research. It's just that we have overdone it.

And we continue to invent entire new disease categories, such as premenstrual dysphoric disorder (PMDD). We once knew it as PMS, and it was claimed that 75 percent of women experienced it to one degree or another. The drug companies, in a flourish of chutzpah, renamed a major antidepressant (Prozac) already on the market and promoted it just for this. So now women are given Sarafem, which is the exact same drug as Prozac. Do you want to take medicine to avoid a few days of irritability, bloatedness, or weight gain when the side effects can include nausea, tiredness, dizziness, and loss of sex drive? Beware.

We persist in assaulting the body as well. A British medical journal recently addressed surgery to reconstitute the hymen for proof of virginity, more common right now in other countries but a perfect fad for future young American women, considering the renewed obsession in some conservative circles with the benefits of abstinence till marriage. Of course, the hymen surgery is entirely based on the myth that all women have hymens before their first experience with intercourse, and that a torn hymen results in heavy bleeding. If you are a woman, did you bleed heavily after your first intercourse? Probably not, and neither did most other women.

Equally absurd is labial reduction surgery for larger than "perfect" labia. Yes, this is extreme and uncommon, but it exists and that's frightening. Can't we just accept our bodies the way they are?

Shockingly, the one area where medicalization and modern medical technology haven't gone far enough is birth control. American women have among the fewest choices in birth control of any industrialized society in the world. One reason is our intolerance for side effects: We are unwilling to make sacrifices for new technology. Birth-control methods that have been successful in Europe are not marketed here, because at the slightest hint of side effects we call in the lawyers, and the product disappears. That's certainly what happened with Norplant.

The complex interplay of politics, morality, and science also has impacted all American women. That's why the morning-after pill, available over the counter in some countries, is just now coming on the radar here.

No advanced technology comes risk-free, and we have to understand that to move forward. The IUD is one of the best birth-control methods there is, yet because of lawsuits surrounding one particular model many years ago, most OB/GYNs do not promote or insert them.

Abortion continues to be the hottest arena for religious and political intrusion. I think all Americans agree that any abortion is a traumatic event, but that's where reasonable discussion ends. Some people say there is never a justification for abortion—even in cases of sexual assault—and the abortion issue seems destined to be in our courts for years to come.

But no laws will prevent the unpreventable, and legislation on such things as abortion and drugs has historically made matters worse. Laws do not decrease behaviors that have been with humans throughout history. Banning something just makes the practice more dangerous. Women will have abortions whether they are legal or not. Unfortunately, illegal abortions kill women. The price is too great just to satisfy the moral leanings of one segment of our society. Decreasing the rate of abortion—not making abortion a criminal offense—is where appropriate public policy begins.

Other countries with more open dialogue about birth control and sex have less sexual mayhem. Their kids delay initiating sex longer, have fewer STDs and unwanted pregnancies and—no surprise here—fewer abortions. Which begs the question: Why do we think we will get to the same place by closing off discussions about sex and access to information about it?

As with so many other issues related to women's bodies, injustices have been done. It's past time to assess how we got so far down the wrong road with something so valuable. Women must fight to regain control of their bodies. And men must support them in this fight.

Pregnancy and Delivery

Q: My first baby was born by cesarean section. I wanted a natural labor for my second child, but the doctor wouldn't let me try. Is there anything I can do to assure a natural delivery if I get pregnant again?

A: Did your doctor specifically tell you why he or she would not attempt a natural delivery? Did you ask for specifics? If not, you should have. Sometimes people need to be persistent with their doctors to have complete, detailed conversations about whatever issue is on the table at that moment.

There is a certain kind of uterine incision that precludes a woman from ever having a vaginal delivery following a C-section. During labor that scar could rupture. If your doctor didn't make that incision during your first delivery, then you have a good 65 to 70 percent chance of a successful vaginal birth, based on what I've read in obstetrical journals.

It was once accepted wisdom in the obstetrical community that a C-section barred the possibility of any future natural deliveries. No more.

Some doctors may hesitate to do a vaginal delivery with you because of your history, yet you don't have much to lose by trying it, and your chances for success are overwhelmingly good.

I know an obstetrician whose C-section rate is around 7 percent, but many doctors have rates of 20 to 30 percent. So get the facts beforehand and be choosy. These rates are published in hospitals, so everyone knows who does what.

Finally, make sure your expectations about a vaginal delivery are realistic. It does not "define" you as a woman; you will not see life differently because of this experience. In the end, when the baby is ready to come out, you want your doctor to do whatever is best for you and the baby.

Q: My pregnant daughter has just been diagnosed with Bell's palsy. It's affecting both sides of her face, and I'm scared about her health. She is just at thirty-six weeks pregnant, and she wants a C-section because this is so stressful and painful. The obstetrician said no. Right now she's being treated with cortisone. Will she be all right?

A: Bell's palsy is a paralysis of the facial muscles due to a constriction of the nerves that serve these muscles. Having both sides of the face affected is very unusual, though. It almost always causes unilateral paralysis.

DID YOU KNOW?
EAT RIGHT AND YOUR BABY WILL THANK YOU

Bizarre as it seems, women who starve themselves during pregnancy can have fatter kids who become adults with an obesity problem. How can that be? Well, if a woman is pregnant and she's not getting enough nutrition, her body says: "This woman lives in a society where there isn't enough food." And the body programs the baby so that when the baby does eat, it lays down more fat as an insurance policy. So, at the risk of repeating myself, the message is: Be smart about what you eat and how you eat. Your child will thank you.

We think it may be a postviral syndrome, and in most cases it resolves itself on its own. But until it does, it can be very scary and is sometimes mistaken for a stroke. One difference is that a stroke usually spares the forehead muscles, but Bell's palsy involves them.

The facial nerve goes through a very tight tunnel, and if that nerve swells, it becomes constricted. Just as carpal tunnel syndrome—another nerve-entrapment condition—is exacerbated by pregnancy, pregnancy may increase fluid retention and keep the facial nerve swollen.

The cortisone shouldn't cause any problems. It is the standard treatment for Bell's because it relieves some inflammation.

Her neurologist should be monitoring her nerve function for any signs of residual damage, which would call for more aggressive action. Otherwise, as I said, most of the time this gets better by itself. I agree with her doctor about refusing to do a C-section, although many OB/GYNs will do a C-section today if the patient asks for one (see next question).

Q: I am twenty-seven and six months pregnant. I know this will sound like heresy to some women, but my doctor has given me the option of having a cesarean, even if it's not medically necessary. Can you tell me the pros and cons of a C-section?

A: Your doctor is on the cutting edge of a whole new way of thinking about C-sections, and he's not alone. One survey has shown that many obstetricians would choose this delivery method for themselves and their spouses. I'm not one of those doctors, but I can sure understand why women would make this choice.

While many women would jump at the chance to skip the pain of labor and delivery, probably the biggest reason to consider a C-section is rectal and bladder incontinence. Because women are living longer and having fewer children, this quality-of-life issue has become more prominent, and an elective C-section is a very real option for many patients, according to a report in the *New England Journal of Medicine* in spring 2003. The *NEJM* report cited a recent study in South Australia showing that disorders of the pelvic floor, including stool and urine incontinence, are strongly linked to aging, pregnancy, and instrument-assisted delivery.

Of course, this is not a simple subject. There are pros and cons for both the mom and the fetus. The baby has much less potential for fractures and nerve injuries with a C-section, but one of the big risks for the mother with a C-section is death. This is rare, but the risk is several times higher than it would be with a vaginal delivery, according to the *NEJM* report.

Q: I had an emergency C-section six weeks ago, and, fortunately, I gave birth to a healthy baby boy. However, because of complications from the surgery, I ended up bleeding into my abdomen for three days. As a result, I had about two quarts of blood in my belly. Is the blood gone by now? The doctors don't want to do more tests to find the source or the amount of bleeding. Will there be any adverse effects?

A: When a baby's vital signs start to look bad during labor, we tend to be conservative by being radical. We don't want to take a chance with the baby's life when a C-section is an option.

The doctors move quickly, and, during such a crisis, blood vessels can be cut. I've seen this happen in a simple procedure like a tubal ligation, when the doctor isn't even hurried. Blood vessels are sometimes in places where we don't expect them, and these kinds of mishaps happen.

At the end of a surgery, the doctors blot everything, look carefully, close up the patient, and everything seems fine. Her blood pressure returns to normal, and suddenly, unexpected internal bleeding begins. The doctor has to decide if the benefits of doing another surgery outweigh the risks of waiting to see if the bleeding stops. A second surgery adds greatly to the trauma of the C-section, which is itself a major surgery that should not be undertaken lightly.

Now that six weeks have passed, the bleeding must have stopped. Like any cut, this one has healed over. The blood that did leak into your abdomen has been or will be absorbed back into your body and boost your iron levels.

Any swelling in your abdomen is due to the fact that you had a baby only six weeks ago. It takes a good six months for your body to settle down.

One problem you might face down the road is a tendency to develop adhesions. An adhesion is weblike scar tissue that can occur in the abdomen and cause tummy aches. I think your risk is low, though.

Other than that, you're a lucky young lady with a healthy baby.

Q: I'm eight weeks pregnant and I'm thirty-eight. In 1997, I had an excellent pregnancy and a healthy child, but last year I had a miscarriage.

I'm having a lot of back pain, which has me worried. I work in a day-care center, and I'm constantly bending to pick up toddlers. Could the back pain be a signal of another miscarriage?

A: The back pain you describe is not a symptom of an impending miscarriage. Your pain is linked with the motion of bending and lifting, and of holding a heavy load, a toddler, and probably a squirmy one at that. A miscarriage might be accompanied by back pain, but it would feel cramplike and would not be associated with your movements.

Although you've had one miscarriage, the odds of your having another are only slightly elevated. Having one miscarriage is fairly common, and it doesn't mean that you are prone to them. Since you have had a terrible loss, it's only human for you to fear a recurrence, but the odds are very low.

Mention the pain to your doctor, of course. You may also want to see a physical therapist to learn a few back-strengthening exercises as well as the best way to avoid back strain when lifting objects or kids.

Q: My wife and I are expecting a baby and we're thinking about having the blood harvested from the umbilical cord. What's your opinion about doing this?

A: Medicine is doing and will continue to do amazing stuff with stem cells. Stem cells in the cord blood are used in the same way that bone marrow is used for illnesses such as leukemia or other aggressive cancers. The cord blood is used to treat mostly blood diseases like leukemia and anemias. There is a possibility in the future that nonblood diseases may be treatable.

As for your question, the stem cells could prove valuable to your family down the road if there's a history of some cancers, immune disorders, or serious anemias where genetics are a factor. However, if that's not the case, your chances of needing these cells are very slim. One child in 2,700 might need this transplant. And this process isn't cheap. Depending on where you live and how many blood banks provide this service, your cost could vary from several hundred dollars to more than a thousand. There is also the annual storage fee to consider, though it's usually modest. You should ask your insurance company if it covers any of these costs, because some do.

If you don't have a family history of certain diseases, you might consider donating the blood to a public blood bank, which would use it for whoever needed a transplant and was a good match. However, you would need to give the blood bank plenty of notice about your intent and also find out if you would be responsible for any costs.

The key to all of this is preplanning, because the blood has to be harvested within fifteen minutes of delivery.

Q: Can you explain why some women have postpartum depression and some don't? I'm expecting a baby in a few weeks, and I've wondered what the likelihood is that I might have to deal with it.

A: Postpartum depression (PPD) is very important and often under-recognized, and many doctors now categorize the new-mom depression as "baby blues," postpartum depression, or postpartum psychosis, depending on the severity of the depression.

In general, PPD occurs in about one in ten women, but often it is not diagnosed, because many women feel guilty about expressing any negative feelings after having a baby, and they believe they should be able to take care of everything themselves. However, when they realize what a big job it is to take care of a new baby, depression can set in—and yet they may not acknowledge it.

One study gave us a little clarity about this issue. It found that women with twins versus women who have only one baby had much higher rates of postpartum depression, which implies that the actual physical stress and trauma of taking on responsibility for a new life can tilt many women toward depressive feelings. So, take that one step further with new moms who may only have one new baby—but have one or more other young children at home—and you can see how overwhelming day-to-day life could be.

Of course, this depression also can affect first-time moms who deliver only one child, and it can occur in women who have suffered miscarriages or recently weaned their baby from breast-feeding. A woman's age, economic status, and ethnicity do not seem to be factors.

PPD has many symptoms, including excessive crying, feelings of sadness, headaches, overeating, or lack of appetite, lack of energy, no interest in the baby or excessive worry about the baby, feelings of worthlessness, extreme fatigue, inability to perform basic daily functions, and hyperventilation.

While the exact cause isn't known, PPD is often a passing phenomenon—it usually lasts about four to five months. But it has to be mentioned to your obstetrician, because if it goes untreated it can get worse, and, in extreme cases, a new mother can harm herself and/or her baby. The usual treatment is medication and/or therapy.

One of these days we will get over the stigmas related to mental health, and people will more readily acknowledge signs of depression and other illnesses. But we're not there yet.

Q: I used Retinol on my face for the first eight weeks of my pregnancy, but stopped as soon as I found out I was pregnant. I also took vitamin A for a few days before I got the news. Now I'm scared. I have mentioned this to my doctor, and she doesn't seem concerned. Should she be?

A: I think the odds are overwhelmingly good that your baby is OK, though this is a good time to remind everyone: If you are trying to get pregnant, be very aware of what you are doing to your body in the way of medicines—both prescription and over the counter—and supplements.

As for the Retinol, which is another name for natural vitamin A, I can't imagine there was enough absorption to cause a problem. Yet Accutane, which can cause birth defects, is a synthetic variation of the vitamin A molecule. Of course, it's a pill, so blood levels will be higher. If the vitamin A pill was beta-carotene, that's never a problem. Beta-carotene is found in vegetables, and your body makes vitamin A from it.

Very, very early on, if the mother does ingest a potentially dangerous substance, the body is likely to reject the fetus.

Q: I don't know if my problem is physical or mental, but since my baby was born eleven months ago, I don't feel anything when I make love. This is my first child, and I'm forty years old. He weighed ten pounds at birth, but I didn't have an episiotomy, because he was born very quickly, and I tore during the delivery.

DID YOU KNOW?
VIOLENCE AGAINST MOM

While statistics vary widely, the issue of violence against pregnant women is getting increasing attention among medical researchers. One report, published in *The Journal of the American Medical Association*, found that violence during pregnancy could be more prevalent than preeclampsia (pregnancy-induced toxemia), gestational diabetes, or premature separation of the placenta.

A: When it comes to the nerves related to sexual function, we know a lot more about men than about women. We know how the nerves run near the prostate, so we do prostatectomies on men in a particular way to avoid them. But we know a lot less about how the nerves along the cervix connect to the vagina and the clitoris, so we may be damaging these nerves without knowing it.

It is possible that childbirth can cause trauma to the nerves connected to sex organs. There are newer tests that measure sexual nerve function, so I suggest that you tell your gynecologist about your lack of feeling. If the doctor's response is a shrug of the shoulders, then look for a doctor who will take you seriously.

Eleven months is enough time for you to have healed. But it should be said that most women routinely experience loss of libido following delivery. The stress, fatigue, and distractions that come with a new baby can easily throw off a mom's love life. You and your husband need to have an intimate, honest, nonjudgmental discussion about this.

Q: I just lost my baby because of preeclampsia. The doctor said I could die if they didn't induce the baby immediately, but all of this seemed to come out of the blue. Is it possible I didn't get the right care during my pregnancy?

A: Your experience with preeclampsia is very typical. If you were to ask most women who've experienced this, they would say it occurred suddenly— which makes it all the more scary, of course.

Preeclampsia and eclampsia occur in about one in twenty women during pregnancy, often during first pregnancies. The first signs are a rising blood pressure and protein in your urine. There's usually a lot of edema and swelling, too. In a small percentage of patients with that problem, a woman can go into full-blown eclampsia, with seizures, bleeding, and kidney failure. It's usually fatal if untreated.

If an expectant mother is headed for eclampsia, a doctor will do a C-section to terminate the pregnancy as quickly as possible. In your case, I have no reason to think you received poor medical care.

We don't know the ultimate cause of this, but one study has linked it to a defect in the placenta. Genetics, a multiple pregnancy, diabetes, and preexisting high blood pressure can be risk factors.

One other recent piece of research worth noting makes a link between how long before pregnancy a woman is exposed to a man's semen (vaginally or orally) and the success of that pregnancy. It seems that if a man's semen is familiar to a woman's body, the sperm and the baby may be more easily accepted by her immune system. An Australian study compared women with preeclampsia and those without, and fellatio had been practiced by more than 80 percent of the women without the condition versus 44 percent of those with it. It seems that the longer a body has been exposed to the partner's semen, the better.

Q: We are trying to have a baby girl. Does a vinegar douche before or after intercourse have any effect on determining gender? Also, someone once told me that sexual abstinence for seven to ten days helps conceive a girl. What can you tell me about that?

A: The simple sex science lesson is that men produce an X chromosome and a Y chromosome. Women produce two X chromosomes. If during fertilization, an X sperm joins the X egg, the result is XX, a female baby. If a Y sperm joins the X egg, the result is XY, or a male.

X and Y chromosomes have different characteristics from each other, so much effort has gone into studying how to support the characteristics of one over the other in order to get a girl or a boy. To have a girl baby, you want to encourage the X sperm and discourage the Y sperm. Obviously, people trying for a boy would want to do just the opposite.

The X and Y sperm swim through different substances at different speeds, and there are technologies that take advantage of that to separate X and Y sperms, concentrate either one, and then artificially inseminate them to improve the odds of conceiving a boy or a girl. This is expensive.

As for do-it-yourself methods, including abstinence and the vinegar douche, there's no evidence they work.

I have five sons because I kept trying for a girl. I've seen so many parents go through this, and fortunately their focus on the baby's gender disappears in the first millisecond after they see the new baby. You also find out very quickly that raising a girl or a boy almost never matches expectations.

Here is the deal: You have a 50/50 chance of getting your little girl. If you get a girl, you'll believe that whatever method you used was the right one. If you get a boy, you'll blame whomever first told you there really was a way to get a girl. Just don't name the baby Sue before you've got him/her in your arms.

Q: When she was fifteen years old, my daughter had an aortic valve replacement to treat a heart defect. She will be twenty-three this summer, and she wants to have a baby.

The valve works perfectly. But one concern is that her aspirin therapy would have to be discontinued during pregnancy. Her cardiologist is not 100 percent for it, because of the risks to her, but he says that he knows from his experience that if she wants to get pregnant she will. Have you heard of women with valve replacements having children?

A: I can understand your worry, but here's the bottom line: Many women with heart problems have children. And the cardiologist is like the plumber who warns you not to overwork the garbage disposal he's just replaced. He's doing his job.

What's important is that your daughter is totally open and honest with her obstetrician and makes sure the two doctors talk to each other. Then they can provide her care as a team, because your daughter is in a higher risk category than is the typical healthy pregnant woman.

The aspirin keeps her blood thin to reduce the risk of clotting around the replacement valve. If she remains on the aspirin, she faces an increased risk of excess bleeding, especially during labor and delivery. I don't think she would have to be off aspirin for her entire pregnancy, but obviously the medications plan has to be worked out by her doctors.

Q: My baby is due very soon, and there's one question that worries me. Over the long-term, will my baby be affected by a difficult delivery or by drugs that I might need during delivery?

A: I find this subject both intriguing and frustrating, because it is a topic that has challenged scientists for many decades, and it is also ripe for abuse by medical quacks. Who could forget the story of the ten-year-old girl who was smothered to death by a blanket while going through "rebirthing therapy" to wipe out the memories of her original birth, as if it were the cause of her current emotional problems?

There is no doubt that a difficult delivery can be traumatic, physically and medicinally, but the question is whether a baby is affected by that trauma—from drugs or forceps or bruising—as it grows up.

Swedish researchers studied a group of American women who needed at least three doses of barbiturates or a morphinelike drug during the ten hours before delivery. The children of these women were five times more likely to become drug abusers as adults than those born to mothers who didn't use medications during labor, according to a report in *Epidemiology*. However, this does not prove cause and effect.

While it's possible that exposure to medications in the uterus could increase the risk of a child becoming prone to drug use, I wouldn't take this as gospel, because there are many other factors that have to be considered, including genetics. Perhaps women who are genetically more sensitive to pain pass those genes to their kids, and that leads to a propensity toward drugs to ease that pain.

At the time of the delivery you need to trust your doctor to do what's best for you and the baby. Talk to your doctor about your concerns, but try not to dwell on them. Remember, too, that many expectant mothers share these same worries. You are not alone.

Q: I have taken Zoloft for depression for three years, and I want to get pregnant. Besides talking to my gynecologist and therapist, what else should I do?

A: You want to live your life to the fullest, and for you that includes a baby. I understand that. But you are right to be concerned.

The first thing you want to do is make sure that your two doctors communi-

---

DID YOU KNOW?
HELLO KIDS, GOOD-BYE SEX

Most couples with children don't need a study to tell them what a survey of five hundred women revealed: The frequency of lovemaking drops dramatically as soon as a little one is on the way.

On average, the couples made love ten times per month prior to pregnancy, five times a month during pregnancy, and less once the baby was born. Two-thirds of the women said they were too tired or stressed for sex once that baby was in the bassinette.

By the way, just in case you were wondering: Intercourse during pregnancy will not harm the fetus. So, if that's your only reason for abstaining, make a date with your husband.

---

cate with each other and that you know how each of them feels about this. One young woman I know talked with her therapist at length about this, and they were in full agreement that there was a bigger risk to the mother-to-be if she went off her medication during the pregnancy. She continued her meds and ended up delivering a healthy baby while staying healthy herself. Right now we think Zoloft does not increase the risk of birth defects.

Also, go to The People's Pharmacy at *www.drdean.healthcentral.com;* it has a lot of current information about drug interactions and contraindications.

I can tell you that no adequate studies have been done on pregnant women taking Zoloft, only animal tests. As you can imagine, testing pregnant women is very tricky. We can't send them home with a new drug and say, "Let's see what happens."

However, there is a growing number of "pregnancy registries" being run by hospitals, universities, and pharmaceutical companies to track the experiences of pregnant women around the world who are taking prescription drugs for everything from epilepsy to psychosis. If you get pregnant, you should consider participating, because the more information these registries have, the more beneficial they will be for other mothers-to-be in the future. Check out *www.fda.gov/womens/registries* and *www.otispregnancy.org.*

Q: The first time I was pregnant, I had a miscarriage in the fifth week. The second time, I gave birth to a healthy baby boy who is now three. Since then I've had two more miscarriages at thirteen weeks. I am thirty-three years old, and I do want to have another baby.

I've been to three obstetricians who specialize in high-risk pregnancy, and each one gave me different advice. The first one prescribed aspirin and folic acid, and was going to put me on heparin as soon as I got pregnant. The second doctor completely disagreed and told me to keep away from the first one. This doctor said that I should just keep on trying.

The third doctor referred me to a specialist in autoimmune disorders. I am now going through very expensive blood tests to see if I have natural killer cells that are causing the miscarriages. Have you heard of this? Or should I go back to doctor No. 1 or No. 2?

A: It is a true immunological miracle that a woman's body does not automatically reject the growing baby and instead carries it to term. If a mother needed a kidney transplant, her body would reject a donor kidney from her child, so how does she get away with not rejecting a fetus?

This type of question led to the recent and controversial hypothesis that immunological problems are the cause of as many as 80 percent of "unexplained" miscarriages, including failure of implantation. The woman's body may be rejecting her own protein or that of the man—treating the protein as if it were an invader. Lots of fascinating research is going on, and a lot remains to be done.

Research on this is tough to do, though, because we can't pull out all the stops in experimentation on pregnant women and babies. So we are left with many unknowns. You are doing the right thing by seeking out different opinions and pursuing additional information.

Though there are no right or wrong answers, I tend to agree with the second doctor, who told you to keep trying. That's because you have had one healthy baby. Not to diminish the trauma of going through three miscarriages, but I do think you should continue to try for a baby the old-fashioned way.

I would not yet label you a habitual aborter. However, if you are so unfortunate as to have three miscarriages in a row, then you should be evaluated for more aggressive approaches. As you have found, there is disagreement on this

DID YOU KNOW?
MORE AND MORE SINGLE MOMS

If you are a single mom, you are not alone. Unmarried women delivered one-third of all the babies born in 2001. This number has inched up over time, as married women have fewer children, and the number of unmarried women grows. Single-mom babies hit a record high of more than 1.3 million in 2001, although the birth rate among unmarried women of childbearing age (fifteen to forty-four) actually declined slightly between 2000 and 2001. On a related note, a recent study by University of Washington economists found that single moms are more likely to marry the father if the child is a boy. And, sadly, fathers of sons born out of wedlock work more hours and spend more money on their families than do the fathers of girls born out of wedlock.

point, and some doctors start testing after two. For women over thirty-five, the American College of Obstetricians and Gynecologists recommends testing after two consecutive miscarriages.

Most women are shocked to find that almost one-half of the embryos in women's bodies are probably rejected within the first few weeks following fertilization. Research has shown that a genetic defect is often the cause. When this happens, a woman supposes she is having a heavy period and never knows that she was pregnant.

In my opinion, starting on heparin isn't necessary yet, and may never be. Since you're already doing the blood tests, you can always make use of those results later on if you need to.

Q: Can the complication at childbirth known as placenta abruptio be caused by inducing labor, and are there any long-range effects that we need to watch for in our baby? So far, our little girl seems fine.

A: Your baby's current good health is the best sign of all. Placenta abruptio, or premature separation of the placenta, has nothing to do with labor. It is the separation of the placenta from the uterus, and the risk factors for it include high blood pressure, smoking, drinking, or drug use during pregnancy. But it also can occur without any of these factors.

The part of the placenta that should rest against the side or upper part of the uterus peels away, and you get some bleeding. And that little part that peels away is not supplying oxygen to the fetus, but in this day and age, we handle that complication pretty well. We're finding that infants are fairly tolerant of a wide range of oxygen levels during birth.

There was a time when women could bleed to death from this complication, which is why every mother should get good prenatal care. A good obstetrician can manage it successfully.

Q: My wife is four weeks pregnant. She hasn't seen a doctor yet, because we don't have our insurance worked out. How crucial is prenatal care? Does it need to begin immediately?

A: As you may have noticed in previous questions, every woman needs prenatal care. There is nothing more significant in predicting the future health of the mom and the baby. And if you go by the book, prenatal care should begin immediately. You don't want to waste any time.

Now, is immediate prenatal care "crucial"? The odds are that even without prenatal care, everything is going to be OK, but your baby's health isn't something you want to you take bets on.

There are important blood tests that need to be done, and your wife needs information about drugs, nutrition, and vitamins, because they can have an impact from the very beginning of a pregnancy.

Early care also establishes a baseline on your wife's weight and blood pressure before these things begin to change. Without seeing a doctor during her first trimester, she won't have a complete picture of how her system is changing. The trends, whether they are up, down, or stable, are important information, especially for something like preeclampsia, which is a rare but dangerous, sometimes fatal, disorder of pregnancy that often strikes without warning.

Anyone who doesn't have insurance should go to a public clinic. This may not be your first choice, but you can always move to the doctor of your choice once you have insurance.

Q: I want to have a baby, but first we need to deal with my husband's vasectomy. I've heard the reversals can take up to a year to work, and that they sometimes don't work at all. If he has the surgery, will he start producing sperm right away, or do I need to be patient?

A: Take a deep breath and throw out any timetable you already have.

Under "normal" circumstances, a young and healthy female just doing what comes naturally with her unaltered man can take about six months to become pregnant. So, when you throw a vasectomy reversal into the equation, you have to assume it will take at least that long, right?

In a postvasectomy man, sperm may show up in semen right away, but if the vasectomy happened many years before, the testicles may have turned down the action and be slow to kick in. His sperm count can be measured right after the procedure to give you some information on that issue.

If you both check out as physically healthy, you can expect a better than 50 percent pregnancy rate following his operation. But don't underestimate this surgery. It is delicate and expensive, and you want a doctor with really good hands and lots of experience.

One other option to consider is in vitro fertilization. The doctors can fertilize your egg by using sperm that they extract from your husband's testicles—yes, postvasectomy men have sperm in their testicles. This process—intracytoplasmic sperm injection or ICSI—is called "ick-see" for short.

During natural conception, as hundreds of millions of sperm attempt to impregnate a woman, only one is the front-runner that achieves its aim. But with reproductive technology, we can take one sperm and, with a very fine, needlelike device, inject it right into the egg. Many doctors consider this a better, more direct option.

Q: What do you think of using a midwife for delivery? My wife is all for it, but it makes me a little nervous. The woman she would be using has delivered lots of babies, and our baby would be delivered in a hospital with doctors nearby.

A: Studies have shown definitively that a midwife-attended birth is a safe birth, but it's important to be clear that midwives do not handle high-risk cases.

Women with risk factors like toxemia or diabetes must have their babies delivered by obstetricians. And any women with any risk factor should not make the mistake of seeking a midwife's care because she wants to avoid a cesarean section or induced labor.

Research on the safety of midwives was confusing at first, because those who opted for midwives were healthier, upscale women who naturally have healthier pregnancies with fewer complications. But the best research today finds that for the routine, healthy delivery midwives are a very acceptable alternative. Until recently, midwifery was an underground profession. However, the decision to license and regulate the practice has been well-received. Along with regulation come training standards and protocols for care. Regulation is not automatically a bad thing.

Legitimizing midwives has given pregnant women an option, and many obstetricians now have midwives in their offices.

Improvements in medicine are responsible for lowering the death rate of U.S. infants from 169 per 1,000 births in 1900 to the 6 per 1,000 births that it was in the last decade. Similarly, 6 to 9 mothers died for every 1,000 live births; today, there are approximately 8 maternal deaths per 100,000 live births. Modern medicine has been a savior in many ways.

However, some folks are still so blasé about deliveries that they don't even bother with midwives. That's a stupid and dangerous thing to do.

Q: I am two months pregnant, and I work full-time in a busy advertising agency. At what point in pregnancy does a stressful job become dangerous to the fetus?

A: It sounds like you want to quit your job right now. Well, I'm sorry but I can't give you the ammunition you want just yet.

Overall, stress increases certain risks to the baby, but it's not straightforward, and the suspicion is that stress early in pregnancy is less significant than stress later on.

Pregnancy's demands on your body are not as great now as they will become. Right now, the fetus is a little tiny thing, and your body can provide everything it needs.

Stress is harder to gauge than something like smoking, where I can tell you just what percentage of risk you are taking with your baby's health. That's because the definition of stress and how it is experienced varies tremendously from person to person.

Gathering data on the relationship between a stressful job and pregnancy is a challenge, because you have to compare women from the same socioeconomic group who have a range of jobs. You can't go into an office building and compare the obstetrical health of the woman lifting boxes in the mailroom to that of the CEO, because they come from different socioeconomic backgrounds, they have different habits, and their family histories are probably different, too.

So, while some obstetricians would advise you to take some time off once you're six months pregnant, some women, even women in high-stress jobs, work right up to the birth of the baby, and the baby is just fine.

Your life is about to change in a profound way, and if job stress is getting to you now, it's likely to get worse once the baby arrives. Unless you plan to be a full-time mom, you may want to start looking for a different line of work.

Q: I'm three months pregnant, and I'm confused about the dangers of drinking too much or too little water. At the beginning of my pregnancy, I was cramping, and the doctor said dehydration might be the cause and that I should drink more water.

Yet I heard about a professional athlete who dropped dead from drinking too much water. How much water should I be drinking each day?

A: I've never heard of a pregnant woman dying from drinking too much water, or too little for that matter. But there's a simple way to know that you're drinking the right amount: Your urine should be lightly colored—not too pale, and not at all dark. If it is dark, you aren't drinking enough water. If it's pale, you're probably drinking more fluids than your body needs.

Fatalities related to drinking water occur in people who go to extremes, such as athletes who drink excessively before marathons. As we run, blood flow shifts from the stomach to the muscles. As we sweat, the body conserves fluid by turning off urinary excretion.

A person who has drunk to extremes can be left with a pool of water sitting in his or her stomach. When the race is over, and the blood shifts back to the stomach, all that water, all at once, becomes absorbed. Too much of it can cause swelling of the brain and death.

Pregnancy Tests

Q: I'm twenty-four weeks pregnant, and, because of complications, I had an ultrasound at fifteen weeks and seventeen weeks. How accurate are ultrasounds at telling the sex of the baby? And what are the chances the ultrasounds harmed my baby?

A: By seventeen weeks, the accuracy of an ultrasound is very good, and, of course, the bigger the baby grows, the higher the percentage of accuracy. But I know of a doctor who claims he can detect a baby's gender from an ultrasound at twelve weeks.

An extremely modest baby might twist itself into a position that makes a sighting impossible. And mistakes do happen, but they are rare.

Most of the initial concern about ultrasound stemmed from the fact that it was done on almost every pregnant woman, although it had not been subjected to careful analysis. We have since done exhaustive studies and found that ultrasound appears to be safe.

However, there are still some concerns about the routine use of it. These are sound waves, and fetuses' cells are different from adult cells and could possibly respond negatively to this type of energy. So far there are no known problems.

Nowadays, the main concern worldwide is the use of ultrasound to determine gender, which, in turn, can lead to gender abortion, which has a profound influence on gender ratios in many countries. I think most people on both sides of the abortion debate would agree that gender is a poor reason to have an abortion.

Q: My wife is forty-two and had a miscarriage last year. She is sixteen weeks pregnant now and was just beginning to relax and enjoy the experi-

ence. When she had an ultrasound, we saw an active baby kicking his legs, but now we've been told the amniocentesis indicates the baby has Down syndrome. We're trying to get the information we need for making educated decisions. How reliable is the testing?

A: Blood tests and ultrasound alone do not give enough information to determine if a baby has Down syndrome, but amniocentesis has a 99 percent accuracy rate. I know you're hoping that the test is wrong, and labs do make mistakes. Obviously, you should verify the results.

These technologies are developed to give parents an option, but the option—abortion—is very upsetting. Accept the fact that right now you have deeply mixed feelings and you won't be able to come up with a decision that feels absolutely right. You will have guilt if you go in one direction and fear if you go in the other.

This is a time for clear and honest communication between you and your wife. A good counselor can help you two talk it through, but it is ultimately up to you two alone.

Whenever this topic comes up on my show, I get tons of faxes from the parents of children with Down syndrome telling me what lovable, wonderful kids they have. Parents often say that these kids have much more pleasant personalities than do "normal" kids.

However, I don't want to downplay the severity of the situation—or the demands on a family with a Down-syndrome child. Down syndrome is caused by an extra chromosome in the fertilized egg and can result in mental retardation that is most often mild to moderate and only occasionally severe. Kids with Down syndrome also have medical problems: About half of them are born with heart defects, they often have vision and hearing deficiencies, and thyroid disease and gastrointestinal troubles are possible.

Obviously, caring for such a child can be a lot more challenging than raising a healthy child. Seek out all the resources you can and talk to the parents of some children with Down syndrome. For Web sites, see our Resource List on page 199.

Q: I'm fourteen weeks pregnant, and a recent blood test shows that I've lost my immunity to the rubella virus. What concerns should I have about my baby?

A: If a pregnant woman becomes sick with rubella—German measles—during her first trimester, her baby has a 25 percent chance of having a birth defect. You are now beyond your first trimester, so chances are very good that your baby is in the clear if you haven't been ill.

Thanks to vaccines, we no longer have major outbreaks of rubella, which causes babies to be born deaf, blind, and mentally disabled. And since rubella is no longer commonplace, you are unlikely to have been exposed.

Because immunity can wear off, as it did in your case, it's a good idea for a woman to be tested for rubella antibodies when she is planning to conceive. Once she is pregnant, it is too late to be vaccinated.

Talk to your obstetrician or to a public health expert about precautions you should take. It has been recommended that a woman in your situation stay away from day-care centers and sick people.

And after your baby is born, talk to your doctor about getting yourself vaccinated against rubella.

Q: While I was pregnant, I used a steroid hand cream for eczema, which my obstetrician told me was safe to use. In my eighth month, I saw my dermatologist, and he told me I shouldn't use a steroid cream during pregnancy.

My baby was born in July, and he has cerebral palsy. Do you think there is any relation between the hand cream and his illness?

A: No. We do recommend against the use of any hormones during pregnancy, even something that you rub on, because it can be absorbed through the skin. Your dermatologist was probably following the general medical guideline of opposing all drugs during pregnancy except for those with excellent safety records or those that must be used to protect the mother's health.

Of course, we are not going to do drug trials on pregnant women to find out if drugs are safe or not. However, in real-life situations, some pregnant women are treated with huge doses of oral steroids for life-threatening diseases. The medical literature reports that these mothers do not disproportionately give birth to children with defects.

I understand that you want to turn over every rock to find out why your child is impaired, but I feel very secure in telling you that it had nothing to do with the steroid skin cream.

Fertility and Infertility

Q: I am forty-eight and I'm going through menopause earlier than I thought I would. I haven't had hot flashes or any other symptoms, but my doctor says that blood tests show that my ovaries have stopped producing eggs.

I have yet to have a baby, but I still want one. I don't have a partner at the moment, and I would rather not use an egg donation when I do decide to get pregnant. Is there something I can do to produce an egg one last time?

A: Your timing is excellent in at least one sense, because we now live in an era when postmenopausal women in their fifties can get pregnant. But I would encourage prospective parents to think long and hard about the wisdom of such a decision. Having a teenager as you push seventy may not be as much fun—or as easy—as you think.

Nevertheless, fertility clinics are the experts here, so that is where you should start. They will review your options. We can stimulate your ovaries to produce eggs, fertilize them, and implant them, and, voilà, you are a member of an exclusive menopausal-mom club.

If ultimately you need to use an egg donor and get sperm from a sperm bank, maybe you'll consider making the world a little bit better by adopting a baby instead, one who's already here and needs a home.

Who needs labor, right?

Q: I had in vitro fertilization, and the doctor implanted six embryos. I'm nearly three months pregnant, and three of the embryos survived. I've been advised to do a reduction to two embryos. My husband and I are struggling with this. Any advice?

A: This whole issue of selective reduction of embryos can be very upsetting to some people, especially if they see it as an abortion. Let's suppose that all six embryos had survived, and you did not have selective reduction. It's not likely that you would end up with even one live baby. Yet some people think you would be better off with six dead babies versus two live ones, simply because they don't believe in abortion.

Reducing the embryos from three to two is a more difficult decision. There would definitely be a statistically verifiable advantage, but by the same token, unlike carrying six babies, your chances of successfully delivering three healthy babies are still pretty good.

The Edell Report
Are You PID Savvy?

I'm afraid that too many women between the ages of fifteen and twenty-five who get pelvic inflammatory disease (PID) don't know much about it. And yet they are the ones most likely to get it.

PID is an infection of the reproductive organs and the leading cause of infertility in women. Anyone who has gonorrhea or chlamydia can transmit PID during sex, but it can occur naturally, too. Douching can raise your risk for PID, so don't do it. Ever. PID can be life-threatening, so know the symptoms:

- *Dull pain or tenderness in lower abdomen*
- *Burning or other pain when you urinate*
- *Nausea and vomiting*
- *Bleeding between menstrual periods*
- *Fever and chills*
- *Pain during sex*
- *Increased or changed vaginal discharge*

When in doubt, talk to your gynecologist.

You need to ask the doctor: "Give me the odds of what happens if I were to carry three babies versus two." Then you're looking at real numbers, and you can make an intelligent choice.

One other thing to keep in mind is that a pregnancy with three babies will most likely mean delivery of three premature babies, and with that come certain risks.

I'm amazed at how many prospective parents are surprised when they find out they may be carrying more embryos than they counted on. It seems that they are so excited by the in vitro technology that they don't hear the warnings.

If this presents an ethical conundrum you and your husband can't resolve on your own, you might talk to a clergyman or someone else who may be able to help you reason it out.

Q: I had two abortions when I was in my twenties, and now I'm thirty-nine and about to get married. What effect could those abortions have on my chances of getting pregnant?

A: A normal abortion should not affect a woman's fertility unless something untoward happened. If you had an infection in the uterus from the abortion, that could definitely affect your fertility, but, in general, we don't think that therapeutic pregnancy terminations affect fertility if you've had only a couple of them.

Q: My husband is twenty-seven, and I'm thirty-one, and we haven't been able to conceive after trying for six months, so I'm looking at the possible reasons. My husband's father was exposed to Agent Orange in Vietnam before my husband was born. Could there be a connection?

Also, my menstrual cycles are irregular. Do women always ovulate fourteen days before their periods, or is it really halfway? For instance, if I have a thirty-two-day cycle, do I ovulate fourteen days or sixteen days before my next period?

A: First of all, it's highly unlikely that his father's exposure to Agent Orange has anything to do with your husband's fertility. Some chemicals can affect sperm production, but sperm are constantly renewing themselves, so, as time passes, the damaged cells are replaced with new cells.

The much more obvious reasons for not being pregnant yet are 1) six months is just not enough time to give yourself a chance to conceive, and 2) your irregular cycles.

QUIZ

By what age does a woman have all her eggs?
A) twenty-six years old   B) at birth   C) eighteen years old
D) puberty
(B: at birth.)

The average, healthy couple conceives after six months of unprotected intercourse. That means a lot of people conceive at nine months, and a lot of people conceive at three months, and everything in between. A couple isn't given a diagnosis of infertility until they have had unprotected intercourse for a year.

Ovulation is signaled by a rise in body temperature, an increase in mucus, and, for some women, a little abdominal pain called *mittelschmerz*, which occurs with ovulation about two weeks before every period in a twenty-eight-day cycle.

Ovulation almost always happens fourteen days before the beginning of a woman's period. The day she begins to bleed is counted as Day One. In the perfect, regular menstrual cycle—a twenty-eight-day cycle—the fourteenth day before the next period is also the fourteenth day after the last period, so ovulation occurs midcycle.

A lot of women think that no matter how long their cycles are, they ovulate on Day Fourteen. They don't. They ovulate on the fourteenth day prior to the next period. So, if you have a thirty-two-day cycle—four days longer than a regular twenty-eight-day cycle—you would actually ovulate on Day Eighteen, which will be fourteen days before your next period starts.

Obviously, it is critical to know when you ovulate, then you'll know which days you and your husband should be having sex for your best chance to conceive.

If you haven't conceived in a year, and you're having intercourse within a day or two of ovulation, then your husband can go for a fertility test, which is a very easy experience for a man. If he's OK, then you will be tested.

Q: **My wife and I are in our thirties and have been trying to have a baby for two years. We have both had fertility testing, and everything checks out OK except my testosterone, which is at the bottom end of the scale. I've been tested several times and get the same results.**

Unfortunately, because I am still within the normal range, my HMO won't recommend hormones. Don't you think that supplementing my testosterone will help us conceive?

A: Absolutely. Since your borderline testosterone level has been consistently documented, you should be treated. What is there to lose? The most worrisome side effect of too much testosterone is prostate cancer, which is not an issue at your age.

If you were my patient, I would definitely put you on testosterone and see what happens. Unless one of you has an unusual fertility problem, this should take the struggle out of making a baby.

Q: My daughter saw an advertisement for egg donors in her college publication, and she is thinking about doing it. She is interested in the money, of course, but she also feels that it's like donating blood. She has healthy eggs that she would like to share. How do we find out if the clinic is reputable? What are the risks to her?

A: First, let's be clear about the meaning of the word "donate." Getting paid for giving eggs is not donating.

Egg harvesting is usually done by fertility clinics, which are mostly aboveboard. However, some clinics have been embroiled in scandals and lawsuits over ownership of eggs.

Taking out ads in collegiate publications or college towns, with their populations of young women in need of money, is a common practice for a fertility clinic. But you should be able to investigate this facility through a professional association. One such group, the American Society for Reproductive Medicine, has a list of member doctors and an office in Washington, DC. They share statistical information with the government's Centers for Disease Control.

You might call a gynecologist in your daughter's area to find out what they know about the clinic.

I'm not aware of any physical troubles related to harvesting eggs.

Women are paid about three thousand dollars for eggs, a lot more than guys are paid for sperm. Of course, "acquiring" sperm is fairly easy, for obvious reasons, and is a lot more fun than "acquiring" eggs.

A woman first has to take medication to boost her egg production above normal. Then the eggs are harvested through a puncture into her abdominal cavity. So there is more to the process than some might think.

When people tell me they object to selling organs, I bring up this egg-selling practice. Is it the size of the organ that's at issue?

I think it's a wonderful thing when women help out other women who are family or friends. Otherwise, I have to admit that egg selling bothers me. As a parent, I think I'd tell my kid, "I'll give you three thousand dollars not to do it."

Birth Control

Q: I have been taking Metabolife, and I am also on Depo-Provera injections for birth control. I was doing fine until I heard a doctor on television who said that some women on birth control pills who were taking Metabolife had gotten pregnant. Have you heard of this?

A: Although I haven't heard these reports about Metabolife, it certainly is possible for herbs—as well as pharmaceuticals—to interfere with contraceptives. We have concerns that some antibiotics, for example, can interfere with the way birth control pills are metabolized in the liver, potentially decreasing their effectiveness.

Even something as seemingly harmless as grapefruit juice has a profound influence on drug levels in the body. Drinking the juice with pills will elevate the levels of many medications. Sometimes that's good and sometimes that's bad.

The Edell Report
Ready for the Morning After?

One of these days, the majority of politicians will realize that unintended pregnancies lead to unwanted children, abortion, and all kinds of expensive social problems we'd like to fix. Until then, I encourage anyone who worries about accidental pregnancies to go to the Emergency Contraception Web site based at Princeton University: www.not-2-late.com.

This site is full of information that anyone who wants to avoid a pregnancy or an abortion should know about. It's a thorough and helpful site, and it's not affiliated with any drug manufacturer. It has everything you need to know about the most effective pill, Plan B, as well as a clear explanation of which birth control pills can be used as potential pregnancy blockers.

And, most important, with just your zip code or your phone area code, you can get information on where to get the morning-after pills in your town or city. Plus, if you need a prescription, this site will steer you to Web sites that can provide prescriptions for a very modest charge.

Because Depo injections bypass the liver, they might not be affected as strongly by pills, which are absorbed and go to the liver first.

While I don't think it's very likely that Metabolife would interfere with Depo-Provera, there are interactions we just don't know about.

You should be suspicious about any over-the-counter herbs, and don't buy the argument that they are safe just because they are natural. Any substance that is powerful enough to affect disease is powerful enough to have side effects. To make things worse, we're way behind in research on herb interactions with other medications, but we do know of some popular herbs reducing the effectiveness of prescription drugs.

In general, you need to take a look at what you think Metabolife is going to do for you. I don't believe that taking pills is the way to lose weight or to get healthy.

There are more than a million abortions a year in the United States, yet there is still little publicly promoted information about morning-after pills for those times when the condom breaks or you were simply carried away by the moment. In fact, most women don't even know that the name is a misnomer; you can start some of these pills up to five days after intercourse, though sooner is always better.

So, please, if you are a woman and you don't want to face a pregnancy— or an abortion—talk to you doctor about having a stash of pills in your medicine cabinet. Or, if privacy is an issue, buy the pills on the Internet.

If you are offended by this information, that's your right. But please don't call me to claim that taking these pills is the same as having an abortion, because it isn't. These pills are designed to prevent conception by blocking the release of eggs from a woman's ovaries—so we're not talking about a fetus here. For women who consider this an important issue, please take a second look at the facts.

Q: I have two little babies, and I'm nursing. I need a birth control method that won't interfere with my milk or with intimacy with my husband. I don't want to rely on nursing as birth control, because that's how I got pregnant the second time.

I recently heard about a specially treated lens that reacts with your saliva when you're fertile. Does this work?

A: You're talking about an ovulation microscope, or saliva fertility test, and I don't think this is really what you want. This system is designed primarily for couples who are trying to have a baby and want to know when the woman is most fertile. A drop of saliva is put on a lens, the sample is allowed to dry for several minutes, then it is viewed under a microscope. If a certain pattern is seen, the woman is ovulating or is just about to start. As a contraceptive device, this process makes me extremely nervous.

I highly recommend an IUD. Because of a bad IUD model and junk science, IUDs were slammed in the American market many years ago. As a result, young American women are not hip to this method, which is very popular and successful in Europe. It has been ranked No. 1 in satisfaction in a survey of women who use birth control.

A doctor puts it in, and that's it. You don't even know it's there. The IUD concept supposedly came about because camel drivers put pebbles in the camels' uteri to prevent pregnancy. A foreign body in the uterus seems to stimulate secretions that prevent implantation and even fertilization.

Any natural birth control method, like the lens, rhythm, or Billings, requires you to track your ovulation and prevent pregnancy by avoiding intercourse during fertility. Saliva can indicate fertility, as can changes to your temperature and your vaginal mucus.

To be successful, you have to be very careful. Women ovulate reliably two weeks before the start of their periods, but no woman can predict into the future exactly when her period will happen. You may regularly have a twenty-eight-day cycle, but if for just one month your cycle is twenty-six days, you'll ovulate two days earlier than you expect. The unreliability of timing is one of the drawbacks of natural birth control methods.

That unreliability has just been underscored by remarkable research that challenges all the conventional wisdom about fertility. One small but impressive study found that almost 25 percent of women are capable of ovulating several times a month. This is common in animals, and may account for the fact that there are cases of women delivering fraternal twins of different gestational ages.

As you noted, nursing—which is the most widely used method of birth control in the world—has a high failure rate. It works best during the first six months or so, when you're breast-feeding five or six times a day. As soon as the baby starts eating, and you cut back on feedings, ovulation can occur. But you don't know you've ovulated, because your period will come after ovulation. Unless, of course, you're already accidentally pregnant.

Using the rhythm method can be a great opportunity for improving intimacy, because it's a great opportunity to increase your sexual creativity. So many people think that intercourse is all there is to sex. But there are a variety of sexual gratifications that will not expose you to pregnancy. If you don't limit yourselves to intercourse, you can have some fun during that fertile time of the month.

Q: What's the main difference between Depo-Provera injections for birth control and Lunelle? I currently use Depo-Provera and like it.

A: You're lucky, because Depo-Provera has not been ideal for everyone. Breakthrough bleeding and loss of menstrual periods are two potential side effects.

Probably the biggest difference between Lunelle and D-P is timing. Lunelle is a monthly injection, the D-P injection is every three months.

Another big factor for some women may be estrogen: D-P does not have it, while Lunelle is a combination of estrogen and progestin. D-P is a progesterone-like hormone called medroxyprogesterone acetate.

QUIZ

What percentage of women between the ages of fifteen and forty-nine practice birth control in the United States?
A) 57 percent   B) 44 percent   C) 66 percent
D) 76 percent
(D: 76.4 percent, according to the most recent research; the first choice in contraception is the Pill.)

Fertility also may be an issue for you. It returns much more quickly with Lunelle than D-P (on average, three months versus ten months). Both can cause erratic periods or stoppage, but this is less of a factor with Lunelle.

Both birth control methods are highly effective (about 99.7 percent), unless you don't get the shot within the allowed time frame, and both may cause weight gain.

Lunelle and D-P have other pros and cons, and you should talk to your doctor about which one is best for you. However, if you were to switch, you would have to wait about three months before starting Lunelle.

Q: I started taking birth control pills when I was sixteen, because of infrequent periods. Now that I am twenty-two, I stopped taking the pills, because I want to get pregnant and because I was having breakthrough bleeding. Well, I quit them twenty weeks ago, and I still have not had a period. My doctor is taking a wait-and-see approach, and that is making me anxious. Do you agree with his approach?

A: Yes. The most common causes for stoppage of a woman's period are heavy exercise, dieting, weight loss, and stress. If you don't have accompanying symptoms, like acne or hairiness, which could be signs of hormonal disease, wait-and-see is a reasonable policy.

The pill itself can be a cause of temporary amenorrhea (no periods). It can take six months for a woman to begin ovulating when she stops taking the pill, and you are still within that range.

It is also possible that the pill was masking a gynecological problem, which is likely in your case, because your periods were irregular to begin with. The pill provides the hormones to regulate your periods; then, bingo, you go off the pill, take the hormones away, the original malfunction is unmasked, and your periods stop.

Don't stress about getting pregnant, because stress may affect fertility. On the average, it takes six months for a young healthy couple to conceive. Even a year is reasonable.

Enjoy this time. You have an opportunity to have fun, and it also seems that a good sex life increases fertility.

If you haven't conceived after another six months, ask your gynecologist about inducing ovulation.

Q: I took a morning-after pill (Preven) within forty-eight hours of unprotected intercourse, but I got pregnant anyway. I'm thirty-four, I already have children, and this pregnancy is unplanned. If I decide to continue the pregnancy, could the morning-after pill do any damage? Also, we were told about a CVS test. Is it worth the risk, and could you tell me something about it?

A: As with all birth control methods, the morning-after pills do sometimes fail. Their window of effectiveness after intercourse is generally 72 to 120 hours, but they don't work all the time, and progestin-only pills like Plan B work better than those with a combination of progestin and estrogen. In general, the sooner you take either pill, the better.

Next time you see your doctor, ask him or her about Plan B. It requires a prescription in most states, but that's changing quickly; check the Internet for the latest information. By mid-2003, California, New Mexico, Washington state, and Alaska allowed you to get this emergency contraception directly from some pharmacists without visiting a physician or a clinic. (For a pharmacy directory, check out the Web site *www.go2planb.com*). Legislation is in the works in many other states, and the manufacturers of both Plan B and Preven hope their products will be approved for over-the-counter sale sometime in 2004.

As of mid-2003, Preven could only be obtained with a prescription.

Planned Parenthood has twenty-four-hour online pharmacies in several states and also offers a morning-after pill at its clinics. And one Web site, *www.not-2-late.com,* offers specific guidance on how to turn many birth control pills into emergency contraceptives. For more information, see our Resource List on page 199 and a related Edell Report on page 178.

Neither of the morning-after pills—which are basically megadoses of birth control pills—seem to have negative effects on the fetus, should a woman conceive in spite of the pill. The effect is similar to that when a woman doesn't know she is pregnant and continues taking birth control pills for weeks or even longer.

In the earliest stages of a pregnancy, very few cells are present. Hormones affect the growth of thousands of cells, but they don't alter the very few cells and the DNA of an early embryo, which is what's really at work in the very beginning of a pregnancy.

The CVS (chorionic villus sampling) test, like amniocentesis, is used to detect birth defects, primarily Down syndrome. The risk of having a baby with

Down syndrome is 1 in 1,250 for a twenty-five-year-old woman and jumps to 1 in 300 for a thirty-five-year-old woman, but of course this is a statistic. It's not as if a woman's risk makes a leap on the day she turns thirty-five. At thirty-four, you are right on the cusp.

The advantage of a CVS test is that it can be done as early as ten weeks, and therefore allows for an earlier abortion if that's what you choose to do in the case of a positive result. CVS has a 2 to 5 percent risk of miscarriage.

Fibroids

Q: For the last four months, my girlfriend, who is thirty years old, has been taking about a thousand milligrams of acetaminophen a day for fibroid pain. I know that acetaminophen can be harmful to the liver, and I'm worried that she has been taking too much for too long.

She doesn't have insurance at the moment, so she is waiting a while before seeing a doctor. I think this is a bad idea. What should I say to her?

A: Fibroids are benign muscle growths in the uterus, and age thirty is a little young to have them. She should be sure that they are the cause of her pain. Blaming fibroids for pain that actually has another source is a common mistake. So it's important for her to see a doctor and get a diagnosis.

Acetaminophen is Tylenol, and a couple of 500 milligram tablets a day is not a lot. Unless her liver is compromised in some way, the Tylenol isn't harmful, but neither is it the best drug for easing pain that is related to the menstrual cycle.

Aspirin- and ibuprofen-type drugs—NSAIDs (nonsteroidal anti-inflammatory drugs)—have specific actions that may relieve menstrual pain. However, the trade-off is that NSAIDs are rough on the stomach, and, as you said, Tylenol can be rough on the liver.

Anyone with a history of hepatitis or with a habit of abusing alcohol should stay away from Tylenol. In addition, the long-term use of combining NSAIDs with Tylenol can lead to kidney trouble.

Once your girlfriend sees a doctor, and the fibroids are confirmed, the doctor can test her liver enzymes to make sure she's not harboring a chronic liver infection and is in the clear for taking Tylenol.

Also, please encourage your girlfriend to be wary of a pelvic pirate who wants to rip out her uterus at age thirty because of fibroids. Surgery (a myomectomy) is now available that removes only the fibroids. In this day and age, fibroids do not mean an automatic hysterectomy. Plus, there are medications that will shrink fibroids specifically, but they are most often prescribed for women who are getting close to menopause.

Finally, the newest treatment is a nonsurgical method called uterine fibroid embolization, which chokes off the blood supply to fibroids. She should talk to a specialist.

Q: I had a hysterectomy to remove fibroids about two years ago, and I haven't been the same since. The doctor did not take out my ovaries, because I was thirty-nine at the time, but right after the operation, I went into menopause anyway.

My doctor talked me out of a myomectomy because of the risk that the fibroids would grow back. Was he right about this? I am filled with regret.

A: Doctors can be a little too quick to do hysterectomies, and while most women are satisfied when the surgery relieves their health problems, your story is an important one for women to hear.

Early menopause following a partial hysterectomy—one that leaves the ovaries behind—is suspicious. It may be that the arteries from the uterus to the ovaries were damaged, and needed hormonal signals are impinged. We don't yet know enough about those connections.

Since your uterus was removed, I'm assuming that evidence of fibroids was found, but I want other women to be aware that before undergoing a hysterectomy, they should have a definite diagnosis and should know all the treatment options.

Fibroids are benign uterine growths that sometimes cause symptoms and sometimes don't. You would be amazed at the number of women who are surprised when the doctor finds fibroids during an exam. You'd also be amazed at the number of doctors who blame a woman's symptoms on fibroids when the cause of the symptoms is something else.

Cramping and heavy bleeding are symptoms of fibroids, but they are symptoms of other problems, too. Fibroids can be treated with hormones, but they do grow back if the hormone therapy ends.

A myomectomy is a procedure that removes only the fibroids. Women who choose a myomectomy can then wait to see if the fibroids return. Sometimes they do, sometimes they don't.

I encourage anyone struggling with a treatment decision (see options in previous question) to get several opinions and to always consider the source of the opinion. Gynecologists are surgeons, and surgeons tend to come up with surgical solutions: they cut.

Breast-feeding

Q: The nipple piercings I got a few years ago did not heal well. I had scabs that wouldn't go away, and I was in constant discomfort, so I removed the jewelry. In the future, when I have a baby, will I be able to breast-feed?

A: Breast milk comes out of the many separate ducts that are in the area of the nipple. Breast-feeding women will tell you that separate little droplets of milk come out all over their nipples.

So, if piercing knocks out some of the ducts, a woman has ducts to spare. However, extensive scarring could block a large number of ducts and impact breast-feeding.

Most women with pierced nipples are able to breast-feed. You won't know until you try.

Q: I had a baby boy last month, and I am breast-feeding. How long after birth does the cervix close enough so that I can safely have intercourse? My obstetrician says three weeks. Do you agree? I'm waiting for the green light.

A: If you had had any birth complications, like a tear, your doctor would tell you to wait. But since your doctor already gave you the green light, I will, too. The general advice is to wait three weeks to a month.

Very often, guys are the ones asking me this question, and I let them know that their partner should not be pressured into having sex before she's ready. Well, you sound ready. Do go easy this first time, though, because your body might be a little bit different.

Most breast-feeding moms have fairly depressed libido, and we think this might be nature's way of spacing pregnancies.

Q: I am breast-feeding. Can I continue to take Prozac? My psychiatrist is concerned about me going off my medication at this point in my life.

A: Most likely, yes, according to one study published in *The American Jour-*

nal of Psychiatry. The focus was sixteen nursing infants whose mothers were taking Paxil, and the serum levels of Paxil in breast milk were found to be below a detectable level; no adverse side effects were noticed.

Prozac is fluoxetine, and this molecule is very similar to Paxil's molecule, paroxetine. I think that what's OK for one would be OK for the other.

However, I don't know all the details about you that your doctor knows— your history, your general health, what your diet is like, or what other drugs you take. You should ask your obstetrician to talk to your psychiatrist and see if they are in agreement about this question.

The Parents Network at the University of California in Berkeley recommends calling the Lactation Institute of UC San Diego or UC San Francisco's pharmacy schools with questions about breast-feeding and medication. Universities in other states are also likely to be good resources.

See the question about antidepressants and pregnancy on page 163 for more information on this topic. We don't test drugs on pregnant or breast-feeding women, so once a drug has been approved for the general population, we have to cautiously, gradually, extend our knowledge of its effects on these other, more vulnerable, populations.

Q: I am a nursing mother who is in the middle of an oral herpes outbreak. What can I do to get rid of it, and how can I avoid putting my sweet, seven-month-old daughter at risk?

When I'm not pregnant or nursing, I load up on Zovirax at the beginning of an outbreak. That seems to tone it down. I tried the acyclovir cream, and it didn't do a darn thing.

A: The dab-on cream called Zylactin might work by coating the sore, but creams aren't going to have the effects of a systemic drug like Zovirax, which directly attacks virus growth. And I'm not sure how much Zovirax actually ends up in the breast milk.

Don't go out of your way to smear your baby with wet kisses, but herpes is everywhere; and I don't think you can really do much to protect her from it in the outside world. You are not too likely to pass herpes to her, but if you did, it wouldn't be horrendous.

Newborns can be seriously harmed by in utero herpes. But at seven months, your daughter has had exposure to a lot of things. You don't sterilize your nipples, and she's picking up germs there. I wouldn't sweat it.

Most of us have the herpes virus in our systems. Some people acquire it at a young age, but the older the population, the higher the percentage of folks who have contracted the herpes cold-sore virus, which is almost identical to the sexually transmitted one.

Q: I am breast-feeding my three-month-old baby, but I've had a dairy allergy my entire life. Dairy causes me to make a lot of mucus and get a postnasal drip. Do I need more calcium to pass along to my baby?

A: First, let's talk about dairy allergies, and then about calcium.

Very often people mistake reactions to foods for actual allergies. Dairy, in particular, is unfairly blamed. Back in the sixties, the Mucusless Diet Healing System, a fad from early in the century, was resurrected and became all the rage based on the idea that milk causes mucus, sinus infections, and runny noses. Well, when we finally tested the idea, it turned out to be false.

This is not to deny that some people are truly allergic or even lactose intolerant, but even some of those folks can eat something like yogurt and do fine.

So, I want you to see a good allergist, to find out if you are indeed allergic to dairy.

Now, about your calcium questions: Vegans, who don't consume any animal products whatsoever, are able to get adequate calcium, so you can, too. Dairy is not the only source of calcium. It is also found in leafy green vegetables.

If you are deficient in some minerals, your body actually becomes more efficient at absorbing them. In other words, you usually absorb a tiny, single-digit percentage of iron from your food, but if you're iron deficient, your body holds on to more of the iron. The same is true with calcium.

Just be sure to eat a lot of leafy green vegetables, and take a cheap calcium supplement, like Tums.

Your breast milk is fine. Your body makes sure that your baby is getting enough calcium. Even if you were totally depleted of calcium, your body would pull it from the calcium stores in your bones to get it to your baby.

Q: My five-month-old son already has his two bottom teeth, and he bites a lot when I nurse him. What can I do, because this is getting really painful?

A: The two of you will work this out through give and take. On your son's part, stimulus and response will teach him. He will find that when he bites, Mom goes "No!" and pulls away. He'll figure out that biting isn't getting him what he wants.

Your adjustment will be that your nipples will toughen. When women first start to nurse, they are shocked by how hard those little suckers can pull. Over time, especially when babies get teeth, the tenderness lessens.

A lactation consultant can tell you how to treat your breasts between feedings. The consultant can teach you exercises to toughen your nipples and tell you about salves to soothe and heal them.

La Leche League and lactation consultants are underutilized; they are the folks who know. Doctors aren't taught anything in medical school about breast-feeding, and most pediatricians answer questions about it by the seat of their pants. Anything I know, I learned from being a father and from reading.

Hang in there. Your baby will lighten up eventually.

For a related question, see page 233 in chapter 5.

PMS, PMDD, and Menstruation

Q: I'm looking at an ad for Sarafem, which is marketed to women with PMDD—premenstrual dysphoric disorder. The ad says Sarafem's active ingredients are the same ingredients that are in Prozac. Is this true?

A: PMDD is PMS with a new name, and Sarafem is Prozac with a new name. "Fem" is for "female," of course. Are you confused yet?

For severe cases of menstrual dysphoria, double-blind studies have shown the Prozac molecule can offer relief. However, I assume that in order to sell the drug for other symptoms, and to disassociate it from depression, the drug companies felt they needed a snappy new name for the same product.

For women with severe PMS, for whom everything else has failed, I think Sarafem is worth a try. If it causes problems, or if it doesn't work, women can just stop taking it. But I'd much rather see women try other solutions first— exercise, a low-fat diet, fish oil and vitamins, herbs, therapy. Anything safe is worth a try.

For treating depression, anxiety, and compulsive disorders, people take selective serotonin reuptake inhibitors (SSRIs) like Prozac for years and years. For PMS the use is intermittent. So it's a much more benign therapy.

What I would hate to see develop is what happened with Viagra. The drug company made a promise to market only to people who needed Viagra for impotence, but they ended up pushing it to everyone. Now it's a recreational drug.

I don't want that to happen with Sarafem. This is for women who really

DID YOU KNOW?
DOES THAT PANTY LINER "BREATHE"?

A recent study found that women who use panty shields are doing their vulvas a favor if they buy a style that comes with a "breathable" back sheet. If the panty liner isn't permeable, the microclimate of the vulva becomes warmer and humidity goes up. The more air your vulva gets, the cooler it stays.

---

have problems and have exhausted all other resources. To me, the world will not be a better place if every woman with PMS/PMD pops pills every month.

Q: My fifteen-year-old daughter gets periods that are so severe she has to miss school once a month. Ibuprofen doesn't help her and neither does her swimming. I'm not comfortable putting her on birth control pills, because I don't want her to take hormones at such a young age.

Her doctor has two recommendations: Tylenol with codeine, or gin. He actually told me to make her a gin and tonic. I had to laugh. He laughed, too, but he said gin works for some women. Can you give me a better option?

A: Gin, as in Tanqueray? Well, I agree with you, I don't think it's appropriate to send a kid to school reeking of gin.

Ibuprofen can be prescribed in much higher doses than the over-thecounter version. Ibuprofen is a nonsteroidal anti-inflammatory drug (NSAID), and this class of drugs is linked to the chemical cause of painful periods. NSAIDs are often fabulously effective.

Swimming may not be the right exercise to relieve this kind of pain. We think that the effect of exercise on body-fat metabolism is linked to its success in reducing menstrual pain. A swimmer's body may hold on to fat. A swimmer will have a higher amount of body fat than will a runner who does the same amount of exercise. It seems that the cold water signals the body to retain its padding.

So a different exercise might afford your daughter some relief. In fact, extreme exercise has been known to stop a woman's periods altogether, which is certainly another way to eliminate pain for a while.

Looking down the road, these terrible periods sometimes disappear with a first pregnancy.

Discuss your concerns about hormones with her doctor. Along with your concerns about her health, you may also be afraid that putting your daughter on the Pill implies permission for her to be sexually active. That's understandable. Once you have all the information, I suggest you have a heart-to-heart talk with her.

Birth control pills do work, though, and the doctor does not have to identify it as a birth control pill. He can just say, "Here's your prescription. Take one a day." They really can relieve difficult periods, and he may have some information that will reassure you about their safety.

By the way, many doctors now offer women a break for several months from the inconvenience of having periods. It's very simple to do with birth control–like medications that are taken every day. Some women are doing this simply to reduce the hassle in their lives, others to avoid the pain that comes with their period, and, finally, for some the reason is a one-time special occasion, such as a wedding or honeymoon.

I do wonder what the consequences would be to a woman's health if she were to take hormones to stop her periods for years and years. We have not tested the effects of this on a large group of women over a long period of time. That kind of research is absolutely necessary before we have tons of women flocking to their doctors for hormones. So far, though, it seems safe. And I have a feeling that if guys had periods, this would be routine.

Seriously, though, a major claim that medicine can improve on the design of the human body requires major proof.

Pap Smears and Exam Procedures

Q: I have some questions about Pap smears. Is it normal for the doctor to insert his fingers to determine speculum size? Should another woman be present during the examination if the doctor is male? Should a gown be worn during the examination? Also, is a breast examination necessary for a twenty-one-year-old?

A: Your questions sound like you think the doctor's behavior was suspicious. Of course, I can't know for sure, so this is something you'll need to decide.

Normally, a doctor does not insert a finger during a Pap smear, because the lubricant that he should put on his finger can alter the cells and the result of the Pap smear.

So, in general, we use the speculum first, do the Pap smear, and then do the internal examination, using a finger in both the vagina and, often, the rectum.

The one exception to usage of a finger prior to the Pap smear would occur if the doctor was concerned about the presence of a hymen in a virgin.

As for having another person present during an internal examination, it's good practice and quite routine these days, especially if the gynecologist is a male. Most doctors want someone there, just to protect themselves.

Yes, a gown should be worn in an exam. No one should be made to lie naked on a table during a gynecological examination.

Deciding if a breast examination is appropriate for a twenty-one-year-old is a tough one. Breast cancer is extraordinarily rare in someone your age, yet patients accuse doctors of not doing thorough exams, so some doctors may include breast exams with all physicals.

Obviously, you have some doubts about the practices of your doctor. If my answers add to your concern, find another physician. And you may be more comfortable with a woman doctor.

Q: After my annual Pap smear, I received a note in the mail saying I have "reactive cells." The note adds that the cells are not cancerous, but that the doctor wants to see me in three months. What are reactive cells?

QUIZ

Which element in their food are some postmenopausal women less likely to perceive?

A) salt   B) spiciness   C) bitterness   D) sucrose
E) all of the above

(D: sucrose; this change in taste perception was reported in a recent study in the British Dental Journal. Obviously, one possible result is an increase in a woman's preference for sweeter foods.)

A: I know those notes cause concern, but you don't have anything to worry about.

Reactive cells imply an irritation on the cells, like an infection or inflammation. We used to call these "precancerous cells," which is a horrible name—"You don't have cancer, you just have precancer."—"Oh, thank you, doctor."

These are not precancerous cells, but some early studies did find that among a thousand women with reactive cells, there was ultimately a slightly higher rate of cancer. However, more recently I saw a study in an obstetrics journal that found that women with reactive cells are no more likely to have cancer than women with regular cells.

We just play it safe. So, check back with the doctor in three months, and make sure you continue to get your Pap smears regularly and as recommended.

Q: After a recent Pap smear, I received a card from my doctor asking me to call to schedule a colposcopy. When I called, I asked the nurse if she could tell me what a colposcopy is. She said, "No."

So, I asked for the doctor to call me, and she said he wouldn't need to, because I would be coming in anyway. Should I get a new doctor?

A: No, but call the nurse back and tell her you won't come in until either she or the doctor tells you what a colposcopy is. It isn't anything to worry about, but it is a reasonable request to want to know about a procedure you are about to have.

Your Pap smear probably shows a slight abnormality. A colposcopy is an examination of the cervix with a tool called a colposcope that shows the surface of the cervix in high magnification. It's a microscope. The doctor also might take a biopsy of the cells of your cervix.

Q: My mother is ninety-three years old and healthy. She had a hysterectomy well over forty-five years ago, yet when she saw her doctor to get her cholesterol level and heart checked, he gave her a Pap smear and a mammogram. Does a ninety-three-year-old woman, especially one who's had a hysterectomy, need these tests? She was really traumatized.

A: I tend to agree with you that your mother doesn't need these tests, but not all doctors would agree.

The argument for doing Pap smears on younger, post-hysterectomy women is that although they have no cervix—it was removed with the uterus—they can contract cervical cancer, because often a little bit of cervical tissue can remain. The incidence is very low, though, and it's unlikely that a woman your mother's age is at risk.

The research on breast cancer rates extends only to the sixty- to seventy-year-old age group, so I don't have data. It's possible her doctor feels that if she did have a breast lump, he is morally and legally responsible to find out and to treat her. If he found and removed a malignancy, she might live to be a hundred and three.

It seems to me that communication between your mother and her doctor is amiss. She has every right to refuse tests and treatment that she doesn't want, especially tests that traumatize her. Talk to the doctor about it.

Menopause and Estrogen

Q: **I'm a very active sixty-five-year-old woman. I was on hormone replacement therapy for sixteen years, because my mom had osteoporosis and breast cancer, and I have had thinning bones. When all the bad news started coming out about the dangers of HRT, my doctor stopped that treatment, and now he's suggesting I take a selective estrogen receptor modulator—specifically, Raloxifene. What do you think of this advice? And, by the way, my bones have thickened.**

A: Your doctor is suggesting what is called the "new estrogen" or "designer estrogen." As you noted, Raloxifene is a SERM (selective estrogen receptor modulator), and it's the first one approved by the FDA.

You are not in a situation that allows for easy answers. We don't know for sure, in terms of large, long-term studies on healthy women, but it seems to make sense.

If you are headed for an estrogen-sensitive breast cancer, it may help reduce your risks, but we don't know if you are headed for breast cancer. Having a mother with the disease increases your risks, but not to a huge amount. I think you'd probably be surprised if you looked at the real numbers.

What we don't know, because you're a healthy woman right now, is if we give you these drugs, will they prevent breast cancer or the thinning of your bones? There is literature to suggest that we can reduce the risk for thin bones and breast cancer in the shorter term with these substances (early research shows Raloxifene produced about a 2-percent increase in bone mass after two years of use), but possibly increase the risk for cancers in the long run.

We are awaiting the results of long-term studies, and we may be unpleasantly surprised, as we were when the long-term studies came in on hormone replacement therapy.

I don't see grave harm in taking the drug, but, to be smart, you might want to talk to a medical geneticist and find out exactly what your risk is for breast cancer.

At your age, I think you'd be blown away at how low it is. Because you have reached the age of sixty-five you have lived through years when many women have gotten breast cancer. So your risk is a lot lower in that regard.

Q: A book I read on menopause recommended natural progesterone for both the symptoms of menopause and osteoporosis. Do you think this is a good idea?

A: I make no distinction between natural progesterone and regular progesterone; progesterone is progesterone, and, as you know, we are going through a very questioning period right now about the use of any hormones in menopause. Why be a guinea pig?

The two main hormones in a woman's body are estrogen and progesterone, and they work in tandem to enable fertility and ovulation. Before the big brouhaha over hormone replacement therapy (HRT) during menopause, we were giving women both estrogen and progesterone because we found that estrogen alone could cause uterine cancer.

The addition of progesterone did not help with the side effects we now see with HRT, and neither hormone is now recommended routinely for menopause. Talk to your doctor about whatever symptoms of menopause are troubling you,

DID YOU KNOW?
RELIEF FOR THE HEAT

Paxil has joined the list of antidepressants that are showing good results among postmenopausal women suffering from hot flashes. Since Paxil can reduce depression and anxiety—which also can come with menopause—it is sure to have its believers. Prozac and Effexor have done well in studies, too.

The Edell Report
Breast Milk but No Baby?

This may sound strange, but a common question on my program comes from women who are lactating but shouldn't be. Often, they have galactorrhea.

This happens in approximately 20 to 25 percent of women—and men can have it, too. The list of possible causes is staggering, but what is most astonishing is that 20 percent of the galactorrhea cases may be caused by medications and herbs, according to a report in American Family Physician. *Everything from anise and fennel to Valium-like drugs and blood pressure medicines can produce a milky breast discharge.*

Other causes include hypothyroidism, pituitary growths, neurologic disorders, breast stimulation, nicotine, poorly fitting sports bras, and illicit drugs like marijuana, amphetamines, benzodiazepines, and opiates.

You need to get an explanation for any breast discharge. It is rarely breast cancer, but that is a possibility you don't want to ignore.

because there are alternatives for treating hot flashes, vaginal dryness, and osteoporosis.

Miscellaneous

Q: No matter which vaginal deodorant I use—Summer's Eve, feminine deodorant spray, or regular baby powder—it doesn't prevent wetness. I occasionally have discharge. How can I control this?

A: Stop using all those products. They are not deodorants, they do not stop wetness, and talcum powder has been linked to ovarian cancer.

Your genitals should not be absolutely dry. Vaginal discharge is normal, unless its source is an infection. At this point, those products may have given you an infection. Please, stop using them and make an appointment with a gynecologist if you haven't seen one recently. He or she can explain what is normal for a discharge and check for any infections, of course.

Q: I have had three children and I now have problems with both urinary and fecal incontinence. What can you tell me about it?

A: Kegel exercises are the best treatment for urinary stress incontinence, the type where laughing, sneezing, and bending cause you to lose urine. This is a risk that comes with vaginal deliveries, and it can be a real nuisance.

If you do Kegels correctly, they are very effective at strengthening the muscles that constrict the flow of urine. Contracting those muscles also will contract the rectal muscles, so Kegels will help you strengthen both areas. You can feel the pressure the exercise exerts on the muscles by inserting your finger into your vagina, or you can buy a device that you can insert to help you feel the physical effects of your efforts.

DID YOU KNOW?
WHEN THE VULVA BURNS

Women who have chronic vulva pain—burning, soreness, stinging— that hasn't been linked to a disease or infection should ask their doctor to do tests for vulvodynia, which is also called vulvar dysethesia. The diagnosis is controversial, and it's not simple to reach. First, it requires ruling out many other possible causes of the pain, from undiagnosed yeast infections to a variety of diseases. And treatment isn't straightforward either, but it is possible to improve the condition with antidepressants, lidocaine jelly or ointment, pelvic floor exercises, and sex therapy. And sometimes doctors recommend surgical removal of parts of the labia. If it seems your doctor doesn't believe your symptoms are real, find a gynecologist who is up to date on this topic.

Once you get the hang of it, this is an easy exercise that can be done anywhere, anytime, because no one can see what you are doing.

To identify the right muscle, start by urinating in the toilet, then force yourself to stop in midstream. The muscle that stops the urinating is the one you want to work on. With Kegels, you squeeze for five seconds, then relax them for five seconds. Do this twelve times, repeating the process at least eight times a day.

Just as any other muscle is strengthened by regular exercise, you've got to do your Kegels regularly to get results.

Aside from the exercises, an array of options like pills, injections, and operations is available. A urologist who specializes in female urinary incontinence is the best person to advise you on treatment.

Fecal incontinence is a little more complicated, and I recommend that you seek care from a gastroenterologist or a colorectal surgeon.

Fortunately, incontinence is now out of the closet, and there is tons of information on the Internet.

Resource List

For free publications, organization referrals and general advice on everything from eating disorders to breast-feeding, call 1-800-994-WOMAN (9662) or go to the Web site for The National Women's Health Information Center: *www.4woman.gov*

For information and to order health packets on a variety of topics, visit the National Women's Health Network: *www.womenshealthnetwork.org*

The North American Menopause Society provides the Menopause Guidebook online in English or Spanish: *www.menopause.org/consumers/index.html*

For pamphlets on a variety of topics, go to the Web site of the American College of Obstetricians and Gynecologists: *www.acog.com*

For the Centers for Disease Control Reproductive Health Information Source, go to *www.cdc.gov,* click on "Health Topics A-Z," and scroll down to "Reproductive Health."

For more information about toxemia, pregnancy-induced hypertension, preeclampsia, or HELLP syndrome, see the Web site for the Preeclampsia Foundation: *www.preeclampsia.org/*

The Center for Young Women's Health Web site (from Children's Hospital in Boston) is designed for girls and women ages 12 to 22. Easy-to-understand information is available on everything from birth control to scoliosis: *www.youngwomenshealth.org*

For facts about various causes of birth defects, go to the Organization for Teratology Information Services: *www.otispregnancy.org*

La Leche League International has everything you need to know about breast-feeding: *www.lalecheleague.org/*

The Web site for the FDA's Office of Women's Health will help you learn more about the impact of various prescription drugs during pregnancy, and you may be eligible to participate in a Pregnancy Registry: *www.fda.gov/womens/registries/*

For fibroid informational brochures and research updates see the National Uterine Fibroids Foundation's Web site: *www.nuff.org/*

For both wacky and substantial information on everything from the perils of douching to the Tampon Safety and Research Act of 1999, go to the Museum of Menstruation and Women's Health: *www.mum.org.*

Information on all fertility-related issues is available at the InterNational Council on Infertility Information Dissemination: *www.inciid.org/*

For information on Down syndrome studies and news, go to the Web site for the National Down Syndrome Society: *www.ndss.org.* Another site, *www.ds-health.com,* was created by pediatrician Len Leshen, who has a DS child.

For detailed information about emergency contraception in English, Spanish, French, or Arabic, go to the Emergency Contraception Web site, *www.not-2-late.com,* or for access to emergency birth control, call Planned Parenthood at 1-800-230-PLAN or go to *www.plannedparenthood.org/ec/*

Subscribe to e-mail bone health updates at the National Osteoporosis Foundation website: *www.nof.org*

For related questions and answers also see chapters 1, 2, 3, 6, 7, 8, and 10.

Chapter 5

Smart Medicine
for Your Children

My mother was a worrier. I spent my life as a kid asking her, "Mom, why do you worry so much? I'm OK." Well, after raising five sons—and answering thousands of questions from worried parents—I know how she came to be that way.

The undeniable fact is, once you have children, the worry never really ends. As I write this, our eight kids range in age from seventeen to thirty-five, and, in any given week, there is something going on in their lives that causes me concern, even anguish: a job change, a new relationship, something as small as a cold. The issues can vary dramatically in scope, but it is natural that we will worry—both mothers and fathers.

However, there's some scientific evidence that women worry more than men, and the questions I get tell me that, too. I am also concerned that many parents have become almost obsessive about their children. Worry is good; trying to protect your child every second of the day is impossible and can have negative consequences, and parents need to tackle that head-on.

Too many parents in our society are seeking perfection, and this is a problem, because there is no such thing. Those who seek perfection—in themselves or their children—are doomed to disappointment. Every child can't go to Harvard or Stanford, very few children always make the right decisions, and the student with a constant string of straight As isn't necessarily going to be the most successful—or the happiest—adult. But I'm amazed how many parents haven't yet figured this out.

I'm not saying it's a bad thing to care about our children's welfare or potential for success, and we should want to do what's right for them. But that's not always easy or clear; there are many forces that have an impact, from the behavior of other kids and their parents to the marketing messages our families face every day. Plus, there are people who will take advantage of our worry, who want to capitalize on our expectations. It's enough to make a parent crazy.

I think that the biggest problem in America today is that we take way too much for granted. And curiously, it seems that even though we are much more informed about a multitude of subjects than our parents were, we oftentimes seem less confident.

How else do we explain the fact that so many of us try to plan every single minute of our children's lives practically from the time they are toddlers? That so many of us just assume that our child is the blameless one when there are disagreements among kids? That our child needs Ritalin? That the teacher is the enemy? And how to explain the rush to the doctor for *every little thing?*

Yet, some folks are playing with fire when it comes to major diseases. My mother wouldn't let me go out and play when I was a kid, because of the fear of poliomyelitis. That was a big scare, and I can understand her reaction. But somewhere along the way, many parents forgot about the devastating effects of diseases that we vaccinate our children against today, and have joined the bandwagon against basic vaccinations. How many of you have seen a case of whooping cough or polio? Do you really want to risk having that reintroduced to the population? Every child in the United States should be vaccinated, and every health insurance program should cover the cost.

Americans are inconsistent about their children's welfare in other ways, too. I frequently come across moms feeding their kids organic vegetables and running to the health food store to buy expensive "natural" supplements for their children. Yet some of these women, by choice, did not breast-feed them, a nurturing act that is so important, so positive, and so simple. Our dismal breast-feeding rates astound me.

I have strong feelings about many national issues about children, some of which you may disagree with. We prescribe way too many psychotropic drugs for our children. The use of Ritalin is out of control. I also think circumcising newborn males is barbaric and medically unnecessary. We need to reduce the number of abortions without bringing the government into the private lives of women, and I think our drug laws are aggravating the issue of teenage drug abuse.

Some of the most serious problems our children face have to do with our educational system. We must make school reform our highest priority in every community. Education has been found to reduce social problems and drug abuse, and it improves the health of all individuals who have access to it. It is the most profound antidote we have to many of our childhood, teenage, and adult ailments, psychological and physical. Yet most teachers continue to face oversized classes with inadequate supplies and little support from parents.

Raising kids to be both psychologically and socially healthy is no picnic, as every generation of parents deals with a different set of issues. Where my parents struggled with such things as long hair and drugs, today's parents of teens struggle with tattoos and piercings—and drugs. It's a delicate balance. You cannot completely control your children. They have to grow up and learn to be individuals. By the same token, you don't want to be so loose as a parent that you allow them to fall into any number of traps waiting to snare them.

Your pediatrician is an important asset, and communication with that doctor is important. He or she is your resource for good, objective information about your children. While all adults have the right to explore whatever beliefs they choose to, I implore parents not to inflict extreme beliefs on their children. The panoply of unusual medical and spiritual beliefs can harm children, and adults who suspect children are at risk have a responsibility to report it.

Few would argue that these are stressful times—in the United States and in the world. But many parents lose sight of the fact that if they are stressed, their children are likely to be stressed, too, no matter how much a parent may try to conceal that. Parents who can relax around their kids, who know when to stop what they're doing and share an unplanned moment, and who will make every effort to talk to their children and laugh with them, will see the results for years to come. It's a relatively small investment with huge potential for returns.

Babies and Toddlers: Big Worries and Everyday Problems

Q: My two-year-old has recurrent ear infections, so his doctor is recommending that he get tubes. At the moment, my son is on prophylactic antibiotics, but he has an infection anyway. He always recovers just fine, but could recurrent infections cause a hearing loss? I remember having a lot of ear infections as a child, and I seemed to outgrow them. I have read that it's kind of iffy whether the tubes really work. Everyone tells me, "Go ahead, it's done all the time," but that doesn't mean it's the best thing, right?

A: Yes, it's done all the time, but this may turn out to be as overused as the tonsillectomy once was. You are right to be skeptical.

We're not even sure that the prophylactic antibiotics help much, and yes, almost all kids do outgrow the infections. Sometimes you just have to wait them out. It's similar to having a fibroid that you wait out until menopause.

However, giving specific advice on this is very difficult. The general guideline is to insert the tubes if the child frequently can't participate in the normal activities for his age, if infection is extending to other parts of his body, or if he is in danger of a hearing loss.

Hearing loss occurs in only a very small percentage of cases. Infections were much more dangerous in the old days, when they could spread to adjacent skull bones. Nowadays, that seldom happens, because of the effectiveness of antibiotics.

I would not tell you to ignore your doctor's advice, but if you bring up your reluctance, he is likely to back off, because he knows that this is a no-man's-land.

The tubes work by draining the ear. If you decide to do it, don't worry. It is a very common surgery, and eventually the tubes fall out and the holes heal up.

For more resources in books and online, see pages 263 and 264.

Q: I have a thirteen-month-old who, for the past three weeks, has had three- or four-day bouts of fever spikes up to 102 or 103 degrees. I can barely control them, and I'm scared. We've been to the pediatrician several times, and the doctor is finding nothing wrong with her. What would you do now?

A: In the med school pediatrics course, students probably spend more time on this than anything else. Once the flu and other common childhood infections are ruled out, doctors go down a long list of things.

The Edell Report
How Will This Medicine Affect My Child?

I don't know why some people get stupid about their kids when it comes to over-the-counter medications, but they do.

The current child-testing legislation has had a limited impact on pharmaceutical companies, so only 25 percent of drugs on the market today are tested on and labeled for children. And some parents don't seem to pay attention to any labels, even those with child-based information on them.

One drug alone—acetaminophen, the primary ingredient in Tylenol and many other over-the-counter medications—is linked to about twenty-seven thousand accidental childhood overdoses a year, some of them fatal. Because of that, an FDA panel has recommended improved labeling for any products with acetaminophen, and the Pediatric Research Equity Act was expected to be signed into law by the end of 2003. This requires pediatric-specific testing of certain drugs by manufacturers.

So, no matter what you are giving your child, read the fine print carefully and, when in doubt, ask questions. Never assume you know what the appropriate dosage is. It can vary from year to year in a child's development.

Eventually you can get into territory called "fever of unknown origin"—FUO—or fever without source. And under this heading, we have another long list of conditions that will eventually answer the question about the origin of a fever. It's a matter of being logical—and patient.

For example, if it's not an upper-respiratory bug, it may be an ear infection. And if it's not that, it could be a urinary tract infection. And if it's not that, it could be a . . . and we go right down the list. In my experience, your daughter's illness is unlikely to be something serious.

You should know that there is ongoing debate in the medical community about how to approach FUO in young children, with physicians divided about the appropriate amount of testing and treatment. In part, that's because fever is quite common in children between three months and three years. Many parents of young children find this hard to believe, but a temperature of 103 is not actually that difficult for a kid. A temperature of 103 degrees would knock down you or me, but kids can do pretty well at that point.

Many parents do overreact to fever, but I'm not telling you that you shouldn't take your daughter to the doctor. When is the fever so high that your child should see the pediatrician? If it's a fever of 101, a child can have it for a couple of days before you go to the doctor. If it's a fever of 105, the child must see a doctor right away. Remember, fever itself is usually not dangerous, but the underlying cause may be.

The most important thing to look at is: How is your child doing? If she has become lethargic or if there has been any change of consciousness with the fever, of course you rush to the hospital. In fact, you don't want to let it get to that point. You do need to pursue the source of these recurring fevers, and I would press the doctor on what step he or she wants to take next. I just know that it will be something that afterward will make you say, "Is that all it was?"

In the meantime, make sure to give your daughter fluids, because the body loses more water when it has a fever, and dehydration can be dangerous.

Q: A TV newsmagazine recently reported that infants who are constantly held and who sleep in the same bed with their parents turn out to be very well adjusted.

Everywhere I go, I see parents lugging their infants around in car seats like sacks of potatoes. I never see them pick the kid up out of the seat. What is your opinion on this type of physical relationship?

A: I share your concern about the babies I see living in little boxes and other "containers." They get carried to the car in plastic boxes, put into plastic car seats and set on tables, in boxes, as if they were paperweights. When they aren't in little plastic playpens, they're hanging from door frames. Taken altogether, that just doesn't feel right.

However, before we go any further on this subject, let's not throw out all baby seats with the bathwater. Car seats are lifesavers, and no child should be in a car without one. One of the most dangerous places a child can be in a car is on someone's lap. And a child, even in a car seat, should never be in the front seat.

As to your question, there have been lots of experiments on babies and touching, and, not surprisingly, children respond to touching just the way most of us do. Premature babies in a hospital who are held and cuddled, for example, cry less and are calmer than the babies who aren't held, and leave the hospital sooner. Other studies have advised that a crying baby can be calmed just by being in a pack on your body, even if all you are doing is cleaning the kitchen. The contact alone seems to be helpful.

The power of touching plays out among all the animals that we have tested. A wise professor of mine was part of one of the classic research projects on rats. The researchers were injecting rats with a hormone to study its effect. At some point they realized that the reactions they observed were not the rats' responses to the hormone, but to being picked up and held for the shot. As a control, they picked up some rats without injecting them and that group had the same response as the group that was getting the hormone.

When it comes to sleeping, there is some controversy. In many cultures it is routine for babies to sleep with their parents. Yet some studies show a risk to the baby. You can injure a baby if you roll onto him or her, and they can be smothered. Other studies have found these are rare occurrences. I think wanting to be close to one's baby is a natural response. Just look at primates sitting around, holding their babies, sleeping with their babies. It is not a surprise that some parents want to do that, too.

Q: Can my three-year-old use a nasal spray? He often wakes up with mild congestion. Should I just let it take its course? Usually, by late morning, most of his stuffiness is gone.

DID YOU KNOW?
WATCH THAT SIPPY CUP

It may be incredibly convenient; it may be your child's favorite possession. But beware: The plastic-lidded cup that parents everywhere depend on for their child's comfort and relaxation could be harming speech patterns and encouraging cavities. However, before you create chaos in your household, ask your pediatrician what he or she thinks about this topic. That's because not all experts agree just how bad sippy cups can be, according to a story in *The Wall Street Journal*.

A: I think this is a borderline situation. While I have no problem with the occasional use of nasal spray by kids, it is not generally recommended, simply because the use of nasal sprays can quickly lead to dependence, and there is some absorption into the bloodstream; it varies by the medication. Waking up with mild congestion is fairly normal; when you lie down flat, fluids in the body are distributed in such a way that the fluid pressure in your feet is the same as it is in your nose. Since your nose is very delicate, it swells when this happens. When you stand up, gravity slowly drains that fluid, and the night-time nasal swelling goes away.

I'd let your son's stuffiness go away on its own, though you can try a simple saline spray, available at most drugstores. This is nothing more than a salt-and-water mixture and it can be very effective for both kids and adults dealing with congestion. If the congestion becomes an all-day occurrence, allergies may be the cause, and they would require a very specific type of inhaler or nasal spray. Your pediatrician may handle this, or you might be directed to a specialist.

Q: Our family takes an annual outing to Yosemite National Park. This year my granddaughter will be eight months old when we go. Our destination is Tuolumne Meadows, which is at 8,600 feet. My daughter-in-law, who is a physician, seems hesitant to take the baby to that altitude. I heard that a baby got seriously ill at 16,000 feet. How high is too high?

A: At higher altitudes, many of us initially can have nausea and headaches, but I don't think 8,600 feet is high enough to cause any problems for the baby. The air in airplane cabins varies, but it's equivalent to something you would find

---

QUIZ

How much does a newborn have to weigh to be classified officially as "low birth weight"?

A) 3.5 pounds   B) 4.5 pounds   C) 5 pounds

D) 5.5 pounds

(D: about 5.5 pounds—or less than 2,500 grams; the number of low-birth-weight babies born in the United States is on the rise, because so many women are having twins and triplets.)

at 5,000 to 8,000 feet outdoors, and we certainly don't banish babies from airplanes. So, breathing air at another 600 feet of altitude shouldn't be a big deal.

In some parts of the world, people routinely live at 16,000 feet, but they are acclimated. The situation you heard about could happen if a baby was suddenly brought to that altitude. Sports docs warn adults that exerting themselves above 10,000 feet, depending on their physical condition, can bring on altitude sickness. The body has to adapt to high altitudes by making more red blood cells to carry more oxygen. That takes time. You and I would die within a few minutes if somebody dropped us on top of Mount Everest.

Climbers can survive at the summit, because they carry oxygen. Some make it without oxygen, but only if they take the time to acclimate at a base camp, they are in extraordinary condition, and they are genetically predisposed to handle this. At extreme heights, besides altitude sickness, a rapid heart rate and increased respiration stress the body to compensate for the lack of oxygen.

Again, I wouldn't worry about 8,600 feet, though I wouldn't make this into a family dispute. If your daughter-in-law feels very strongly about this, back off. Tuolumne Meadows is one of the most beautiful places on earth, so I'm sure you will want to visit it again when your granddaughter is old enough to remember the trip.

Q: My three-year-old is obsessed with his penis. He constantly pulls his pants down and touches himself. I've told him that this is inappropriate to do in public and that he should go to his bedroom or to the bathroom if he has to touch himself. So, he is in his room a lot, "playing the privates game," as he calls it. Is this OK?

A: "Playing the privates game." That's cute.

You did exactly the right thing. You say, "We don't do this in public," and send him to his room. Don't make a big deal about it, because if you do, he will do more of it. In time, his fascination will disappear—for a while. Since he's a guy, it will probably reappear in a decade or so.

I have never seen this be a sign of a serious problem, though sometimes a lesion is irritating the child. But that doesn't sound like this situation.

Touching just feels good, so at this age both boys and girls rub themselves. Even fetuses show sexual activity. I've kept a fascinating article about female fetuses observed on ultrasound "masturbating"—that is how it is described—to what, some researchers propose, is the point of orgasm.

Keep on handling this lightly, and he will lose interest.

Q: I have a little girl who is almost two years old, and I am filled with fear about something bad happening to her. I don't hover over her, but I'm very careful; I frequently imagine the worst possible scenarios. For instance, when I'm at the supermarket, I feel anxious that someone will snatch her from the cart. When my father watches her, I worry about what would happen if he had a heart attack. Is it normal to have all these fears all the time?

A: Yes and no, but since you are worrying about your worry, it's time to do something about it.

First of all, I'm not surprised by your feelings, especially considering the world events that have enveloped us these past few years. We are bombarded with scary news all day long, and that can lead to stress and anxiety. Add to this mix the fact that radio, television, and magazines are all constantly planting ideas in our heads not only about all the bad things that can happen but about what it means to be a good mother. You can see why lots of parents are on edge.

Unfortunately, your anxiety is making your life miserable. It's robbing you of having fun with your little girl, and while you, of course, want to take some normal precautions, your constant worry can never guarantee absolute safety.

I'm reminded of how early awareness of sudden infant death syndrome (SIDS) caused some women to stay up all night checking on their babies' breathing. SIDS is extraordinarily rare, and yet it has received a ton of media coverage over the past several years. This makes it seem common, and it is hard to ignore. But mothers need sleep in order to be good mothers.

I want you to make some changes in the direction of increasing the fun and relaxation you have with your baby and reducing your anxiety. Find a way that

---

QUIZ

What's the average age of girls when they show readiness skills for using the "potty"?

A) twenty months   B) twenty-two months

C) twenty-four months   D) twenty-eight months

(C: *twenty-four months; boys are a bit slower to get the concept—their average age is twenty-six months.*)

DID YOU KNOW?
BE ALERT TO WATER HAZARDS

Just because you don't have a pool, don't assume your child is safe from drowning. More than a hundred children die each year in the United States from other water hazards, including bathtubs, five-gallon buckets (if a toddler falls in headfirst, he probably can't get out), spas and hot tubs, even toilets. Be aware, because even a small amount of water can be a killer.

works for you—meditation, exercise, or even joining a parents' group or seeing a therapist who has expertise in these matters. You need to talk to your partner or spouse about this topic, too. They can be a part of the solution, but only if you are talking to them. Internalizing your feelings is not good for your long-term health.

Q: When my two-year-old son doesn't like what's going on, he drops to his knees and bangs his head on the floor really hard. He also smacks himself in the head with his hands. He's a very bright boy, and other than this, he's a pretty happy guy.

He's the middle child, in between his three-month-old baby sister and his four-year-old brother. When his sister was born, he ate less and talked less than before, but it's the head banging that really scares me, because he's hurting himself. He cries and holds his head, and says it hurts.

How concerned should I be? And should I run to him and hug him because he hurt his head or should I ignore him? I've tried both.

A: Young kids are constantly challenging both parents and doctors, and it can be difficult to assess just how extreme certain behavior is.

There are kids for whom head banging is a compulsive disorder. These children have to wear helmets to keep from hurting themselves. In serious cases, the child is put on medication and goes through aversion therapy.

If your little boy does not have other symptoms—other behavior problems beyond the head banging—I would assume that he's having plain old-fashioned tantrums, which is what a kid does to get attention or because he is too young to understand and handle his complex feelings of rejection, jealousy, and anger.

Medical experts have all sorts of opinions on how to cope with this. Most often, pediatricians recommend that tantrums be ignored. Making a big deal about them gives a child reason to keep having them. Head banging does hurt, and I've seen a kid realize on his own that he's gone too far and doesn't want to do that to himself anymore, especially if he doesn't get anything good from it.

Do try to keep him on a carpeted floor when he starts to carry on. You could try saying something like, "Remember, that hurts. You don't want to do that." Also—and I know this is a challenge for anyone with three young children—try to find some time each week for at least a short outing for just the two of you; and do the same with the four-year-old, if possible.

I'm pretty sure this will pass, especially once you are consistent with your response. But make sure your pediatrician is in the loop on this situation, and ask for his or her advice, too.

Q: **I work in a day-care center, and one of our little boys—he's almost three—is a master at holding his breath when he wants something, and sometimes it gets scary for just a moment. Of course, we have mentioned this to his parents, and they have experienced the same thing at home. What should I know about such behavior? Is it possible he could hurt himself?**

A: The good news is that this probably won't last much longer. The bad news is that occasionally this can be dangerous.

This behavior actually has a medical name, breath-holding spells or BHS, and it usually happens after the child cries because he or she is upset, has been startled, or has suffered some minor injury. Then the baby or toddler becomes silent, and their skin often changes color quite quickly; this period can last from seconds to more than a minute before the child begins to breathe normally again. In extreme cases, the child may lose consciousness. As you said, this can be scary.

We used to think this was purely driven by willful behavior, but we now know it's not that simple. For some kids, this may be genetic, and the BHS is an automatic reaction. Of course, it takes an expert to determine whether the child needs treatment.

According to a report in *Pediatrics*, one study found that BHS can begin as early as six months and usually ends around thirty-seven to forty-two months, though it can go until age seven. But that's very rare. The same study, which followed ninety-five children for up to nine years, found that about a third of the kids would do this at least once a day, but, on average, BHS happened about once a week.

Just to be safe, the next time this little boy is in one of his spells, try to note how long it lasts and give that information to the parents. Of course, if the child should pass out or have any other unusual behavior, make sure the parents know about it.

Parents should also talk to their pediatricians about the best way to respond to their children if they have BHS. Understandably, some parents react more negatively to kids who have this.

Remember, this too shall pass.

Q: My twenty-nine-month-old granddaughter doesn't talk at all yet, and has poor motor control. But what worries me even more is that she sometimes abruptly stops walking, gets a glazed expression, and then shudders and continues on her way.

A pediatric neurologist did a workup on her, and now she wants to do an MRI. The baby's parents backed out of one scheduled MRI already, because they don't want to put her under general anesthesia. How can I convince them that this is important? What will the MRI show?

A: Sometimes parents get so scared they don't realize they may be hurting their child by not following their doctor's advice. You are in a difficult spot, but you must persist.

An MRI (magnetic resonance imaging) can reveal any bleeding, tumors, blockages, or nerve damage in the baby's head. MRIs are wonderful, because they catch images of tissue. Regular X rays only show us bone.

The neurologist is recommending the next logical diagnostic step because the growth and development evaluation didn't turn up enough information. The doctor's recommendation and your concern are right on the mark. You have to encourage the parents to follow through, because the MRI will show invaluable information. The child has to be anesthetized because patients must lie totally still during MRIs, and young children just can't do this. Anesthesia in a child is routine and completely safe. Putting off a diagnosis is not.

Take care with your approach to the parents, because, sadly, a grandmother's wisdom is often resented.

You want the family to pull together as a team to get the best care for your granddaughter.

Q: What would cause a urinary tract infection in a seven-month-old girl? I hate seeing my little daughter in any pain.

A: Far and away the most common germs to cause urinary tract infection (UTI) are E. coli bacteria coming from the colon. Other germs from the colon are sometimes at fault, too. Cross-contamination during a diaper change is a likely source of contact.

Diapers and soap can also cause an irritation at the opening of the urethra that would compromise local immunity and let germs in more easily. We used to have a theory that girls have shorter urethras that allow germs to enter more easily. That was disproved by exposing baby girls to bath water loaded with germs. They didn't get a lot of infections.

UTIs in females even may be linked to how a baby is handled right after delivery. Babies who are whisked into the hospital nursery as soon they are born, rather than handed right over to their mothers for a time, have their whole systems, including their genitals, exposed to tougher species of germs. A baby who stays with her mother and meets her mother's germs before being introduced to the hospital's germs, is much less likely to get a urinary tract infection. About one to two percent of infants have UTIs, and the rate is even higher in low-birth-weight babies.

Your baby's infection probably began with one of these common causes, but children with urinary tract infections should always be checked for any urological abnormalities. The abnormalities are rare, but they can result in serious kidney dysfunction down the road.

Your daughter should also have a urinalysis to identify the germ and to make sure it's not a nasty, recurrent type.

Be scrupulous with her diapers and with cleansing. You don't want to let her get irritated. When she is older, she should be taught to wipe front to back, not back to front, when she eliminates.

Q: My three-month-old son has had a clogged tear duct for about two months now. The pediatrician said it should go away on its own. He gave me some erythromycin eye drops, but they seem to make it worse. Should I take my baby to a specialist?

A: Your pediatrician is right—this does usually resolve itself. But since it's still clogged, I think it's reasonable for an ophthalmologist to examine your baby. He or she might give you a similar answer, but I can understand that you would want to hear it from a doctor who specializes in eyeballs.

Pediatricians are primary care doctors for little kids, and they do play the role of gatekeeper in today's managed-care environment. They try to keep parents from using up specialists' valuable time.

The tear duct—which is called the lachrymal duct—is between the corner of the eye and the inside of the nose. When it is blocked (which can be congenital), tears overflow onto the child's cheek and can cause irritation. A gentle massage can help to speed up the process of opening it; however, it sounds like you are past that point.

In the past we treated clogged tear ducts aggressively, giving the child anesthesia and poking open the tear duct with a tiny prod. Often, this treatment turned out to be premature, because we later found that the duct opens on its own.

I'm not surprised that the drops aren't useful. Since the duct is closed, how can they get in there? Also, in my experience, an infection is rarely present, so erythromycin drops are unnecessary.

Q: My four-and-a-half-month-old godson has about thirty brown spots on his body. The specialist who examined him says these "café au lait" spots are Elephant Man's disease. The doctor was very optimistic about the baby's treatment, and says that when he gets tumors they will just remove them. Is this really that straightforward and simple to treat?

A: Most people would be frightened by something called Elephant Man's disease, which is more accurately called neurofibromatosis (NF) or von Recklinghausen's disease. In fact, we don't know for certain that von Recklinghausen's disease is what ailed John Merrick, who was known as the Elephant Man. Also, while the disease can be very nasty, it is seldom disfiguring. The occasional case of major disfigurement generates much negative publicity.

The spots are flat—if you rub your finger over them you won't feel a thing—and are the color of coffee with milk. If a child has more than a half dozen, the chances of having NF go up. Most cases are so minimal that patients are well into adulthood before they become troubled enough to seek a diagnosis for what they thought were just moles or lumpy skin.

The café au lait spots themselves are not the problem. But they are an indicator that the typical tumors may be present. They look totally different from the spots, and they don't look like moles either. They can range from small bumps under the surface of the skin to large, distinctive lumps that hang from the body.

The tumors grow from the lining of the nerves and are rarely malignant. Their growth is unpredictable, however, and if they happen to grow on the nerves as they pass through bone, they can distort the shape and growth of the bone. These are the cases that make the disease frightening.

A lot of kids have these café au lait spots, so parents should keep an eye out for them and know how many there are. Neurofibromatosis is a genetic disease, but the line of inheritance is not crisp and clean. The spots and tumors are not moles and are not passed on by parents who have moles.

The National Neurofibromatosis Foundation, which has chapters in every state, can answer a lot of your questions. For more information, see the Resource List on page 263.

Q: The soft spot on my three-and-a-half-month-old daughter's head is considerably smaller than is most kids', according to her pediatrician. Upon his referral, we have seen two neurosurgeons, and they each told us something different.

The first one said that if all three of the plates in her head begin to fuse, she would have to have surgery. The second doctor, a pediatric neurosurgeon, said that it doesn't matter when the plates fuse or when the soft spot disappears, that surgery was not necessary and that the other neurosurgeon was incorrect.

Whom should we believe? Could the fusing put pressure on her brain and cause brain damage?

A: I'd put my trust in the pediatric neurosurgeon. Obviously, because the baby's brain is growing, you don't want the plates in her head to fuse prematurely, and they usually don't. They can, however, fuse in a lopsided way, causing a kid to have a healthy but funny-shaped head. Some folks blame the put-babies-on-their-backs guidance, which resulted from concerns about sudden infant death syndrome.

Well, now people seem to be jumping at unnecessary neurosurgeries to avoid this lopsidedness or flatness. I think that's overkill. The literature I've read says that your baby is too young for you to be concerned about this, and the results of the surgery aren't very noticeable, anyway.

For the time being, keep an eye on her condition under the guidance of the pediatric neurosurgeon. I applaud you for pursuing this with a subspecialist, and I'd follow that doctor's advice.

Q: **After my four-month-old granddaughter became limp and lifeless, she was hospitalized and diagnosed with infant botulism. We understand that it affects the nerves so severely that it causes paralysis. At first, she was so weak that she couldn't open her eyes. The doctors say she might be sick with this from five days to ten months. It sounds awfully scary. What could have caused this illness? And what do you think her prognosis is?**

A: Your granddaughter's prognosis should be good. What's very important is that she has been diagnosed, because now she can get the right treatment. Infant botulism is uncommon, so it's not an easy diagnosis to make.

The good news is that the toxin produced by botulism wears off after a while. It is very unlikely that her recovery will take a full ten months.

The botulism bacteria and spores are not the problem as much as the toxin that the germ produces when the bacteria grows. The toxin is one of the world's most powerful poisons—experts say a gram could kill one million people. It paralyzes muscles, and people die because they can no longer breathe.

The botulism organism is all around us, mostly in soil. We eat it all the time, but our stomach acid kills it off before it can grow. But if we take in the toxin, it can be fatal. Improperly canned fruits and vegetables and improperly stored homemade and commercial foods traditionally have been responsible for most deaths from botulism toxins, and babies now account for most cases of the illness. ·

The organism can be present in honey, and since babies are particularly vulnerable because their stomachs can't handle it, we recommend that they not eat any honey during their first six months to a year.

This is one of those curious germs that has proved to be both a health boon and a health worry. The very thing that makes botulism so dangerous—the paralysis it causes—can be put to positive use when we are in control of it. A doctor I know invented the use of Botox—the botulism toxin—for treating crossed eyes. We paralyze the muscle that is pulling the eye the wrong way by injecting it with very, very diluted Botox. We can relieve wryneck—a twisted neck caused by a spastic muscle—in the same way. A Botox injection can also help people who sweat too much, because it paralyzes the sweat glands. And, most notably for the past few years, we inject Botox into wrinkles and frown lines to paralyze those muscles and smooth the skin.

Kids and ADHD: This Is Out of Control

Q: My sister's seven-year-old is really difficult to be around, and he can't seem to stand still for even twenty seconds. I know the teachers at his school have called my sister in for conferences several times, but she's yet to see a doctor specifically about his behavior. Should she?

A: Yes, your sister should talk to her child's doctor. But if you're thinking this child needs Ritalin, you won't have my automatic vote of support just because his behavior isn't perfect.

In fact, we don't yet have enough scientific evidence to support the massive use of Ritalin and other psychiatric drugs on kids. Other countries do not prescribe these drugs to 5 to 10 percent of their young population. Why do American children seem to need this pharmaceutical help?

Many physicians like myself feel that there is a spectrum of personalities among children that is entirely normal. But because of the constraints in the school systems, and because some people aren't sure of their parenting skills, the drugs have become an easy solution to a variety of behavioral problems. However, no parent should put his or her child on Ritalin just because a school says it is necessary. This should not be a teacher's decision nor a principal's decision—though some school districts feel it is, and parents are finding the fight can take them to court.

As you might expect, most schools don't have staff capable of focusing on kids who disrupt classes, learn differently, or are simply more difficult to handle than others. And when the teacher sends a note to the parent about a child's behavior, the frustrated and concerned parent immediately goes to the pediatrician, who often does not have the time or resources to adequately assess the child but does have a prescription pad right there on the desk.

Thus, we find a staggering number of kids on Ritalin and other psychotropic drugs. Yes, in many situations, they do seem to help kids focus and stay on task. But these are amphetamine-like medications, and if you've ever taken a drug like that, you know that even the most boring task can become tolerable. Yet that may be stifling other, more important and creative parts of the personality.

There are many creative geniuses in history who, if they lived today, would be diagnosed with attention deficit hyperactivity disorder (ADHD). If we had drugged them, we might not have benefited from their creative outputs. Kids who are ADHD are more likely to grow up and own their own businesses. They are not the kinds of kids who want to sit in front of a computer terminal all day long. Making these kids more manageable might make everyone's life easier in the short term, but in the long term, those children could pay a price.

If your sister consults a doctor, make sure the doctor does lots of assessment tests before reaching a diagnosis. Your sister may need some help and some education on how to handle a child who is a little bit different. I don't think parents have been given enough behavioral strategies for such children. It's also possible your sister has yet to figure out some parenting issues, such as setting basic, consistent rules for her child. If that's part of the problem, it's not too late to start, but she has a lot of work ahead of her.

Q: I'm very concerned about what my daughter expects from her toddler in the way of good behavior. Her daughter, who is almost three, is constantly on the move, which seems very normal to me. My daughter thinks she might be hyperactive. What can I do? By the way, this is her first child.

A: First-time parents in particular can be overwhelmed by the activity of a young child, but both new and experienced parents have been caught up in all the chatter about ADHD. Unfortunately, your daughter's expectations for her child are similar to those of many parents.

Three-year-old kids are supposed to be rambunctious and curious. A three-year-old who can sit quietly for an hour is rare indeed. But a *Newsweek* magazine survey done several years ago found that one in four parents does expect a three-year-old to be able to sit quietly for an hour, and 51 percent expected a fifteen-month-old to share toys with other children.

QUIZ

True or False? The drug Ritalin is now listed among the "Drugs of Concern" by the Drug Enforcement Agency, along with cocaine, LSD, Ecstasy, and more.

(True: Teenagers are using Ritalin (methylphenidate) in growing numbers as a recreational drug. One study by Indiana University showed that 6.8 percent of the ninth graders who participated in a survey reported using Ritalin illicitly at least once.)

Folks, let your children be children; these are unrealistic expectations. And the experts say that "unrealistic expectations can create frustration on both sides, and can lead to abuse and neglect."

In fact, 61 percent of the surveyed parents who had children under seven "think spanking is an appropriate 'regular form of discipline.' A third of the parents even believe spanking 'helps children develop a better sense of self-control.' "

Well, we have lots of strong evidence to the contrary. These unreasonable beliefs about kids' capabilities are at the core of another major problem: the attention-deficit-disorder epidemic. I think it's time we learned about how kids really behave, instead of how we think they should behave, and start treating them accordingly.

Asthma, Arthritis, and Other Chronic Diseases: What We Know, What We Don't Know

Q: There is a history of diabetes in my family, although I don't have it myself. Does this make my four-year-old a more likely candidate for juvenile diabetes? Are there signs I should watch for?

A: Even though diabetes can run in families, it is so inconsistent that I wouldn't worry too much about this. Both of my grandmothers were diabetic, and it hasn't shown up in our family since then. Juvenile diabetes is different from the kind of diabetes that you get later in life, which is usually associated with obesity. At this particular point, while it is smart to be aware of frequent urination, fatigue, and other general symptoms that would make you consult your child's doctors anyway, I wouldn't look for any specific signs.

Type I (juvenile) diabetes is caused by a lack of insulin, which is why these cases are treated with insulin. Adult-type diabetes has to do with the resistance of our cells to the insulin that is present in our body.

Q: Can children really get arthritis? My five-year-old granddaughter is currently being treated for this, but I'm skeptical.

A: Children definitely can have arthritis; it's called juvenile rheumatoid arthritis. We usually think of arthritis as an old person's disease, but it isn't. In fact, if you ever hear the term "growing pains," always be skeptical, because there's no such thing. If a child's joints hurt, there should be an explanation. While not all such cases are juvenile arthritis, of course, they certainly can be.

Make sure your granddaughter is being seen by a rheumatologist, who specializes in childhood rheumatic diseases.

Q: My two-year-old son has had a really nasty cough for six weeks. After looking at an X ray, an allergy/asthma specialist diagnosed a sinus infection. This same doctor wants my son to be tested for allergies. My husband and I are very torn. We don't want to put him through the tests. Also, I've heard from various sources that a two-year-old is too young for allergy tests.

A: He is young for sinus problems, and we can't say with certainty that allergies are the cause. However, by identifying his allergies, the doctor may be able to help him. I know you don't want to upset your son, but the few pricks involved in the allergy tests aren't very bad considering that they might prevent future infections. Swollen tissues in the nose clog the openings to the sinuses, which then get inflamed and infected.

The tests aren't dangerous, and they will give you some information. He might be allergic to something at home that you can easily eliminate from his environment. The more informed you are about your child's health, the better.

Occasionally, a chronic cough is a sign of low-level asthma, which can be tricky in a child, though there are things we can do for it. Soon, you should know a lot more.

Kids and Surgery: Be Smart, Be Informed

Q: My daughter just turned six, and she has a congenital heart defect, so she'll require open-heart surgery. We have met with surgeons at two different university hospitals, and we're having a difficult time picking a surgeon. What should we consider when making the decision?

A: I bet you're having a difficult time! When you're looking at heart surgeons at a university hospital, you're probably looking at people who are all equally qualified.

When I talk to people about how to pick a surgeon, I tell them that Americans are very poor at judging quality physicians. When we do surveys about the things people value the most in their doctors, the No. 1 thing is that the doctor talks to them about nonmedical things like "my roses and my dogs and my kids." People love that; they love to feel friendly and close.

I can see where that could be important when you are picking a pediatrician, but if my child needs heart surgery, I don't care if the doctor has the personality of an oyster. A doctor with good hands and experience is whom I would trust to do the surgery. And by experience I mean more than ten cases. You should also make sure that the doctor you're talking to will be the one actually performing the surgery.

I strongly believe in the training of younger doctors in teaching hospitals when I say that, but it's important to give you this advice. In many teaching hospitals, the chief surgical resident will do the operation. In most cases, he or she is perfectly qualified, especially with the attending doctor standing right there during the operation. If you object to that kind of a thing, just remember that they're not using your child as a guinea pig. This is how they learn.

University hospitals, even with the system I just mentioned, have lower death rates and higher success rates than the average hospital. The outcomes are better, because a lot of brains are involved in one case.

Since the surgery to be performed on your child is usually fairly routine open-heart surgery—though I know it's not routine to you—I would say the quality of the institution is just as important as the surgeon. You want an institution that has a lot of experience handling heart surgery for kids.

All things being equal, if I were you, I'd go with the comfort level you feel with the doctor and the institution. If your child just happens to have to stay in the hospital a little bit longer, you'll be happy you picked a more communicative doctor.

If you want to take one more step, talk to a pediatrician or two and ask them what they would do if their child were facing open-heart surgery. Ask them to whom they would send their child.

Finally, there's new research related to children and surgery that all parents should know about. Sometimes the tiniest patients are ignored—or undermedicated—because they can't articulate their needs. All they can do is cry, and sometimes that's what they are doing when the gas mask goes on their face.

But it seems that trauma for a child, especially a young child, at the start of anesthesia could mean behavioral problems and even nightmares after the surgery. If a child is given a mild liquid sedative about twenty minutes before they face a gas mask, they are relaxed and much less likely to remember anything that happens after that. Talk to the anesthesiologist in advance if you have any concerns.

I'm sure your child will be fine. The surgery is as routine as an appendectomy was in my day. I hope that puts any anxiety you may have to rest.

Q: My fourteen-year-old son was born with mild Treacher Collins syndrome; he has a very minor hearing loss and he needs braces.

We are asking ourselves if, along with the orthodontia, he should also have surgery to draw his jaw out to change his appearance. We've already met with the cranial-facial panel of doctors at the local children's hospital. The surgeon would actually cut the jawbone and use a little screw mechanism on the side to crank it forward.

My son has terrific self-esteem. He's very athletic, and he's got everything going for him. How do we go about making a decision like this, to put our boy under the knife, to take the risk of surgery? Whom can we talk to?

A: This decision is an especially tough one, because the surgery you're talking about is primarily cosmetic—plastic surgery—and the patient is a child.

Treacher Collins syndrome is a birth defect that occurs in about one in ten thousand births. The child has underdeveloped cheekbones and jawbones. In more severe cases, breathing, eating, or hearing are impaired. Of course, repairing the jaw in a child who cannot eat or breathe freely would not be cosmetic surgery.

The first person you should talk to is your son; a kid should be given a chance to feel the best he can about himself. You can also tell him that braces can bring the jaw forward, but it takes a long time to accomplish that. Surgery is quicker but more traumatic.

Be sure that you have a full and clear picture of the specific risks and benefits from the surgeon, and, once you do, I recommend that you sit down and do a basic decision-making list. In separate columns, detail the pros and the cons, both medical and quality-of-life issues, and discuss them. Realize that whatever decision you make, it will be mixed; you will have doubts, which is OK, because decisions are rarely perfect. If the answer were so obviously right or wrong, the choice would be easy.

This is major facial surgery, so if you decide to have it done it will be tough while he's in the midst of it, but my instinct is that after it's all over, he and you will be happy about going through with it.

Q: My four-month-old son was born with a severe case of hypospadias. The doctor wants to repair it. I thought it would help to do some additional research on the Internet, but I scared myself by reading about all the complications that can result from this surgery. What can you tell me about it? Is it usually successful?

A: Yes, it is usually very successful. But you are smart to go into this with a full understanding of the benefits and risks, because complications can happen with any surgery. And this particular surgery does have its opponents.

Hypospadias is a birth defect in which the opening of the urethra is on the underside of the penis rather than on the tip, so the child's urine may just come out at an angle, or it may come out at an opening anywhere along the underside of the penis all the way down to the base, where it meets the testicles.

This condition is fairly common, and in the hands of someone with a lot of experience, the repair is routine. The urethral reconstruction can require a skin graft using the foreskin. One possible complication could be a blockage caused by scar tissue.

I do want you to get facts from a skilled and reputable doctor. One question to ask is what age is best for doing the surgery. You may well have the luxury of time to make this decision. The surgery could be more difficult in an infant. After all, an infant has a teeny, tiny penis, and a repair later on may be less technically difficult. But it could be more traumatic because the child is older.

Whether or not to repair hypospadias is actually controversial. Except in severe cases, the repair is cosmetic. No one sees an infant urinate anyway, and, as a boy grows, he will modify his aim as needed. Some people say that's not so bad.

The Internet can be friend or foe. Resist fixating on the worst that can happen and focus instead on what's most likely to happen. And, in general, always seek out reliable medical sources. Look for the experience and credentials of the sites' experts.

Q: I have a fourteen-year-old son who insists on being circumcised. He is the only one out of a class of thirty kids who is not circumcised. I told him that all boys are born the way he is, but he says he doesn't care. He threatened to run away. What can I do to change his mind?

A: Circumcision on a boy this age is plastic surgery, because there is no medical reason to do it. You can tell him that when he's twenty-one, he can make this decision and that's OK. But at this age it's not appropriate—and it's not his choice.

The number of boys who are circumcised varies from region to region in the United States. In the West, two-thirds are left intact. But that's obviously not the case where you live, and you need to be supportive while stressing that he doesn't have to be like everyone else. In the South and Northeast, one-third of boys are left intact; in the Midwest only 20 percent are left uncut.

You might explain to him the sexual advantages of not being circumcised. You have to decide if he, at fourteen years, is old enough to hear about this. You could also relate this situation to that of tonsils, and all the operations that doctors have done over the years that have turned out to be unnecessary. Point out that, like circumcision, tonsillectomies were a medical tradition that turned out to be wrong.

Sometimes kids can't see beyond their own neighborhood. Tell him that in most of the world boys are left intact. Tell him that when he travels and goes out into his life, he's going to feel very differently.

My heart goes out to you, because you took a chance and a risk by not having your son circumcised. I did the same thing, and it hasn't been an issue with my sons, in part because where we live, the majority of kids are left intact.

Q: My son is fourteen months old, and he has a severe case of tongue-tie. The bottom of his tongue is attached toward the tip of his tongue. Our physician doesn't seem too concerned about it. I am really concerned about it, because it doesn't look right. I'm also concerned about his speech when he gets older.

A: Your concerns are reasonable. If anything, we tend to be less aggressive these days with this than we once were, and there are many reasons for this.

We see kids who have a very prominent frenulum of the tongue, which is what it's called, and they do OK. Their speech and swallowing both work just fine. However, other kids do seem to have problems that need to be addressed, and snipping the frenulum is an easy procedure.

Because your son is so young, I'm not sure how aggressive you want to be just yet. The person who could give you a really good read on this as your child ages and starts to talk is a speech pathologist. They're part of the medical care system that, in general, is underutilized. They know much more about this kind of thing than the general pediatrician.

Keep in mind that this is something that can be fixed at any time. If you notice your child having difficulty speaking, then you may want to consider treatment. This also can improve with time; the frenulum can begin to recede a bit. Of course, if your child is developing a speech impediment you don't want to wait until he's fourteen years old to help out.

Q: I have a twenty-month-old daughter who has a bump on her right eye. We first noticed it when she was about a year old. It's right on the corner of the eyelid. It isn't red or inflamed. For several months the pediatrician just thought it was a cyst, but it never went away, and we finally went to a pediatric ophthalmologist. They said it was a dermoid cyst.

The doctor wants to have it removed, because, he said, if she bumps into something it could disperse. Am I getting good advice? Could this come back?

A: My thirty-year-old son had one of these when he was younger. It was in that same location, and we eventually had it treated, mostly for cosmetic reasons. He could do weird things with it, like pop it out and make it look gross— always when we had company for dinner.

A dermoid is a very interesting cyst that's congenital and considered benign. It's like skin turned inside out, and it can have a strange composition, with hair, even teeth, bone, and other things. They can occur anywhere in the body. Also, they can rupture with trauma, and the contents can be very irritating to surrounding tissues, but, in my experience, this is very rare.

Still, if it's a dermoid and it's noticeable, I'd have it removed. But there's no need to rush, and you want to make sure the doctor is an expert. This is something an ophthalmological plastic surgeon should take care of, because the eyelids are tricky. Obviously you wouldn't want a pediatrician to tackle it.

I doubt that there will be a noticeable scar when she matures, because folds of the skin at the corner of the eyelid should cover the incision.

Autism and Other Syndromes

Q: My twelve-year-old daughter is autistic. She has very delayed language and speech. We still don't always understand everything she says and, in general, she leads a frustrating life.

I know you don't believe there is a link between autism and vaccines, but I saw a program on television that brought up some really interesting points about autism and the measles, mumps, and rubella (MMR) vaccine.

They showed slides of autistic children's cells with these measles virus-type things—little, black, spidery-looking things—in the cells of their intestines. The children who were not autistic did not have this. Don't you think this is significant?

A: I am sure her life must be very frustrating for you, too, and I can understand your desire for an explanation as to how this could have happened to your family. But there's one big problem with that report you saw: Those spidery-looking things may not be measles particles. The interpretation of histological slides is not nearly as simple as a TV program would make it look. In fact, those slides are very difficult to understand.

My disbelief in the possibility of a link between autism and vaccines goes beyond opinion. It is based on the fact that research on this very important subject repeatedly finds no conclusive evidence of a connection. It is based on the fact that the MMR vaccine saves countless lives, and yet people allow fears and television shows to drive their decisions about their children's health care.

Some of the calls I get about this subject are angry or irrational, and I'm amazed how many folks have been caught up in conspiracy thinking on this topic. I don't blame parents for looking for answers and wanting to find fault with the obstetrician or anyone they can, but sometimes it's just not that simple.

Investigating the cause of cell differences between autistic and non-autistic children is very significant, but let me tell you that, based on science, the vaccine theory is way down the list of suspects. What's at the top of the list are the genetic theory and the intrauterine theory. One recent study tells us that there are elevated levels of certain proteins in the blood at birth—*at birth*—that appear to foreshadow autism and mental retardation later in childhood.

This is a remarkable study. Researchers archived newborns' blood samples at birth and waited to see which children went on to develop autism or mental retardation. None of these babies had yet had vaccines. Clinicians found that, at birth, neural growth factors were significantly elevated in children who later developed autism and mental retardation. Another study found antibodies in the mom's blood during pregnancy in cases where the child was later diagnosed as autistic.

As we continue to turn over stones to discover the secrets beneath them, if we find clues that vaccines might hold some answers, we will certainly look at them. However, when responsible scientists tell us, "We've checked that rock and there's nothing there," we have to move on.

Science has got to concentrate its resources on the weight of the evidence supported by the majority of the experts who have spent their lives in this field. The beauty of science is that if objective evidence shows us that something else is going on, then we can change our minds.

I can't abandon facts, and one of many that I can't ignore is that autism pops up in countries that haven't seen a vaccine in a long time.

Objective reasoning is our greatest gift. It will answer these questions eventually; fear will not. You sound hungry to know more, and I would encourage you to check out the autism sites mentioned in our Resource List on page 263.

Q: When we grew concerned about our two-year-old not talking, our pediatrician told us to take a wait-and-see approach. But we pressed on for an explanation, and our son was found to have autism. Every parent that I know who has an autistic child was told, "Don't worry. Wait and see."

What do you consider an appropriate "waiting" time when people are concerned about the behavior of their young children? This answer won't help me, but it might help someone else. By the way, I knew there was something unusual about my child before he was eighteen months old. He actually had language, and then began to lose it.

A: The average two-year-old knows a few words and can make simple two- or three-word statements, but the range is large, indeed. If a child isn't talking by age three, something is likely to be wrong.

So, while a pediatrician might consider autism in a two-year-old who doesn't speak, he or she also knows the odds are low that the child is autistic, and very high that nothing is wrong and the child is just a late talker.

Unfortunately, we cannot afford to send every two-year-old who doesn't talk for a full neurological work up. Especially since, for the vast majority of parents, this would create totally unnecessary fear, if not panic, and could be traumatic for the child.

As you know, there isn't even a diagnostic test for autism. Like Alzheimer's, it's diagnosed when other things, like unresponsiveness and lack of communication, begin to manifest. Plus, we aren't sure how much of a difference early intervention in autism makes.

And yet, there is a real dilemma. When something is wrong, parents shouldn't just be put off, and waiting doesn't make the problem go away. As you pointed out, the pediatrician is not the only resource. Sometimes, parents have to make discoveries on their own.

I don't want to scare people whose children are late talkers. I wasn't talking at two—but once I started, I wouldn't shut up. My mother always loves to tell that story.

Q: Our six-and-a-half-year-old son was just diagnosed with high-functioning autism. A psychologist who specializes in treating autistic children has referred us to a woman who is a doctoral candidate who uses a combination of electrostimulation and behavior modification therapies and who claims she has almost cured her own grandson. We are skeptical, but we also want to do what's right for our child. Have you heard of this treatment?

A: I sure wish I had optimistic news here. Her grandson's claimed improvement is an anecdote, of course, and has no implications for what would happen with your child. Behavior modification in a traditional sense is surely worth a try, but I know of no electrostimulation therapies that have helped. Just paying a lot of attention to some autistic kids, especially those in the "high-functioning" category, can make it seem as if they are improving. And, of course, one always has to take into account that any disease state, mental or physical, goes through various phases, and some days are better than others. That's called the natural history of disease.

It's easy to give credit to whatever therapies are being used during those periods when the disease actually may be improving naturally. When things happen at the same time, a cause and effect may be automatically assumed, but that's not good science.

In general, we still know very little about how to treat autism, Asperger's syndrome (AS), and other illnesses that fall under the broad category of pervasive developmental disorders (PDD). In fact, children with a PDD can vary tremendously in their behavior, and researchers are still trying to categorize various disorders within PDD. For more information, go to the Web site for the Yale Child Study Center (*www.info.med.yale.edu/chldstdy/autism*), which is conducting the Social Disabilities Learning Project to study many aspects of PDDs.

Q: My eight-year-old daughter told me that she sometimes sees images smaller than their actual size. The example she gave is that several times a day the huge tree on the street corner will appear to be the same size as the much smaller traffic-signal box.

She also has a history of headaches, but she hasn't had one at the same time as these size distortions. What could they be? What kind of doctor should she see?

A: I think your daughter might have a fairly rare condition called the Alice in Wonderland syndrome—named, of course, after the storybook character who saw huge objects and tiny objects. The belief is that author Lewis Carroll based Alice's visions on his own migraine-induced hallucinations.

My best guess is that your daughter has this unusual form of ocular migraine. Ocular migraines do not manifest as headaches, but as a variety of visual distortions.

I don't think you have much to worry about—this is often short-lived—but you should get a firm diagnosis. Have your pediatrician recommend a pediatric neurologist.

Q: My eight-year-old son has Tourette syndrome. In just this last month, he has started to show signs of copralalia—using a lot of inappropriate language, which is causing trouble at school.

We were advised to put him on some heavy-duty antipsychotic medications to control this, but one makes him very depressed and the other makes him paranoid. I don't want to put him through that.

The literature validates that he has a disability, and I'm considering telling the school that they have to just accept him. On the other hand, I want to help him, because his bizarre behavior is already causing him to be ostracized by his classmates.

A: What a tough choice: Put your child on heavy drugs or risk further isolation and misunderstanding at school.

The spirit of the law concerning the rights of disabled people is that society must adjust itself to accommodate the full range of human beings on this planet. The other side of the issue is that a child who can't control his tics and cursing may be disruptive and alienated in the classroom.

According to the law, I think the school will have to accommodate your boy. Having his doctor or an outside respected adult talk to the kids about Tourette might calm things down. I have seen this work very well.

Those who aren't informed about Tourette think that the swearing and twitching are voluntary and a reflection of poor morals. Morals have nothing to do with it. This is a neurological disease that disables the inhibitory parts of the brain, and there's a lot we don't yet understand about it.

The school has to meet you halfway. In fact, as you know very well, when you're around someone with Tourette, you soon learn to tune out the disruptions, and that's what might happen in his classes.

But don't give up entirely on the drugs. The ones he was on may have been the right drugs at the wrong time. They might work for him when he's older. Sooner or later, you are going to want to help him control some of the symptoms. For now, try some other medications. You can always stop them if they don't work out.

Your boy certainly has my sympathy as he moves along through the world. As tough as this is, he is fortunate to live at a time when we talk openly about Tourette. Ten or twenty years ago, people with this disease were doomed to being shut-ins.

Kids and Sleeping: How to Get Through the Night

Q: When I put my seventeen-month-old baby to bed for the night, she sleeps for an hour and then wakes up crying. For the last four nights, we have tried to just let her cry it out, but she gets so upset she vomits. We eventually pick her up to calm her down. What should we do? We're desperate.

A: I'm not too concerned about the vomiting right now. Crying squeezes the chest and abdominal cavities, which increases the pressure in the tummy. This can cause children to spit up. Because the esophageal sphincter is underdeveloped in kids, it just gives, which causes the upchuck.

Since this is at bedtime—some hours after a meal—she's not going to lose a lot of nutrition. And I doubt very much that she's losing too much fluid.

All kids stir in the night and wake up. But the big difference is that some kids put themselves back to sleep and others don't. One thing to consider is that if she goes to sleep with a stuffed toy, a blankie, or a bottle she will probably want that same thing when she wakes up at two A.M. She relies on them to get to sleep, and if it's not there or if it has dropped on the floor, you've got a problem.

If she's used to drifting off with you by her side, with you patting her back, you've got an even bigger problem, because that's what she'll want in the middle of the night. Teaching a baby self-comfort is one of the keys to helping them sleep.

Callers to my show have mentioned the Ferber method, developed by Dr. Richard Ferber, director of the Center for Pediatric Sleep Disorders at Children's Hospital in Boston. This involves sticking to a very rigid schedule that allows crying for a specific number of minutes and then a short period of time when you check on the baby, calming him or her with your voice but not picking up the child. The next crying session goes a bit longer, and so on, until the child gives up on the crying. This works for some parents, but others find it too difficult to let their little critter cry.

Teaching your baby good sleep habits is much more of a challenge than controlling the vomiting. That will take care of itself. In the future, she will be able to cry really loud without bringing up a meal. If you want to know more about Ferber's approach, his book is called *Solve Your Child's Sleep Problems*.

The good news is that with time most sleep problems go away.

Q: I have seven-week-old twins, and I never get any sleep. As soon as I get one settled down, the other one wakes up. They sleep much easier on their stomachs, but I know that puts them at risk for sudden infant death syndrome (SIDS). Do you know how the risk of sleeping position compares to other risks, like parents who smoke? My pediatrician has a different answer from what I read.

A: SIDS is a very rare condition, but we do know that placing babies on their backs to sleep decreases the odds of SIDS even further.

You certainly have my sympathy about how tough lack of sleep can be, but you know yourself that no matter how small the risk, you aren't willing to take it.

So, my advice on this is simple: Keep them on their backs. It is very unlikely that SIDS will strike your babies, but the tragedy would be immense. If your babies were on their stomachs and one of them died from SIDS, your grief would be overwhelming.

Most babies learn to sleep on their back relatively quickly. Until yours do, talk to family members or close friends about how to share this load. You might also want to read *When You're Expecting Twins, Triplets, or Quads,* by Dr. Barbara Luke and Tamara Eberlein, which includes "survival tips" for those first stressful months at home. It's tough being a new mom, and you need to care for yourself as well as your children. You need help.

Q: What would cause a six-year-old to grind his teeth while he's sleeping?

A: Nighttime teeth grinding is usually normal. Compare flapping your wrists around to flapping your jaws, and you can see clearly that the jaws hold a lot a more tension—and even kids can have tension. We've all experienced the type of muscle spasm that jerks us awake just as we're falling asleep. Teeth grinding is another form of spasm. And, of course, if you've ever watched dogs, you've seen how much their muscles twitch during sleep.

Is the child going through an unusually tough time at home or in school right now? Some think children's bruxism—the medical term for teeth grinding—is caused by stress. But there's no proof of that, and the grinding is likely to be a temporary problem, though it can persist in some. If he has an excessively wired, nervous, or anxious personality, the grinding could be a permanent habit.

Make sure that the child has as happy and settled a life as he can, which is what we all want for our kids anyway. And get a referral to a dentist, so he can be fitted with a little bite plate that will guard his teeth at night.

Breast-feeding: The Best Thing You Can Do for Your Baby

Q: Until my granddaughter was switched from breast-feeding to a bottle at age two months, she was a contented baby. Once she started drinking formula, she became a fussy baby. She is three months old now, and she is always fussy.

She is constipated, too, so the pediatrician said we should give her an

ounce of prune juice in four ounces of water. The baby now has screaming attacks. Picking her up to soothe her does not calm her down. She just keeps screaming as if something is really hurting her. Could prune juice be too harsh for her system?

A: I share your suspicion; I would not give prune juice to a three-month-old baby. A three-month-old does not need anything other than breast milk—if possible—or formula.

If you can suggest a second opinion without causing a family fight, I advise you to do it.

Juice is known to cause gastrointestinal upset in babies. Even adults get bloated and gassy after encountering the carbohydrates and sugars in certain juices, and the result is diarrhea.

A baby this young shouldn't need any kind of supplement, even to counteract constipation. We expect variability in bowel movements in tiny babies. Even among breast-fed babies, some go a million times a day, some have a watery stool, and others are more solid. Our adult views about regularity aren't applicable to newborns.

Q: My friend wants to continue to nurse her six-month-old twins, who have been diagnosed with a kidney problem. The babies are doing well, but the pediatrician wants them to eat rice cereal to put on some weight. Can she do both?

A: They are at the age—six months—when introducing solids is desirable. And, yes, they can eat solids and continue to breast-feed. In fact, since breast milk contains antibodies and gives them an immunological advantage for fighting infection, both forms of nutrition would be desirable.

Kids who eat solids before six months of age have higher rates of food allergies and gastrointestinal problems, and they also don't need the calories. Nature sets up infants so they get what they need from breast milk.

Q: My cousin breast-fed her baby for about a month, and then started feeding the baby a homemade formula of barley water, milk, and corn syrup. Is that healthy for the baby?

A: Breast-feeding was the best thing she could do for the baby, and she replaced that with a poor substitute. If you want my official disapproval, you've got it. There is no way that any grain and syrup can provide what the human mother's body makes for her baby. This is dangerous and will harm the baby.

Formula manufacturers are constantly updating the way they make formula, because they discover new nutrients that are in breast milk that they add to their product. It's a very complex mix of protein, vitamins, nutrients, and fat that babies need to thrive. Unless you've studied nutrition, making your own formula is looking for trouble. Even powdered baby formula created by chemists has had tragic consequences for babies' health when the mix of formula to water was wrong. In other words, a baby can get very sick if the formula is too diluted or too concentrated.

What has happened to our ability to think? I don't know if you can reach people who are that far out on the limb, but she must love her baby. See if you can use that to convince her to at least get a pediatric exam for her child.

See more on breast-feeding in the chapter 4.

Parents, Kids, and Food: The Ultimate Can of Worms

Q: I make tofu to supplement my eleven-month-old son's protein intake. We're not vegetarians, but we don't eat a lot of meat. Do you think that's OK?

A: Yes. Be careful, though. If your child consumes large amounts of tofu, he may be exposed to plant-based estrogens, and we still don't know what effect those have on children. So far, research hasn't discovered any serious trouble.

Tofu is almost a complete protein, so it's a decent protein source. As long as your boy eats a variety of foods, he should be fine, and even though he's not eating meat, he shouldn't need a supplement.

Many parents cut out meat to reduce fat in a child's diet. Unfortunately, the American obsession with fat has confused well-intentioned parents who started worrying about their kids' fat consumption just like they worried about their own. Parents shouldn't be afraid of giving kids fat or milk. The vast majority of pediatricians discourage the reduction of saturated fat intake by children. What doctors can't yet agree on is the age at which a child's fat intake should be lowered.

You seem to be on the right track and to be avoiding extremes. Keep in mind that there are no evil foods—there are only bad diets.

Q: My daughter is a small woman who has an eighteen-month-old baby who is in a low height/weight percentile for his age. My grandson has been

a poor eater from birth. As an infant, he had trouble keeping down his formula, and now, at eighteen months, he refuses to taste a lot of food, or he
spits it out. Could there be something wrong with his taste buds, or would
you recommend one of these new supplements?

A: I'm not sure I'd recommend anything. Kids your grandson's age are notorious for throwing food on the floor or back at you. There's usually nothing to
worry about as long as the child is growing.

Small people tend to have small children, and, most of the time, fussy
eaters are not endangering their health. What is usually wrong is that we
expect babies to eat more than they need.

Height and weight are plotted on a curve, and some people are going to fall
on the ends of the curve. However, if your grandson is extremely low on the
height-and-weight chart, and especially if he is losing weight or is not growing, then something is wrong. I can't imagine that his pediatrician wouldn't be
on top of this; ask your daughter what the doctor has said—if you can ask
without sounding like you are meddling.

If something is wrong, it could be due to a variety of problems, from
pyloric stenosis—a narrowing of the opening to the stomach that would cause
him to spit up his food—to lactose intolerance to food allergies.

Generally, we overfeed our babies in this country, giving them a head start
on food and weight problems. Most Americans assume that babies need much
more food than they actually do. The nutritional quality and variety of the
food, not the amount, is what matters.

Studies have shown a wide variation in the amount of calories that kids
consume at individual meals, but their daily total comes out about the same. In
other words, while one kid might pick at food early in the day, another one

---

QUIZ

What is an "acceptable" total cholesterol reading for children two to
nineteen years old?

A) less than 150   B) less than 170   D) 140–190

E) 130–200

(B: less than 170.)

gobbles breakfast and then tapers off. At the end of the day, they've taken in similar quantities.

Many parents—and grandparents—worry meal by meal, but it's more valuable to consider what they've taken in by the close of the day.

Q: My grandchild has all kinds of behavior issues, and whenever my daughter-in-law gives him sugar—soda, cookies, candy—he gets really wired. She won't listen to me and says that I'm crazy and that sugar has nothing to do with his wildness. Who's right?

A: I'm afraid I have to side with your daughter-in-law. Although many of us blame children's bad behavior on sugar, the evidence says quite the contrary, and we've tested this many times, giving some kids real sugar, some kids artificial sweeteners, etc., and observing what happens. It turns out that sugar does not make a difference in a child's behavior.

What does happen, though, is that when kids are acting really wild, it's often at family holidays and other occasions where there's also lots of sugary foods and drinks, coincidentally. If your house is anything like ours, when all the kids get together, they just seem to act more hyper.

I'm not suggesting that sugar is good for children, but it has been blamed for problems that aren't legitimately linked to it. Right now, the only disease that we know is caused by sugar is tooth decay. All the other stuff is a myth.

Finally, this isn't the kind of thing you want to tackle with your daughter-in-law anyway. Bigger issues are likely to surface down the road, so save your energy.

Q: My neighbor is a vegan (doesn't eat any animal-based products), and when she finishes nursing her first child, she plans to put the child on soy milk or rice milk instead of regular milk. Is this OK?

A: No, and this is one case where I would encourage you to speak up, even at the risk of alienating her or being viewed as a meddler.

Tell your neighbor about a flood of childhood malnutrition cases reported on in *Pediatrics,* the journal of the American Academy of Pediatrics.

In one recent case, a twenty-two-month-old child was admitted with severe kwashiorkor; this is a disease that you see in Third World countries because of protein deficiency. His parents, who were well educated, thought he had a milk allergy, because he had chronic eczema. So, he was started on rice milk. Actually, it isn't even milk, it's a beverage made from rice. The child was anorexic, had lost hair, was not thriving at all, and had one of those big bellies you see on TV! Kwashiorkor can kill kids.

Fortunately, the doctors diagnosed the problem and began to feed him what he needed, and he recovered.

In another case, a seventeen-month-old was diagnosed with rickets, which is caused by a vitamin D deficiency. The child was breast-fed until he was ten months old and then was started on a soy health-food drink. The child took solid food well, but his diet included no animal products. Because he was not fed vitamin D–fortified foods and did not spend much time outdoors, he developed a vitamin D deficiency.

The child was normal until nine months and then suffered a complete "growth arrest." He regressed in gross motor skills, and when he was admitted to the hospital, he couldn't crawl or roll over. Once the problem was identified, the child was treated with calcium supplements and vitamin D. He regained his lost skills and began to thrive.

"Milk remains the main source of vitamin D for toddlers. It is prudent to ensure that any beverage given to a toddler in place of milk is fortified with vitamin D," said the researchers in this study. So, parents need to be very careful with kids' diets. You could do more harm than good if you give them health-food beverages, believing they are more healthful than real milk.

So, speak up. Hopefully, your neighbor will thank you.

Q: My four-year-old daughter is really hooked on cranberry juice; we took her off apple juice on the advice of her pediatrician. I heard you say that grape juice might be easier on kids, because it has less sorbitol than apple and pear juices do. How does cranberry juice compare?

QUIZ

Which food is most likely to promote cavities?
A) cheese   B) raisins   C) apples   D) chocolate
E) peanuts
(B: raisins; their stickiness means they are more likely to stay on the teeth and feed the bacteria.)

A: I'm afraid lots of folks have gotten distracted by the issue of sorbitol when they should be looking at the amount of any juice their child is consuming.

First, sorbitol is a sugar alcohol that occurs naturally in some fruit, and, because it is nonabsorbable, it can cause gastrointestinal problems in kids— especially in babies and toddlers. Apple juice, the most popular juice of all, has a high fructose/glucose ratio and a lot of sorbitol.

However, the equally important issue is that too many parents fall into the habit of using juice as a pacifier. In fact, too much juice may give a baby a tummy ache and actually cause her to be cranky and irritable. Many folks are surprised to learn that for a four-year-old, various experts recommend no more than six to twelve ounces of fruit juice per day. That's not a whole lot of juice.

You should also know that fruit juice does not fully meet a child's daily fruit and vegetable requirements, because fiber and other nutrients are lost during the processing. All children need whole fruit daily for a balanced, healthy diet.

That said, one benefit of cranberry juice is that it is tough on the bacteria that want to cling to our insides, especially the bladder. But once your daughter has an appropriate daily juice portion, give her water.

For more information on juices, go to the American Academy of Pediatrics Web site: *www.aap.org*.

Q: What kind of vitamins should my kids be taking? They are five, nine, and thirteen, and all are generally good eaters. I try to serve balanced meals, and we always have plenty of milk and juice in the refrigerator.

A: Based on how your kids are eating, I don't think they need any vitamins. None, zero. Shocking, huh?

Nature did a very good job of providing us with the vitamins and minerals we need through our food. The vitamin industry grossly overstates the needs we have for their products, and while, in the past, it would have been difficult to point to any harm from taking vitamins, we are beginning to see their bad side.

First of all, vitamin pills do not contain the range of vitamins and minerals contained in natural foods, and they may even suppress the body's ability to use natural vitamins. The other issue is that because of the fortification of the foods your child is eating, it is easy to overdose a child. Children are extremely sensitive to certain vitamins and minerals: Iron can be very toxic and is not recommended, and vitamins A and D are fortified in most dairy products, but

DID YOU KNOW?
WHAT PARENTS SAY ABOUT A CHILD'S WEIGHT

Are you being fair in your assessments of any weight problems your children might have?

A recent study from the Centers for Disease Control found that while more than 67 percent of the moms questioned accurately described their children as overweight, more than 30 percent said their kids were "about the right weight." That's disturbing, and so is this fact: Girls were more than twice as likely to be described as overweight as boys, from among all the kids who were heavy enough to be at risk of unhealthy weights. Parents need to remember: Fat children are unhealthy children, no matter what their gender.

---

that amount is sufficient for a child. Many parents mistakenly give children vitamins in addition to a crummy diet, thinking that they are compensating for poor nutrition. They are not helping their children.

Q: Does caffeine stunt children's growth? Or is that just an old-wives' tale?

A: To my knowledge, it does not. Caffeine does have the same interesting effect on children that Ritalin (the drug of choice for ADHD) does. Caffeine and Ritalin are both stimulants that have a calming effect on hyperactive kids.

Occasional ingestion of caffeine in a kid may leave them wired. But if they chronically use caffeine, they become habituated.

Q: My twenty-month-old son is very healthy, but he will not eat fruits or vegetables. He'll eat a little corn, but no fruit at all. He's a meat-and-potato eater. Will he be harmed in any way because he's missing out on so many vitamins during the years when his brain is developing?

A: A meat-and-potatoes guy, huh? Well, it would be best for him to eat some fruits and green vegetables, but he's not going to wind up with a brain problem if he doesn't.

I think you should persist and work on your skills of disguise. The rule of thumb is to present the food five times in a row, and present it when it's the only food around. Be creative. I can't imagine a kid who'll turn down a fruit smoothie. Or maybe he will eat fruits or veggies if they are chopped or pureed in a blender. Try working fresh blueberries or thinly sliced bananas into pancakes, too, or top ice cream with apples sautéed in butter with a little brown sugar.

We have learned that there is a relationship between taste and genetics. People can be categorized into tasters, super tasters, and nontasters, and a vegetable flavor that appeals to one group actually tastes bitter to others. We think this is why some kids avoid certain foods, although sometimes they just turn it down by habit.

Many parents aren't able to get as far as corn and potatoes, like you did, but I'd love to see you go even further, because there are certain phytonutrients contained only in fruits and vegetables.

Also, be very aware of the messages being sent at mealtimes by other members of the family. If a sibling or a parent is talking negatively about some food, the twenty-month-old may pick up on that, too.

Q: My five-year-old has been a picky eater practically since she stopped nursing. Am I doomed to another thirteen years of difficult meals, until she heads to college, when I won't know what she's eating?

A: I can't really tell you what your daughter will be eating when she's fourteen, though a certain amount of junk food is a distinct possibility. But I do have good news and bad news for the parents of neophobic eaters, a.k.a. picky eaters.

First, the bad news: A study that followed healthy children from age two

QUIZ

Which of these juices is the least nutritionally beneficial, based on a day's worth of vitamins and minerals?
A) apple　　B) prune　　C) orange　　D) cranberry　　E) grape
(A: apple; the old apple-a-day maxim just doesn't fly when it comes to the juice.)

months to eighty-four months (seven years old) showed that this behavior doesn't seem to go away. Children who start out picky stay that way. Children who reject vegetables at two months continued to reject them throughout this study. As these children matured, these behaviors began to be played out in other nonfood events, such as a lack of manners and exhibiting disruptive and oppositional behavior at the table. I know a few of you must be weeping at this point, but hang in there.

As if most mothers didn't have enough guilt already, this study showed that a mother's own food-related behavior and attitudes had a great deal of influence on her children. Researchers suggest that mothers try to choose and cook new foods outside their normal selections.

Furthermore, about half of the children in this study were also in day care.

DID YOU KNOW?
MOST TODDLERS AND PRESCHOOLERS DON'T HAVE GOOD DIETS

If your young children are picky eaters, you are not alone. And if your child's favorite meal is fast food, you need to make some changes at your house. According to the Healthy Eating Index (the official measure of how our diets comply with the recommendations of the USDA's Dietary Guidelines for Americans and the Food Guide Pyramid), the proportion of children ages two to five with good diets, on average, is only 27 percent.

Before you blame these statistics on kids whose families can't afford to feed them properly, think again. There's only a small margin between children in families living in poverty and higher-income children. Among children ages two to five, 22 percent of those living in poverty had a good diet, compared with 29 percent of those living above the poverty line.

Both numbers should make us reassess our priorities for all children.

The study says that because of institutional regulations, menus were not varied enough to reinforce "positive sensory experiences" surrounding varied food choices for these children.

Now for the good news. Researchers found there are no significant differences between picky eaters and kids who ate a variety of foods in terms of the amount of food that kids took in and their height and weight. Growth patterns of all the children in the study were normal.

So, it would seem you are facing a few more battles about meals, but I would suggest you pick those battles, especially if you value your relationship with your daughter.

Q: Will my fat child become an obese adult? Both my husband and I are overweight though not obese, and we try to set good examples at dinnertime. My nine-year-old son is already about fifteen pounds overweight, according to the pediatrician.

A: Studies have shown that heavy newborns tend to become fat children, and that fat children tend to become fat adults. Other studies have shown a link between low birth weight and central obesity—a fat stomach—in adolescence.

To investigate the influence of parents' body types on the body types of their adolescent children, Michigan researchers looked at data on 1,993 babies at the time of birth and when they were either fifteen, sixteen, or seventeen years old. The data was collected in the Child Health and Development Studies conducted by the School of Public Health of the University of California, Berkeley. The children's parents were also measured and categorized as lean or fat.

This is what they found: "Heavy newborns became heavier or fatter adolescents only when the mother or father was also fat and, among heavy newborns, the risk of becoming fat adolescents was 5.7 times higher when the mother was fat rather than lean.

"These findings suggest that fatness during adolescence is related to parental fatness, but not to prenatal fatness." In other words, a fat baby born to skinny parents isn't likely to become a fat teenager.

So the efforts to keep women from gaining too much weight in pregnancy or to cut back on a chubby newborn's food don't seem to have anything to do with the child's weight as it grows up.

I was a very heavy newborn, and my parents were of normal weight, and I grew up to be of normal weight. But if this study is on the mark, if, along with my heavy birth weight, I also had had fat parents, the odds of my being fat would have greatly increased.

But please don't throw in the towel about your child's health just because of these patterns. Your child deserves your absolute attention on this topic, and there are several approaches you could take to get him on the road to a healthier body. To start, talk to your pediatrician about coming up with a concrete plan for your son. And if you don't consider yourself knowledgeable about what constitutes healthy eating, make an appointment with a dietitian.

Finally, think about making weight loss a long-term family plan by taking up a family activity such as hiking, bicycling, or kayaking.

Kids, Sports, and Exercise: Be Careful Out There

Q: I have an athletic ten-year-old daughter who fell and bashed her head at school last week. She blacked out for a minute. Afterward she had nausea and headaches, and we called the doctor. He told me the symptoms were those of concussion and said to bring her in if she got worse. She didn't get worse, and the headaches finally went away about three days ago. According to her, she's feeling fine. We're still restricting her to quiet activities. When should she return to sports and other normal activities?

A: The "second-impact syndrome" is important to consider. When an injured kid gets bonked on the head a second time, a very minor hit can have very dire consequences. So we're very cautious about this.

I don't like the fact that she had headaches and your doctor didn't examine her. By definition, a concussion is a blow to the head that renders one unconscious. So, by definition, she had a concussion.

By now, your daughter is probably in the clear, but I'm really concerned that she had nausea and a headache for several days. This can be a symptom of a little bleeding inside the skull, against the brain. It can resolve itself, which may explain why she now feels better.

I suggest you get a specific recommendation from an experienced sports-medicine practitioner about her readiness to run around again.

Q: I know it's not good for a child to lift weights, but I lift weights and I have an eight-year-old son who likes to do what Dad does. Is it OK for

him to do resistance training with his own body weight, such as push-ups and pull-ups?

A: Of course you are right that this attraction is about imitating what Daddy does. Otherwise, what eight-year-old wants to sit still and lift something up and down, up and down, over and over again?

An adult lifts weights in an organized way to make certain all the muscle groups get a workout. Kids are designed by nature to work all their muscle groups just by doing what kids love to do—run, climb, lift, and jump.

He can join you in push-ups and pull-ups, but nothing else. I expect his interest in exercising your way will be short-lived, and it's a good idea for you to let it fade. According to most sports-medicine professionals, once kids hit puberty, they can do a little resistance training, but none of the maximum, all-out stuff. We have no idea what might happen in an eight-year-old, because we have yet to measure the effects in such a young child.

You are in the happy position of helping your son create a lifetime pattern of exercise. Turning toward fitness is a challenge once we have become fat and lazy; it is a mighty struggle for many adults and even kids. Prevention is where it's at.

Kids also need to know that being fit doesn't have to mean spending hours at the gym. I'd be so happy if more people would just get off their butts and go for a walk.

Q: More than once I've heard you challenge the value of sports for kids.

I don't get it, and I'm wondering if I'm missing something. I have two daughters, ages nine and eleven, and they both play soccer and love it. I love it, too, because I feel it's one of the healthiest things they can do, win or lose. I've also seen lots of statistics that show that girls, in particular, will do better in life overall if they participate in sports. How can this be a bad thing?

A: Please don't get me wrong. I think sports are great for kids. It's been well documented that young women who play sports are less likely to get into drugs and they are more likely to delay sexual relationships. And I'd much rather see boys and girls playing a game of softball or basketball than sitting in front of a television for hours on end. Unfortunately, kids who play team sports such as soccer and football are not as likely to maintain their fitness in aduthood as kids who compete in individual sports like tennis and swimming.

Overzealous parents and ignorant or uninformed coaches are my biggest concern. Sports for kids are about fun and healthy exercise, not winning at any cost. Eating disorders, serious injuries, and unnecessary stress can result, and no kid needs that.

I have a problem with sports when they dominate children's lives to the point that there is no room for anything else.

Pre-puberty and Puberty: Too Early, Too Late

Q: My friend's fourteen-year-old son is going through puberty, and the tissue around one of his nipples is swollen and painful. We want to take him to the doctor, but he's resisting, because he's very self-conscious about this. Is there anything he can take for the soreness?

A: Most likely he doesn't need a doctor. This is common—about two-thirds of young boys have these symptoms—but because the problem isn't talked about, people are under the misperception that it's rare or a cause for alarm.

The swelling and soreness—and soreness is actually a good sign, because it implies inflammation rather than cancer; cancer doesn't usually hurt—happen at the peak of puberty because of sex hormones in his blood. The discomfort may last for as long as six months.

Ibuprofen will probably reduce the pain, because ibuprofen quiets inflammation everywhere in the body. It will soothe him mentally, if not physiologically, just to do something about it.

The Edell Report
Swing-Set Mania: What's Next?

Listen, I know lots of diligent parents are keeping their children away from wonderful wooden structures in parks and backyards because the Consumer Products Safety Commission (CPSC) says wood treated with arsenic-based preservatives can be carcinogenic.

Well, I think this is overkill. Our fear of carcinogens is out of control.

Kids are surrounded by enough stress as it is. They don't need to be worrying that some cool swing or slide might cause cancer—and it's ridiculous to discard a relatively new play structure in a public park, especially considering how little extra money there is in most city budgets for things like parks.

The CPSC has made sure that any new wooden sets sold after 2003 will use arsenic-free wood, and that's fine. But I'd rather see a child spend time on any swing set than sitting in front of a television or a video game.

I hope he is also soothed by knowing that he's not alone. If he takes a look around the gym, he'll notice that a lot of his peers are in the same state.

Q: My eleven-year-old daughter started her period last year. Is it a myth that she won't get any taller? She is 5'2" and so am I. Her father is 6'2".

A: Once puberty begins, the pituitary gland is signaled to slow down on the growth hormone, but it doesn't stop entirely. It would be unusual to stop growing at eleven, so I think she'll add another few inches, but at a slower rate of growth.

Age eleven is a little earlier than the average age for a girl to begin her period, but it's not that unusual. Breast and pubic-hair growth are starting earlier and earlier. We're reorienting ourselves to what "normal" is and to how we define precocious puberty. Children who mature too early—earlier than your daughter—can lose inches from their height. Your pediatrician can check her bone age to be sure.

Q: My daughter is getting close to puberty, so the question of menstruation has come up. Should a young girl wear pads and avoid using tampons for any reason? My daughter is worried about keeping up with activities like swimming and gymnastics during her period.

A: If a girl is comfortable using tampons, there is no reason she shouldn't, especially since many women claim that wearing a pad is uncomfortable and not secure enough for an active female.

Some girls are afraid to put in tampons, so, for the first few cycles, they may want to start out with pads. A pad is a fine option by itself or, later on, in conjunction with a tampon.

Toxic shock syndrome is rare but still out there, and it can be caused by too absorbent a tampon. Teach your daughter appropriate tampon hygiene.

Q: My daughter is eight, and she's already developing breasts. She has not had her period, though. The specialist we took her to suggests we give her a drug called Lupron Depot once a month for two years. Otherwise, the doctor says, she might stop growing. Also, my wife and I really don't want our eight- or nine-year-old to deal with having a period. What do you think of this treatment?

A: I think you are right to ask questions. You want to know what you're doing before you put a little girl on hormones. This treatment is the big dividing line among pediatric endocrinologists right now. Some doctors agree with your doctor, and others would advise you not to medicate her.

A few years ago, I was shocked when I read the first research findings that breast development and pubic-hair growth are now so common among eight- and nine-year-old girls—with African-American girls starting a bit sooner than Caucasian girls do—as to be considered normal.

It turns out, though, that while these secondary sexual characteristics— breast and pubic-hair growth—are beginning earlier, the menstrual cycle doesn't seem to. Do not assume that you will have an ovulating nine-year-old running around the house.

If she is not menstruating, she will continue to grow. Once menstruation begins, a girl's growth does slow, because the onset of puberty signals the brain that she is becoming a teenager. You can always have the doctor track her bone growth, and, if she's falling behind, you can decide then whether or not to treat her.

Your little girl faces less danger from starting her period too early than she does from being overmedicated. I urge you to do some research online. Take what you find to the doctor.

Now, precocious puberty does exist, and if your daughter had started her period, I'd be more inclined to recommend treatment.

Q: My sixteen-year-old daughter still hasn't started her period. Is there something wrong? I know that dieting or extreme exercise can delay periods, but she isn't into either of those.

A: She's late but still on the cusp. For a small percentage of young women, sixteen is a normal age for the first period; so, chances are, this is what's normal for her. If she were eighteen, I'd be more concerned.

Still, I would mention it to her pediatrician. Some girls do need hormones to make their periods start, but I think the doctor will probably want to wait for another six months or so without intervening, unless your daughter has some other symptoms. Also, keep in mind that stress is another thing that can delay the onset of a girl's period. And eating disorders are not always noticed by parents.

There's a positive side to a late start: Studies show that earlier menstruation increases a woman's risk of breast cancer. We think the longer exposure to estrogen—say from the age of thirteen until menopause at fifty—is the culprit.

All the Other Stuff That Gives Us Gray Hair

Q: My granddaughter is ten years old and she's still bedwetting. When my daughter took her to the pediatrician, the doctor really didn't seem that concerned and just said to use an alarm clock and some other tricks. Is there a doctor that she needs to see and any tests that should be done?

A: Believe it or not, bedwetting is not that unusual at age ten—although both the parents and kids involved probably feel it is. In general, we like to do a urinalysis just to make sure the child doesn't have a urinary tract infection.

It is considered good practice to do a "minor" urological workup if the bedwetting persists for months or longer, but I often think that's overkill. A pediatrician should know this territory fairly well, when it comes to a specific test. A pediatric urologist would do the tests.

In terms of helping her, there is a lot more that can be done. First, we've had success with a new generation of little electronic sensors that you put in the child's pajamas or underwear when they go to sleep, and it wakes them up when it senses the first drop of urine. That's very helpful.

There also are medications in nose-drop form that turn the kidneys off briefly so you don't make urine during the night. A lot of pediatricians think it is overkill, but it's effective.

Often, when I talk to parents about this, I find out that they aren't even doing the basics—the kids are still drinking a full glass of water or a soda just before they go to bed, and mom or dad can't figure why they're peeing in the bed.

Restricting liquid for a couple of hours beforehand, then insisting the child use the toilet just before bedtime, is frequently all that is necessary to eliminate the problem.

Finally, a lot of kids are just late getting over this hump. I think I was, and some of my kids were, too. It's important not to make too big of a deal about it, because the kids want to be dry—they can't go to their friends' houses, they're very embarrassed—and you'll find most of the time they will cooperate.

So, your daughter should start by being scrupulous about fluid restriction. I'd get one of the newer sensor alarms—you can get them at a drugstore or through the Internet—and that should do it.

If that doesn't work, and this persists another year or so, then your daughter should go back to the pediatrician and explore possible medications if no urological problems are diagnosed.

Q: Our daughter has always been a thumb sucker. We read that it gives her comfort and it's not a bad thing, so we never made an issue of it. But she is now five years old and she sucks her thumb when she goes to bed and when she gets upset or frustrated. The thumb is really dry and scaly and looks the worse for wear. Is she going to outgrow this habit, or should we try to wean her? If we do, what techniques should we use?

A: My kids used to get those really funky thumbs with funny calluses, too. And I'm not sure I could tell you what age that all stopped, but it did, eventually.

I would continue not to make a big deal about it. One study from the University of California, San Francisco, found that kids who comfort themselves with attachment objects like blankets and toys don't have a higher rate of anxiety or neurosis, and may in fact be less likely to be bullies as teens. I think thumbs fall in this category, too.

The habit can spontaneously dissolve, and since she is mainly succumbing when she's upset and at bedtime, I think she is at the beginning of the end.

Like potty training, a battle over thumb sucking is a battle that parents cannot win. As soon as you turn around, that thumb is back in her mouth. So don't spend your energy on a fight over it. But please do ask her dentist about the consequences to her teeth.

If you do want to influence her, use encouragement. You don't want to demean or embarrass her, but talk to her about what big girls do. An appropriate reward if she can quit is to polish her fingernails. You can even go all out and take her to get a real manicure. Another option that seems to work for some kids is to wrap an Ace bandage on the child's elbow before bedtime,

---

The Edell Report
Kids, Marriage, and Divorce

Are you one of those parents who insists on staying in a miserable marriage "for the sake of the kids"? Well, here's one study that says that's probably OK. What's really important is how you relate to your children, not how you deal with your spouse.

The Journal of Personality and Social Psychology *reported on a long-term study of adolescents and parents and siblings that found that young adults tend to be more successful in their romantic relationships if the parents were warm and supportive toward the kids while they were growing up, regardless of the relationship the parents had with each other.*

I've often said to people: If you're in a bad relationship, you're not showing kids what love is, you're not showing kids that you can value each other. I've always felt you should present something real to your child. You're better off getting divorced than exposing your child to the horrors of the yelling and screaming, which usually happens in a bad relationship.

But this study challenges that notion. It says, "Children appear to mimic the way their parents behave toward the children, not the way parents behave toward each other."

using just enough pressure for the bandage to pull the thumb from the child's mouth when she falls asleep. The bandage should not constrict blood flow in any way.

Five is still pretty young. When I get questions from teenagers who want to quit, I take a different approach.

Q: My husband and I hope to adopt a child from Ukraine. Do you think there could still be health implications from Chernobyl?

A: Health issues can be a factor in foreign adoptions, but Chernobyl is probably not one of them. The people in the Ukraine who are at risk for radiation-related health problems like thyroid disease and certain cancers are those who were alive in the region in 1986, when the explosions occurred.

Babies born overseas, and those who have spent time in orphanages, may have higher rates of certain infectious diseases, like hepatitis and tuberculosis. These are not horrible diseases, and are often self-limiting or treatable, but most Americans who adopt have no experience with them. A simple health evaluation and follow-through should resolve any issue.

Adoption medicine is now a subspecialty. Several states have clinics that specialize in health evaluations and immunizations for adopted children and their new families. You will find a listing of some of the clinics at *www.comeunity.com/adoption/health/clinics.html*.

I know that adopting a child is not an easy, straightforward process. With all the unwanted babies in the world, I think it should be simplified.

Giving a child a home is wonderful. I wish you the best.

Q: I am considering the adoption of a baby from a situation where the mother was a drug addict. What special health questions should I be asking? And what likely health problems would be on the top of your list?

A: The kinds of diseases that a drug-addict mother can contract can definitely be passed on to a child. Most adoption agencies are now very astute at screening children for these diseases, and some are more serious than others. In general, the special health questions that should always be asked revolve around a mother's status during pregnancy and how complete the screening tests will be before a decision is made about the child.

Of course, AIDS and hepatitis C are at the top of the list, although that hardly completes it. I think you should involve a local pediatrician in the process, to make sure the right things happen.

DID YOU KNOW?
DANGER IN THE VITAMIN CABINET

I'm amazed how many folks still express ignorance about one of the most common household dangers. So, here it is again: When it comes to kids, treat vitamins just the way you would treat any other dangerous substance. Keep them well out of reach. And one substance that's particularly toxic is iron. As few as three adult iron tablets can poison a child, even fatally. So, don't put vitamins where they are convenient for you. Put them where your kids can't possibly find them.

Q: I like to practice yoga in the nude in my living room. This has become a problem for my wife, because we have a twelve-year-old daughter, and my wife doesn't think she should be exposed to this. And the therapist my wife sees agrees with her. We have been fairly casual about nudity in our household in the past, and I can't see why this is such a big deal. What's your opinion?

A: This is a bit of a dilemma for me personally, because I think our society could be a little more comfortable with the human body. But, in reality, you're playing with fire. Your wife and you no longer share the same philosophy about nudity in your house, and your behavior is not something a lot of twelve-year-olds would be comfortable with—even in their own homes. Do your yoga in your bedroom with the door closed or put on some clothes, if the living room is the only space that works. You can get the benefits of yoga with your clothes on.

Q: We got back some party pictures the other day, and the kids' eyes have those red dots. I thought I heard you say on the radio that these could indicate eye cancer. But everybody's eyes have the red. Is there something else I should be looking for?

A: The reason you see the red-eye reflex in photos is that the flash in most newer cameras actually bounces off the retina—the back of the eye—and it's picked up by the film as a red spot. You know how you can be driving in the country at night and see animals in the darkness as their eyes reflect your headlights—and their eyes appear to be bright dots? Well, it's the same thing in snapshots. These dots in photos are more common today, because the flash in modern cameras is really close to the lens.

Photography aside, occasionally photos will show a child with one eye showing a red reflex and the other showing a white reflex. That's where you have to be wary. If you ever see that in a photo of someone you know, you need to tell them to see an ophthalmologist immediately.

The white reflex could be a sign of inner eye disease. In children, there is a particular type of cancer, retinoblastoma, that often goes unnoticed, with tragic results. The photo dots can be the first clue, and in my career I have had more than half a dozen people who heard my advice and whose children were subsequently diagnosed with eye cancer. But they would not have known about it if they hadn't known what to look for in those family photographs.

Be persistent. Any time a white reflex appears in a photo it has to be explained by your doctor.

Q: My kids love their little squirting bathtub toys. I know that, in between baths, mold can accumulate on them, but my kids suck on them all the time. How dangerous is it?

A: Isn't it amazing what kids will put in their mouths? In fact, there is a school of thought that says it's kind of OK or even good for kids to be exposed to a variety of germs, because it gives their immune system a workout and that may actually reduce the occurrence of asthma and allergies and things like that.

But there has got to be a limit, and funky water in the bathtub might cross that line for me. There is organic matter in that water, like sloughed skin cells, fecal matter, etc., and if it's sitting around in a toy, germs could grow. And, yes, germs can harm us, and thinking of them sucking on it and drinking the water—yuck! Frankly, though, my own germ-conscious upbringing may be showing through, because no one has ever proven that kids get sick from bathtub toys.

I would be crazy to say that your fear is without foundation, because I think sure, there could be infections that kids get that way—but it's the kid's own germs, too, unless you're putting a bunch of kids in there. And gastrointestinal disease is rampant in kids, though pediatricians don't usually take the time to try to find out the source of these infections.

Just to be safe, I'd stick the toys in the top level of the dishwasher about once a week—if they look like they can handle the heat of the dishwasher. The rest of the time, I would flush them with fresh hot water from the bathroom tap just before use. Remember, the bathwater of that day is going to get into their mouths anyway.

Q: We want to buy an older home, but we're afraid of the lead-based paint. I've been reading about what lead can do to kids, and it's very worrisome. Are we asking for trouble, or are we being ridiculous? I know lots of people with kids who live in old houses, and I haven't heard of any problems. I need a level-headed perspective.

A: If you swept up dust from little crevices in an old house and sent it to a lab, you would probably find higher than normal levels of lead. But as long as you deal with the lead in a prudent way, you have nothing to worry about.

Lead is a problem if you ingest it or breathe it, so you don't want to do that. You also want to be sure that your kids do not pick paint chips off the floors and windowsills.

And if you renovate, you will want to take specific precautions to prevent paint dust from flying around. You have to wear a mask to filter the dust, and use a special power-wash process for removing old paint.

The power wash wets the paint dust and knocks it to the floor. This prevents it from volatizing, floating in the air, and being breathed into the lungs. You should never just rub lead paint with a sander.

Before doing any work on the house, find out what the regulations are. You should be able to get information from your local health department. You might want to get a painter's advice before you buy the house, too.

Q: My daughter had head lice, but I didn't realize it, because she had chicken pox at the same time. I saw bumps on her head that I thought were chicken pox, but when I examined them closely, I saw that they were bugs. By then my daughter was totally miserable. How could I have avoided this?

A: Head lice is every parent's nightmare. You're so afraid of catching them yourself that you don't want to hug your kids, you don't want your kids to see their friends, you start wondering about the seats at the movies, etc. Of course, it's usually the school nurse who finds them, and your child is stigmatized when he or she is sent home. Did I mention that I've had personal experience with this?

The fear is real, because we now know that many products on the market don't work. To fight the resistant bugs, malathion is back on the shelves in a product called Ovide.

Some folks also still rely on nitpicking—combing out the nits in the hair—which is very helpful but time-consuming. In some parts of the world (including New York City), professional nitpickers are back in business. These are people who are paid to sit and pick or comb lice out of kids' hair.

Lice can cause minor infections in the scalp in some kids—scratching can cause excoriations that become infected. As far as I know, lice don't carry disease, though, so it's a benign infection.

What can you do to keep you and your kids from having to deal with such a nuisance? Not much, except to teach your children to not share combs, brushes, or hats. And they shouldn't touch other kids' hair, either. Lice has nothing to do with personal hygiene, and it happens to the best of families.

Q: My four-year-old daughter complains that her bottom hurts. I took a look at her anus, and the skin is a little raw. The sore spot is very tiny. Her pediatrician advised using Neosporin. Is that right? What could have caused this?

A: A child's anus can get raw from foods, overzealous wiping, or constipation. In my experience, most often a fissure—a little raw, open area—is the cause of the pain.

Neosporin is soothing, but it contains some very powerful antibiotics, antibiotics that are too strong to take internally. A fissure is not usually caused by an infection, so I don't know that Neosporin is necessary. Also, Neosporin may cause an allergic reaction on her skin.

Take her for another examination if she doesn't heal soon. If she's constipated, address that with fiber. In adults, they are using Botox to temporarily weaken certain muscles that may be holding open the fissures so they can't heal. But I haven't heard of anything like this that's appropriate for kids.

Q: My four-year-old son constantly washes his hands. I'm hoping it's just a phase, because he worries endlessly about germs. He asks about them every five minutes. How can I reassure him?

A: Let me first reassure you that frequent hand-washing is not uncommon in young kids, but I assume you have a concern that your child is leaning toward an obsessive-compulsive disorder.

I'm the first person to say that a little obsession can be a good thing—I'm no stranger to obsession—because without it some things in life wouldn't get done.

We are constantly bombarded with ads about germs, invisible creatures that can make us sick. This could easily push an anxious child into taking an appropriate behavior—like washing after using the bathroom and before eating—to an extreme.

A simple fact that a lot of kids don't know might help him: Most germs are friendly. The body is covered with good germs that keep out the bad ones. To get this message out to the public, one chapter in my first book, *Eat, Drink, and Be Merry*, is titled "Some Germs Are Your Friends." So, you could tell him that washing his hands too much washes the good germs down the drain. But logic doesn't usually help with obsessions, compulsions, and phobias, if that's what he's dealing with.

Much of the time this behavior turns out to be nothing more than an anxious phase for a child; I watched similar obsessions come and go with my own kids. Sometimes children do need professional help for coping with an obsessive-compulsive disorder, but use caution. You do have to watch out that no pediatrician or child psychiatrist overreacts and immediately medicates your boy because he's a hand washer with no other symptoms.

Q: My little boy is fifteen months old, and I know that taking care of his teeth is a very important part of his hygiene. When should he start using toothpaste, and what kind should I buy?

A: Start him early on a fluoride toothpaste, especially if your water isn't fluoridated. Beyond that, the brand or type of toothpaste is not important. He's not too young to begin now, but if he resists brushing, try giving him a toothbrush just to chew on. Even chewing a toothbrush is helpful in abrading the surfaces of his teeth.

Although toothpaste is perfectly safe when used as directed, you don't want him to swallow too much of it, because swallowing fluoride toothpaste results in bright, white stains on the teeth. He shouldn't use a big old gob that leaves him foaming at the mouth. Teach him to use just a tiny dab of paste.

Include tooth brushing in his morning and bedtime routine. And be patient if he does a lousy job, so the task doesn't become unpleasant. Of course, he's not going to brush perfectly, so don't be alarmed when a lot of spots show up if a dentist applies the dye that highlights the teeth that the brush bypassed.

You may also want to introduce him to an electric toothbrush; lots of kids find these fun to use. What's most important is that your son is comfortable learning the skill.

Q: About a month ago, we noticed a red bump on my three-month-old daughter's thigh. Just today, we took her to the doctor, because it has doubled in size in the last few weeks. The doctor says it is a hemangioma. He measured it and said he wants to wait a month before he would do anything. Does that sound right? Is waiting dangerous?

A: No, waiting is the best advice. Hemangiomas are commonly present at birth, and they almost always go away on their own. It's a mistake to operate, unless they are on the face. These can distort a child's features and bone growth.

Hemangiomas are blood vessel tumors that are totally benign. They show up under the microscope as many tufts of blood vessels and capillaries. One of my sons had a beautiful heart-shaped hemangioma on one buttock when he was born, and we hoped it would be permanent. But it disappeared in a few years.

Q: My daughter frequently spends weekends with a friend whose parents are smokers. I'm concerned about secondhand smoke, especially after seeing a television report linking secondhand smoke to asthma. Do I have anything to worry about?

A: The best answer I can give is that I'd let my kid continue to hang out with her friend.

Yes, smoke is a toxic substance, but those studies are talking about the exposure that comes from living or working with smokers for long periods of time. On some days, your kid is exposed to air pollution that is equivalent to cigarette smoke.

So, while I agree with your concern—and parents should always be aware of the health habits of the people our children spend time with—the risk to your daughter ranks low on the list of dangers our kids face these days, while the upset at not being able to see her friend will rank high on her list.

For their own sake, and the sake of their child, I would hope the parents don't smoke a lot around the kids. But, of course, this is a sensitive issue that I think you should leave alone. No matter how well intentioned we are, people never want someone else's opinion on these touchy topics.

Q: Our pediatrician wants to test my three-year-old son for an extra Y chromosome, because he's very big for his age, very active, and his speech is delayed. What are the ramifications of an extra Y? Should my son have this test?

A: Your pediatrician is sharp to put this together. The normal pattern of chromosomes is XX for females and XY for males. There are a variety of chromosomal abnormalities, including missing chromosomes or extra chromosomes. Some of them cause serious physical problems and some do not.

About one in one thousand male newborns has an extra Y chromosome, and your son does have the symptoms of an XYY male—extreme height and energy, and delayed speech. And while some boys with an extra Y do have learning disabilities and can have attention deficit hyperactivity disorder, anxiety alone is enough to cause hyperactivity and learning difficulty.

It was once believed that extra-Y men were likely to be violent. That has been disproved.

Yes, you should have him tested. If the results are positive, you will be able to prepare for special training and support for you and your son if he needs it. But he may not. There are healthy men who are running around with an extra Y chromosome and they don't know it.

Q: The doctor advised us to put our ten-year-old daughter on growth hormones. In three years, she has grown less than two inches, but the doctor doesn't know why. The growth hormone level in her blood is less than half of normal. She was born premature, after just twenty-eight-weeks gestation. By age two she was up to the fiftieth percentile. But I'm five-ten and my husband is six feet. What do you think?

A: Since she does indeed have a growth-hormone deficiency, it sounds to me like she's getting the proper care. But it's a shame that it took this long to detect the problem.

The one thing she should be checked for is early puberty, because that will slow a child's growth. People think that a child who enters puberty early will be tall, but the opposite is true. Puberty signals the body that growth is coming to an end.

You're lucky to live in a time when we are able to manufacture growth hormone biosynthetically. In the past, we could only get it by grinding up the pituitary glands from cadavers, so we had just a few precious drops available each year. Now it's so easy to come by that sports-crazed parents are giving it to their kids to get them into the NBA.

Your daughter will most likely grow and do well. Your doctor should be able to provide you with some numbers on her likely height when she stops growing for good.

Q: For several years my nine-year-old son has had trouble having regular bowel movements. He will go for more than a week without one. He eats regularly, and he's active. I send him to school with a bottle of water, because I've been told he may not be drinking enough liquid. I've tried herbal teas. I don't want to give him laxatives. Is there anything else I can try?

A: This is a very common problem that's fairly easy to address, because aside from a couple of very rare neurological diseases, there are two main possibilities for the cause: Either he is not eating enough fiber, or he has encopresis. A child with encopresis actually withholds on purpose.

Start by increasing his fiber. Give him a whole-wheat cereal every morning and lots and lots of fruits and vegetables. If that doesn't work, he can take a fiber supplement, but I'd much rather see him get the fiber from the cereal and the produce.

Encopresis can be caused by a painful anal fissure that he's not telling you about, or because he is loath to stop what he's doing to take time for a bowel

---

QUIZ

What is the most likely cause of death for kids between the ages of fifteen and nineteen?

A) motor-vehicle accidents   B) firearms   C) drugs

D) other

(*A: motor-vehicle accidents are the cause of about 37 percent of the deaths. Firearms accounted for about 23 percent of the deaths, though male African-American teenagers are much more likely to die from firearms than vehicular accidents.*)

DEAN'S LIST: BOOKS TO HELP KEEP KIDS HEALTHY

Lots of good books have been written about children's healthcare. Here are just a few:

Asperger Syndrome & Your Child, by Michael D. Powers, PSY.D., with Janet Poland

Breaking the Antibiotic Habit: A Parent's Guide to Coughs, Colds, Ear Infections, and Sore Throats, by Drs. Paul A. Offit, Bonnie Fass-Offit, and Louis M. Bell

The Children's Hospital Guide to Your Child's Health and Development, by Children's Hospital Boston

More Than Moody, Recognizing and Treating Adolescent Depression, by Dr. Harold Koplewicz

The Parent's Complete Guide to Ear Infections, by Dr. Alan R. Greene

Parents in Charge: Setting Healthy, Loving Boundaries for You and Your Child, by Dana Chidekel

The Portable Pediatrician, by Dr. Laura Walther Nathanson, FAAP

Raising Your Spirited Child, by Mary Sheedy Kurcinka

Straight Talk About Psychiatric Medications for Kids, by Dr. Timothy E. Wilens

movement, or because he has an emotional aversion to having a bowel movement.

Do some research on the Internet about encopresis, and, if it fits your son, talk to his pediatrician about it.

Q: My three-year-old nephew swallowed a penny. The doctor said to wait three days for it to pass and to make sure he has no breathing problems. We keep checking, but it hasn't come out. Everything is normal, though. He is eating and sleeping normally. Do we need to do anything?

A: If you are sure that he swallowed a penny and it hasn't come out, he needs to have it removed. A stuck coin can hang up at the esophageal-gastric junction and erode a hole in the place where the esophagus joins the stomach.

That's because coins have zinc, which can be very corrosive.

Kids who swallow coins should always see a doctor. And the first thing they will do is find out where the coin is by using an X-ray machine or even a magnetic scanner.

If the coin hasn't been passed, it usually can be removed with a long tool with a balloon on the end.

Resource List

For the latest legislation and the latest research related to children's health issues, visit Medline Plus, which is provided by the U.S. National Library of Medicine and the National Institutes of Health. Type "children" in the search box on the home page: *www.nlm.nih.gov/medlineplus*

Search for definitive information by topic at the American Academy of Pediatrics Web site: *www.aap.org*

The American Academy of Family Physicians has an easy-to-use Web site packed with advice in both English and Spanish: *www.familydoctor.org*

KidsHealth is an extensive, user-friendly Web site with news and general information targeted toward both kids and adults: *www.kidshealth.org*

The American Academy of Child and Adolescent Psychiatry Web site offers helpful information in both English and Spanish: *www.aacap.org*

Call 1-800-221-7437 to talk to a counselor at First Candle (formerly SIDS Alliance) or find out more about Sudden Infant Death Syndrome at: *www.firstcandle.org*

For information about the various forms of juvenile arthritis, go to the Web site of the Arthritis Foundation, *www.arthritis.org*

For information about port-wine stains and hemangiomas, consult the Vascular Birthmarks Foundation Web site: *www.birthmark.org*

Sign up for a free electronic newsletter at the Autism Society of America: *www.autism-society.org*

Are you looking for a special school program for your child because of disabilities or behavioral or emotional issues? Do you need help finding the right program? Check out the Web site for the Independent Educational Consultants Association: *www.educationalconsulting.org*

For the latest asthma research information, or to see about participating in a clinical study, check out the Asthma Clinical Research Network at *www.acrn.org*

Sign up at the Allergy & Asthma Network Mothers of Asthmatics Web site for free online classes that last three to five minutes each: *www.aanma.org*

Neurofibromatoses are genetic disorders that cause tumors and are often linked to learning disorders. For more information, see The National Neurofibromatosis Foundation Web site: *www.nf.org*

The Tourette Syndrome Association Web site has a variety of helpful information: *www.tsa-usa.org/*

For related questions see chapters 1, 2, 3, 8, 9, 10, 11, and 12.

Chapter 6

"Old" Is All in Your Head. Now Where Did I Put My Hat?

When I was young, I used to dream about living to be a thousand years old. After all, who isn't curious about what the future will bring to our lives, and those of our offspring and the world in general. But as I got older, this youthful fantasy faded into reality. I don't want to watch the world I have known become a totally foreign place. And I sure don't want my kids to have to deal with an old codger for a couple hundred years. As for cryogenics—I have no interest in sharing a freezer with anyone, not even baseball star Ted Williams.

These days, as I find my way through the heart of middle age, quality of life is the most important consideration, a longevity philosophy that research shows is more French than American. I'm not as concerned about whether I live to eighty or ninety as I am about making the most of the time between now and then, and I am convinced that's the healthiest way to get to eighty or ninety.

Before I explain how that works, it is important to understand what we really want. When people say they want to live longer, they actually mean that they want to extend that period of life in which they are most happy and healthy, when their faculties and resources are within their control. But life extension doesn't usually happen that way. When we talk about adding years to a life, it means adding years to a normal life, and that includes the final phase, no matter how long that may last and what shape it may take.

As much as we may enjoy reading stories about ninety-five-year-olds who still drive or swim thirty laps in their pool, and the number of centenarians is growing, do any of us really want the last years extended if we are stuck in a nursing home and are blind, deaf, incontinent, or in the throes of dementia? Not me.

Of course, if we can extend our lives an extra five or ten years, and those are useful and enjoyable years free of ill health, that would seem like a plus. Right now, though, we have yet to find a single strategy that guarantees it. It seems that in the whole of the earth and throughout all its history, with everything being perfect, including perfect genes, and a perfect environment, humans don't seem to live beyond a hundred and twenty. Ponce De León's search for the Fountain of Youth may have been among the first efforts in North America to find a magic potion for longevity, but we know this was a hot topic even in the time of the Romans, when it was believed that the goddess Hebe could restore beauty and youth to the aged. Well, folks, there was no magic potion then and there's none now. Not selenium supplements, not coral calcium, not hormone replacement. It is easier than ever to *look* younger, if that's important to you, but no amount of Botox is going to add years to your life.

What we do know that the Romans and Ponce de León didn't is that literally thousands of separate factors determine the day when you and I will take the last breath, and considering that we only know a few of them, and can control only a few of them, I don't think it's healthy to spend your entire life worrying about how long you will live and what ailments may strike you. My life story is a simple case in point.

As I write this, my father is ninety, and my mother is in her mid-eighties, and they've had imperfect health habits throughout their lives. Both were smokers, and both have standard meat-and-potato American diets, and, to my knowledge, they have never gotten one minute of intentional exercise. All in all, hardly models for longevity.

At times I've thought I could get away with murder because of this history—and studies do show I am more likely to live a long life—but I now believe that reckless behavior is stupid.

My parents aside, we do know that people who reach one hundred, in general, did not follow health fads and diets. They do seem to be fairly moderate in their lifestyles, and they also *enjoy* life. But the truth of the matter is that the most important factor is genes. After that, most of the newer studies are finding that lifestyle factors that have to do with our psychological lives may play more of a role than we ever thought. In other words, people who make the most out of life—who go to concerts, read books, play games, have social interactions—have a leg up on those who don't. This, of course, cannot be sold in a pill, and it takes some work.

This does not make us immune by any means, but research has shown that even one of the most high-profile and feared diseases—Alzheimer's— may be thwarted by staying stimulated and maintaining an interest in life.

When I spontaneously find myself in the midst of some major family get-together, and everyone is laughing and having a good time, I realize this is exactly what healthy aging is all about. These are moments you can't go out and purchase, you can't obtain with a fast-food mentality. This is the advice I got from my parents, that family and happiness were things to be culti-vated—built and nurtured over the long term.

What we often fail to understand when we are in our twenties and thir-ties is that, as you get older, there seems to be a general acceptance of hav-ing done things that life offers. Most people, when I talk to them about extending their lives, really don't want to go back and redo what they've been through. They've enjoyed building their careers and building their families and watching their grandchildren grow, and as they retire into whatever life they've created for themselves—whether it's a golf commu-nity or a small town where things are simpler—many people, as they age, begin to accept the ultimate reality of life and the fact that no one will escape death.

The flip side of this aging scenario is one that is on the wane, thank goodness. I cannot relate to those folks who have energy for only one thing, usually a job, and who expect to reach sixty-five and find that everything will be just fine when they "retire"—as if we can postpone living until we reach a certain age. Too often that approach to life leads to alcoholism and depression—and an early death. Surveys have shown that people who live well into their eighties will tell you that the best years of their lives came after the age of fifty—but these are folks who recognized the key ingredients of emotionally sophisticated and stable lives at an early age. They didn't spend their lives watching endless TV or complaining about what "might have been."

Either because of past family experiences or certain personality traits, not all of us are lucky enough to have that insight. I used to have a coworker who was the thriftiest—and least adventurous—person I had ever known. She would never take vacations or do anything else nice for herself. She was single and childless, so it wasn't as if she was preserving her money for family reasons. I was constantly urging her to live life for the moment, but she did not share my philosophy. She had her reasons, and it could be she feared reaching old age without the resources to care for herself. Of course, she should have just told me it was none of my business how she lived her life. Still, in my book, a "healthy" life is one that makes the most of every day. You cannot buy the experience of going to Europe at twenty-eight—or forty-eight—when you are seventy-five, even if you make it to that age and are still seeing the world.

Of course, finances are a reality for every generation, and I don't think that living in debt—or wondering how you will pay the mortgage—is a recipe for a long life. We know more and more about stress, and it's not a good thing. Neither is staying in a bad marriage, becoming anxious every time a word or memory eludes you, or living lean because your kids have told you they expect an inheritance. Divorce can be a healthy decision at any age, most of us will not get Alzheimer's, and you don't owe your kids anything beyond your love and affection.

That said, one smart estate planner once told me that rather than leaving your kids a bunch of dough, give it to them while you're alive, piecemeal, so you can have the pleasure of making their lives a little easier or seeing them do things they might not have done. Not all of us have that luxury, though, and I believe our relationships with friends, siblings, children, and grandchildren are at their healthiest when they're based not on money but on simply sharing time together.

Another important element of healthy aging is one that most of us would still rather avoid. The inevitabilities of life seem to be among the most difficult subjects for us to talk about with our immediate families. While we acknowledge that we have trouble talking about sex with our kids, and about money and sex with our partners, death is probably the most difficult and most avoided subject of all. Get used to talking about it with your kids, and, when the time comes, they will be used to talking about it with you, which will be a benefit to all.

Living a Long Life: What's Important?

Q: My sister and I are close, and we'd like to retire to the same area of the country. Is there such a thing as the "perfect" environment for a long, healthy retirement? I figure there must be some reason so many old people live in Florida and Arizona.

A: Only you can decide what's best for you. I'm a city boy, but I love the country and hope to spend my latter years in a rural environment. I can cope well in the city, and enjoy it, but I've known people who live in the country, and when they come to the big city, they just become one frazzled bundle of nerves. What stresses one person can be much different from what stresses another person.

By the same token, a person who has spent a lifetime being emotionally miserable isn't going to be instantly happy because of a move to a new environment—at least not unless he or she also gets counseling.

Usually, as we get older, we develop a better understanding of what we need and want, of what is in our best interests. Doing things because other people want you to do them, or doing things because you think you *should* do them, is not usually productive or healthy. Focus on what *you* want in your life—and from your environment—and that should help you find the "perfect" environment. If you're still stumped, spend a month or so with your sister in each of your top-of-the-list destinations before you make a permanent move.

You could also adopt the philosophy of one of my favorite bumper stickers: "Wherever you go, there you are." Good luck.

Q: Should I get physicals more regularly once I turn fifty? I don't want to be a hypochondriac, but I don't want to be careless either.

QUIZ

Which lifestyle habit is most likely to contribute to successful aging?
A) breakfast   B) seven to eight hours of sleep each night
C) optimism   D) social contact with others
E) all of the above
(*E: all of the above; of course, lots of other factors may play a role, too, from having a pet to doing crossword puzzles.*)

A: As we age, doctors recommend fewer physicals, but more specific testing, and those tests are constantly being analyzed for their value.

For instance, chest X rays are no longer routinely done, because the people who got chest X rays didn't seem to have lower rates of death from lung cancer. In fact, if lung cancer shows up on an X ray, then it may already be too late to cure you. Not so with the colonoscopy; this test screens for colon cancer and it's considered a lifesaver. It's recommended that anyone with a family history of that cancer get this test at the age of fifty and that the rest of us have an annual fecal occult blood test (also known as the stool test, or the Hemmocult test), at the very least.

When it comes to mammograms, they are essential for adult women of all ages, but they are being supplemented by sonograms in some instances. And researchers have determined that the type of breast cancer cells you have may be more important than how early breast cancer is detected. Does this mean you should stop getting mammograms or get them less often? No, but ask your doctor where he/she stands on the topic.

What tests should be at the top of your list as you age? Regular blood pressure and cholesterol checks can pay dividends. That's because catching high blood pressure or heart disease early on can make a difference in your ultimate risk for serious illness and death. And PSA tests, as controversial as they are, are done beginning at age fifty. Other tests are less important as we age, such as the Pap smear for women. But don't stop any regular tests without talking to your doctor; he or she knows best what your body and your family history dictate.

In general, talk to your physician about how often to have a physical or specific tests. Only he or she will know what "risk" factors might justify certain tests on a regular basis.

People who worry a lot about these things can have too many and, often, unnecessary tests. This can shorten your life, too, because test taking can be stressful, and if you are constantly being tested, the problem of false positives (which can require a more intense—and possibly dangerous—level of testing) becomes a factor sooner or later.

Q: My father's mother lived to be ninety-five, and most of her sisters lived well into their eighties. Can my siblings and I count on such good fortune in our later years?

A: Yes and no. While nothing is guaranteed, a recent study at the Boston

---

The Edell Report
Save Yourself from the Flu!

Each year 20,000–30,000 people, mostly adults over the age of sixty-five, die from the flu, yet only 54 percent of adults, mainly those in the sixty-five-plus age bracket, get a flu shot. This is crazy, because the flu not only kills but can cause debilitation—and Medicare pays for the shot.

The recommended time for a vaccination is October or November, but if you wind up being delayed until December, go ahead and get it. The shot is effective two weeks after it is given, and we never know exactly when the flu season will start.

The main reason people are not getting these shots is that they don't know about them, and their doctor has no incentive to remind them. Medicare reimbursement rates for pneumonia and flu shots are less than half what pediatricians receive for childhood immunizations. So, you've got to watch out for yourself on this one. And if you have someone who provides care for you in your home, make sure he or she has been vaccinated, too.

See more about the flu in chapter 9.

Medical Center and Boston University Medical School, looking at 444 families where at least one person lived to be a hundred, found good news for both the brothers and sisters of the centenarians. The guys were seventeen times more likely to get to a hundred, and the women were eight times more likely to hit the triple digits.

However, this may be the toughest aging concept of all, even though it sounds simple: On average, a thousand people whose parents lived to be a hundred will live longer than the thousand people whose parents died in their sixties. Yet, in both groups, some people will live beyond those ages, and some won't get close.

Some people think, "I have good genes, so I can smoke a pack of cigarettes every day." That's a gamble I would never take. Actually, the more important information to take from your parents' lives is their medical history. There's a reason doctors ask for your family's medical history, and the more complete your knowledge, the better your doctor will be at assessing future risk. In the meantime, take care of yourself.

Q: I'm sixty, in excellent health and hoping to stay that way. What vitamins should I make sure to include in my daily regimen?

A: So many of us fall prey to the idea that there is some magical food or supplement that will immediately transport us to health nirvana. That's naïve and, if you bite, potentially very expensive.

While all the hype and misinformation out there would lead you to believe that vitamins will get you to a ripe old age, that's fiction. We did once think that vitamins were helpful because people who took vitamins seemed to be healthier.

However, a closer look at the studies showed that most people who took vitamins did so because they could afford them. They made more money, because they were in higher social demographic groups, and therefore they took better care of themselves, ate better diets, got more exercise—and could afford to see a doctor whenever they needed to. As you can see, we weren't comparing apples with apples.

The results of double-blind studies—where one group takes vitamins and one group takes a dummy pill—were not only disappointing but also a little frightening. For instance, recent studies on vitamins A, C, and E showed they may do more harm than good. We've seen higher rates of cancer, higher rates of heart disease, and other problems in those who were taking the active vitamins. Part of that may be the fact that the vitamins that are contained in vitamin pills are the result of older thinking and older technology.

We are finding, for instance, that the form of vitamin A and vitamin E

DID YOU KNOW?
LOOKING INTO THE CRYSTAL BALL

The U.S. Census Bureau demographic indicators for 2000 and 2025 show life-expectancy-at-birth averages increasing by about four years, from 76.6 to 80.5 years.

found in vitamin pills is different from the form of those vitamins found in food.

Don't assume that you can eat a lousy diet and take vitamins, and that the vitamins will make up for it. They will not. In fact, eating fruits and vegetables has been shown over and over again to be the best way to get your vitamins, no matter what your age. Adding a simple multiple vitamin, not a megadose, is probably OK, but don't have unrealistic expectations.

Q: Do you think good relationships among adult siblings make for healthier lives? Aren't our spouses and our children enough emotional support? I am part of a big, semi-dysfunctional family that has managed to work up quite a debate on this topic.

A: Most research shows that strong connections to family and friends seem to increase longevity—and I've never met a family that didn't have its occasional bickering, no matter how strong the bonds.

When I compare time spent on a treadmill to time spent enjoying children, tackling family projects, or just taking a walk around the block, it's a no-brainer to me what has more long-term worth. And, usually, the latter is a lot more fun, which is the point, right?

However, if you seldom take pleasure from being with your siblings, you need to step back and assess why that is. Maybe the situation is fixable, and maybe you will need to draw instead on your best nonfamily friendships for the happiness you can't find within your family.

Q: All my friends—we're in our late sixties—are curious about the various anti-aging medicines you see in stores and in ads. Are there any that actually have some value? Are these all human-growth hormones?

QUIZ

In 1900, in the United States, one in 1,500 women lived to be a hundred. Today, that ratio is:
A) one in 350   B) one in 22   C) one in 135   D) one in 40
(D: one in 40; according to the New England Centenarian Study, *90 percent of centenarians are women, 10 percent are men.)*

A: You see the ads everywhere because we have become so neurotic and anxiety-ridden about aging that some of us will buy anything we think might keep us young. In fact, one of the latest fads—human-growth hormones (HGH)—may have the opposite effect.

HGH can cause diabetes, it may make your joints ache, and there is also a risk of cancer. While it might slightly increase muscle mass—and slightly decrease fat tissue—the results are not worth it. If you look at people who have extra growth hormone in their body because of a disease called acromegaly, you will see people with big, thick knuckles, square jaws, diabetes, and tumor growths, among other symptoms. This is serious stuff.

Growth hormone is expensive medicine administered by injection. What the health-food stores peddle—usually amino acid mixtures that purportedly increase HGH output by the pituitary gland—are worthless.

Depression and Other Emotional Issues

Q: My father, who just turned sixty-five and has been divorced for several years, seems to focus more and more on the negatives in his life, in spite of many good things he could celebrate. It's wearing me down, but I also wonder what impact this is having on his health, which is generally good. Could he be dealing with depression?

A: Depression in older people is extremely important to acknowledge, because older folks do not manifest it the way younger people do. You cannot count on seeing a parent in a down mood to diagnose depression. Your mom or dad may simply get more anxious about things. It takes a professional to spot this. See if you can convince your dad to see a psychologist or a psychiatrist, and it would be even better if you can find one whose specialty is geriatrics. Or call his primary care doctor and mention your concerns.

Depression is a common illness among the elderly, especially after someone experiences trauma, such as injuries from a bad fall, major surgery, or the loss of a spouse. It can be effectively treated, but only when it is diagnosed. While there is a lot of debate about the ultimate origins of depression, there are a lot of things you can do, and some solutions don't require medications. Unfortunately, many folks avoid seeing their doctor for depression, because they think medication is the only solution—or they are embarrassed.

Depressed folks often string together a series of negative thoughts. In other words, if one thing goes wrong, they begin to think that everything is going to go wrong, and they get themselves worked into a downward spiral.

You may find that your father is resistant to seeking professional help; there is still a stigma about mental illness in this country that is very sad and dangerous, particularly among older people who may have never had an experience with a psychologist or psychiatrist. It is a brave and wonderful thing to be able to seek help when one is down, and the results can be remarkable.

Q: My mother recently died, and I'm worried about my dad, especially since he doesn't live close to any of his children. We see him about twice a year. He's sixty-eight, in good health, and just recently retired. What should I do?

A: I'm not sure you can do much. First, recognize that the death of a spouse is the most stressful event a person can go through. On scales of stress that psychologists have devised, it ranks No. 1. And death rates for surviving spouses are increased, so your concern is appropriate.

Of course, many people go through this and survive and do well, but it takes time. You have to be patient and supportive and let him know that you are available. I'd also make impromptu phone calls at different times of the day, just to see what he's up to. If he's seeing friends and is involved in activities, he will probably be fine.

Frequently, the children of aging parents come to think that they are better judges of what's good for their parents than the parents themselves. That's a sad mistake, and one to avoid at all costs. Children who want to "take over" while the parent is still capable of independence should first look twenty years down the road and ask themselves, "Would I want my children to treat me this way?"

Q: I don't want to rush my parents to their graves, but I think they're in denial about death. They're both in their early seventies, and generally in good health, but their children—me included—think it would be a good thing if we had some idea about their wishes, should they become critically ill or die suddenly. As the oldest child, I've been asked to get some answers, but they get defensive when I bring up the subject. How can I get them to cooperate?

A: No parent wants to hear their children contemplating their demise. And it's a very scary subject for some folks and a very private one, too. But it's also an important subject, so don't give up.

The Edell Report
The "Other" Aging Fear

Memory loss and Alzheimer's may be getting most of the attention when it comes to "hot" aging topics, but another issue ranks right up there: falling. Fortunately, folks, this is a health issue that can be attacked more easily than dementia. And, as with most fears, if we let it control us, it can have as detrimental effect as the actual event we fear.

The fear of falling is so great among some people over sixty that they can begin to dramatically restrict their activities—even to the point of not going outside. Of course, there is some foundation for this fear: Bad falls can lead to broken bones or worse, as was the case with publishing legend Katharine Graham and diet guru Dr. Robert Atkins, both of whom died from bad falls. But many studies have shown that inactivity can lead to depression and declining health, so the fear of falling is not to be taken lightly.

One pilot program in Boston found that those fears began to lessen after participants began talking openly about their fears, looked at how to fix home hazards, began strength and balance exercises, and set goals for increased activity levels. That makes complete sense to me.

I also can understand why there have been mixed results on studies about the effectiveness of external hip protectors. There are various brands to help protect the elderly who have weak bones and a high risk of falling, but the thought of wearing special underwear padded with plastic inserts makes me feel old. Give me tai chi any day.

The way to bring this up would be to discuss it in terms of what your mom and dad each want to happen should they become seriously ill and are not able to make their own decisions. Show them a Living Will or "power of attorney for health care," which you can get specifically for your parents' state of residence through the Internet for about ten to twelve dollars. If you explain that knowing their wishes will help avoid any major family disputes about appropriate treatments, they might be more cooperative.

I see many people who are thrown emotionally as they face the end of their lives because they've never thought much about death, or have been in denial about it. By the same token, I've come across folks who, when they know they are facing the end, have some of their finest moments. After all, it's a period when you can/should stop worrying about college tuition and the gutters and the lawn. You are free to do, say, and feel things that might have been more difficult before. This is a subject that our culture needs a lot of help with. Facing death does not have to be as horrible as many people think it is.

That said, don't talk to your folks like they are going to die next year. After all, they are only in their early seventies. On average, they have a lot of living to do. If your parents continue to resist any discussion, consider writing a joint letter from the children to them, expressing your love, concern, and desire to make sure their wishes are known and fulfilled.

If none of that works, throw in the towel. You don't need any more stress on this subject, and neither do they.

Osteoporosis, Bad Backs, Hips, Knees, etc.

Q: My mother broke her hip when she was about sixty, but she was never told she had osteoporosis. She's seventy-eight now and has not broken any other bones. I'm a forty-eight-year-old woman who has no signs of osteoporosis, and when my doctor asked me if there was any history of osteoporosis in my family, I said no. But I then mentioned that my mother had once broken her hip, and my doctor insists she has osteoporosis. Can you clarify this for me?

A: I think the medical community has oversold osteoporosis as this horrible, debilitating disease—the scourge of all women. I'm not suggesting it's a good thing, but worrying excessively about it isn't going to help.

A broken hip can be very devastating, because having to put people to bed—especially older people—can lead to other problems, including pneumonia, which can lead to death. That's why we are very aggressive about broken hips, and perform surgery. While it implies a weakness to bones, one can't be sure, because broken hips can happen to anyone at any age.

We are at a very confusing stage with osteoporosis, because we don't know exactly how thin bones need to be before we step in. There are many things that can be done to prevent this disease, though nothing is perfect. It seems to be more common in thin, blue-eyed Caucasian women than women of color. The heavier you are the less likely you are to get osteoporosis. This is possibly because the extra weight causes your bones to respond by thickening up.

Calcium is not the magical cure-all that some will tell you, although adequate calcium is essential to keep bones appropriately thick. Eating too much protein and certain other negative dietary habits, like not getting enough vitamin A and D, can cause bone loss.

Q: The surgeon wants to use a metal-on-metal hip for my mother's hip replacement surgery. He says that the materials have been used in Europe for a while and have just been FDA-approved in the United States. What's your opinion?

A: I have heard good things about the metal-on-metal artificial hip. This is not my expertise, of course, but I would trust her orthopedist. No matter what material is used, for someone suffering with pain, hip replacement surgery can have amazing results.

The weak link in artificial hips is not the materials but how they are attached to the bone. You have probably already heard the terms "cemented" and "uncemented"—which has to do with whether the new hip is glued to the existing bone. Generally, we glue the new joint into the bone, especially in older folks, because we don't want to wait for the bone to grow around it. We want to get the patient up and out of bed fast because there is always the danger of potentially deadly bladder or lung infections developing in an older person lying in bed for a long time. So we are aggressive in keeping these patients in motion.

These hips will last ten years and more, depending on how they're used, and people who have been in pain and are now pain-free absolutely love them.

Q: Ten years ago, when I was forty-nine, my family doctor told me to take two Tums twice a day to help prevent osteoporosis. I'm still doing this, but my son recently questioned the wisdom of this. Could I be hurting my stomach?

A: Tums is a very cheap form of calcium, and, if you need a calcium supplement, it would be appropriate. But people shouldn't take calcium just because they are in their forties, because you can get calcium in other parts of your diet, and extra calcium alone does not seem to help everyone.

Thinning of the bones is not just due to a lack of calcium. In fact, many people who have thinning of the bones have eaten adequate calcium throughout their lives. There are other factors involved, including hormones, exercise, body weight, and genetics.

Tums is not going to hurt you but, of course, it is mostly used as an antacid, so I can't help but wonder if it could impact your digestion of some foods, though there's no proof that will happen. And I am never wild about the idea of taking something like this for a lifetime. Finally, one new study suggests that the risk of food allergy is higher in people who take antacids.

Talk to your gynecologist about this.

Q: I've been a runner for thirty years and I'm now sixty-five. I have some knee pain but not bad enough to take medication. What am I doing to my knees if I keep running 10Ks?

A: Lots of people run because they want to assure long-term good health. Well, unfortunately, many are beginning to pay dearly for this effort.

Avid runners and other serious recreational athletes can face a future of osteoarthritis and other joint problems. So let me repeat what I've said many times on my show: You don't have to run 10Ks to be healthy.

The best evidence tells us that just brisk walking three or four times a week for a half hour will give you most of the benefits that you can expect from exercise in terms of your heart. If you're a professional or you really love your sport, that's a bit different. In that case, the risks may be offset by the pleasure you get from it. But don't be naïve—no body joints are designed to take a beating like this all your life.

And osteoarthritis, we fear, is a wear-and-tear disease. Since you have been running for thirty years and are just now experiencing pain, you've gotten away with murder. "No pain, no gain" is a preposterous concept, yet people still believe it. Before you go any further, you need to find out if you are harming your cartilage or ligaments, or if you have an inflammatory disease, because continued running could be something you will really regret later on.

If you reach the point of extreme pain, you might consider knee replacement. This surgery can produce fabulous results, though the new knee will never function as well as the old one, and there are complications. The joint can loosen, there's always the risk of infection, and it's possible the surgery won't take. Talk to your doctor, should that time come.

Q: I know I'm asking a question that's hard to answer, but I'm hoping you can offer some guidelines on the subject of joint pain that comes naturally as we age. How do we know what's an appropriate amount of discomfort when we wake up in the morning? I'm fifty-six and in generally good health, but I can't help but notice that I'm stiffer when I first get up, compared to, say, ten years ago. At this rate, what will I be like when I'm eighty?

A: When you sleep for seven or eight hours, your body usually stiffens up, so morning pain and stiffness are normal, but it's a matter of degree. If you have swelling, redness, soreness to the touch, or the pain persists throughout the day, then see your doctor.

Of course, arthritis is a common diagnosis for joint pain (the word means "joint inflammation") but most people don't know that there are more than a hundred different types of arthritis, including the most common—osteoarthritis and rheumatoid arthritis.

The ailment that can make you feel old is also one of the oldest known diseases. In fact, signs of arthritis were found in the spine and hip joints of a mummified body of a man that has been dubbed the "Iceman." The mummy is 5,300 years old. The mummy also showed signs of hardening of the arteries. This, of course, undermines the argument that disease is the product of our modern world, doesn't it?

Q: I'm sixty-seven, and I've had chronic back problems for years. I finally got some relief with an epidural cortisone shot, but the doctor says there's no guarantee that the results will last. Can you explain this treatment, and is it legit?

A: This is the best way to use cortisone. Many people fear this drug, because they've heard it can have side effects and, indeed, it can. But that's when you take it as a pill, or when you take shots that are meant to go throughout your body. When cortisone is injected into specific spots in your joints (it's usually done on an outpatient basis at a hospital), it delivers a very powerful anti-inflammatory wallop, and it does not affect the rest of your body, because the formula we use prevents it from disseminating easily.

Some people get amazing results with the very first shot—they literally go from extreme pain to no pain in twenty-four hours—while others have to have several shots. Of course, as with all treatments, it doesn't work for everyone. You can do this many times, and if it makes you feel better, why not? Because cortisone works by suppressing inflammation, the success of the shot tells you that inflammation is an important part of your basic back problem, which could help your doctor make a diagnosis.

Q: Is weight loss a sign of depression in the elderly? My mother has had no recent diagnoses of illness, but I can't help but notice that she's getting thinner and thinner.

A: Weight loss in any adult has to be taken seriously if it's not purposeful. Yes, some people get depressed and eat less and lose weight, but other people get depressed and eat more. If her appetite is the same, and she's losing weight, she needs to see a physician. One of the first signs of cancer is weight loss, and if you ignore this, it can have devastating consequences.

The Heart

Q: My husband, who's seventy-one, was hospitalized for a week after a moderate heart attack. Soon after he left the hospital, we went to the mountains for a long-planned weekend trip, and we had to leave immediately, because he couldn't breathe. I'm scared about what's coming next, but, unfortunately, he's really bad about asking the doctor questions, and he won't let me come with him. What can I do?

A: There are two problems here. One, men. Men hate to go to doctors; men hate to admit they are needy or that they have a problem. Put it in the same category as men not liking to ask directions. Shortness of breath is a very important symptom with heart disease. If he had a heart attack, and he's having trouble breathing at a higher altitude, that could be an important sign of a failing heart. But frankly, if a moderate change in altitude caused shortness of breath, he either has a heart on the verge of failure, or he just got anxious.

He needs to see a physician, and if he won't do it, you need to drag him there and speak for him. This is not a time for couples therapy, because time is of the essence, and his physician needs to know what's going on. If he's angry with you, he'll get over it eventually.

If he's at all cooperative, the two of you should sit down before the doctor's visit and write down any questions you might have. Then you're sure to make the most of the time with his doctor.

Medicine is making great strides with heart treatment, and death rates are dropping, but heart disease is still the No. 1 killer. The most recent statistics show it accounted for 33 percent of all deaths for all races for both men and women sixty-five and older. If that doesn't get your husband's attention, nothing will.

Q: My husband is forty-two years old and healthy, but he lost his father to a heart attack at age forty-three. He also has an uncle who is sixty and has had four angioplasties. So, as you can imagine, he is starting to get a bit nervous.

The Edell Report
Do You Want Resuscitation?

Not too long ago, an eighty-five-year-old retired British nurse had a little red heart tattooed on her chest. It wasn't a statement of love, it was a statement of desire. The heart had a slash through it and was surrounded by the words "do not resuscitate."

I love this story—it's the kind of vignette that I often use at the beginning of my radio show—but unfortunately, the issue of DNR is so much more complicated—and hardly humorous.

DNR, "do not resuscitate," or "pre-hospital medical care directives," all refer to the same thing—medical orders that can be an ethical and legal quagmire for patients, families, caregivers, and hospitals.

At their simplest, they are statements signed by both an individual and his or her doctor that request that no CPR or other resuscitative efforts be used to restart the person's heart or breathing. Seems pretty straightforward, right?

Wrong!

All kinds of issues surround DNRs, including: a "pre-hospital" form may not be recognized at the hospital, should you make it that far; private businesses, such as nursing homes and assisted-living communities,

A doctor on the news the other night was advocating the use of a whole-body CT scan to screen for heart blockages. Do you recommend this or anything else for our peace of mind?

A: Those CT scans you see advertised can pick up some problems, and they are noninvasive. But because it's usually done in a shopping mall, the whole context of your medical history is ignored. They are condemned by most doctors, because they pick up lots of false positives, causing instant high anxiety, and they do not screen for most of the common cancers, including breast and prostate. Plus, when it comes to the heart, CT scans only show calcium in the arteries, and calcium measurement alone doesn't tell you

may have their own rules—and you need to know those; not all family members may recognize a DNR, and, if a hospital is faced with a dispute among family members—and lawsuits are threatened—they are not likely to act quickly; a DNR is not automatically transferable from one state to another; DNR laws vary from state to state; and, finally, not all doctors will automatically respond to your DNR, even if all family members agree, and sometimes that means families have to go to court to have it enforced.

I urge anyone who is seriously ill or has a close family member who is seriously ill to learn everything you can about this subject before you face a life-threatening medical crisis. At the very least, make sure the primary-care doctor has been consulted for his or her views on DNR, and familiarize yourself with the policies of the hospital that is most likely to be involved. And it is essential that all immediate family members know the affected parent or sibling's view on this issue.

Some people fear that having a DNR gives a hospital license to provide substandard care. If you have those fears, get a second opinion from your primary care doctor.

Bottom line: A simple tattoo is not likely to have much impact all by itself.

everything you need to know. Your husband needs something more specific than that.

The best thing your husband can do is to eat right, get exercise, and take care of himself. He is not old enough for a routine cardiovascular workup, but with the family history he has, his doctor will probably order a stress EKG, which will give an electrical reading of his heart under physical pressure. The CT scan is a halfway measure, and halfway is not enough to let him relax. If he were to apply for life insurance, the insurance company would pay for an EKG; they would not rely on the CT scan. The insurance company is going to put up a million dollars on his life, so they really want to know, and the stress EKG is the gold standard for noninvasive tests.

An angiogram is another sophisticated cardiology test, but it requires injecting dye right into the arteries. It allows the doctor to give the arteries an "all clear" or to say, "Uh oh, this one is clogged." These tests can tell if a patient has a normal amount of cholesterol plaque in his arteries for his age, or if he has more or less than normal.

It has predictive value, but not enough to make a person feel complacent about negative results or panic-stricken about positive ones. If he does have a serious blockage, his doctor would take him to the next level of evaluation and consider treatment.

Q: I worry constantly about my dad, who has had three heart attacks in the last twenty years. He tries to watch his diet and get regular exercise — he has a treadmill. How much more can he control about his situation?

A: Beyond whatever program and medications his doctor has prescribed, diet and exercise are the mainstays for preventing second, third, fourth, and

---

QUIZ

What is the five-year survival rate for heart-transplant patients?

A) 45 percent   B) 53 percent   C) 64 percent

D) 71 percent   E) 81 percent

(D: 71 percent; the one-year survival rate for heart transplants is now 85 percent.)

subsequent heart attacks. Often, what is not discussed is the problem of stress. Major studies have found that a combination of relaxation exercises, like yoga, as well as active exercise and diet, are the most helpful in preventing heart attacks down the road.

Some folks, after a heart attack, spend the rest of their lives worrying all the time. That adds extra stress that makes matters worse. So his current mental attitude should determine whether he needs additional help to deal with stress.

If you're worrying about this more than he is, you need to take a deep breath and back off. He doesn't need that. And you don't either.

Q: I have atrial fibrillation that kicks in periodically when I'm under a lot of stress, and that worries me. I've been told not to eat chocolate. It's not the caffeine in chocolate that's a problem, but the chocolate itself. To the best of my knowledge, I haven't had caffeine for a long time. I am on digoxin, which seems to delay my memory. Is there something else my doctor should be doing to treat me?

A: Atrial fibrillation (AF) is a fluttering heart. In other words, the two small upper chambers of your heart (the atria) quiver instead of beating effectively.

As you know, chocolate does contain caffeine, and also theobromine, which is a stimulant and a vasodilator. But, to my knowledge, the small amounts in chocolate are just not enough to do people any harm.

Large amounts of chocolate can kill a dog, though, and the theobromine in the chocolate is the fatal ingredient.

Of course, you should avoid huge amounts of caffeine, but I don't think you need to avoid it altogether. However, you should follow your doctor's orders, and if you're getting along without caffeine, you may as well stay off it. By the way, alcohol can increase your risk, too.

Digoxin comes from the foxglove plant, and is one of the oldest herbal-based drugs around. Vincent van Gogh was given it to treat his mental illness, and large doses of digoxin can certainly affect mental function. I would doubt that you're on a very large dose, though. It's also important to have your blood thinned to prevent clots, which are more common with AF.

Beyond medication, there are a variety of treatments for this disorder, from electrical cardioversion to atrial pacemakers. People with AF can have normal hearts, with no problems in their coronary arteries.

Q: I am a fit eighty-one-year-old who eats two fried eggs almost every morning. Should I be worried about my breakfast ritual? My wife eats toast with butter and she thinks her diet is better than mine.

A: This reminds me of a question I once had from a ninety-four-year-old who was worried about his pack-a-day cigarette habit. There are many people who can eat foods and enjoy habits that kill other folks. And yet, they live a long life. There are no automatic rules to be followed or broken at this age.

In fact, research tells us that when you get into this age bracket, it doesn't matter what you do. For instance, we've never proved that reducing cholesterol levels in older people increases their longevity. If you live this long, your body seems to be used to whatever you've been doing all your life, and you'll do just fine.

And if you and your wife love toast and butter and coffee and fried eggs,

---

DID YOU KNOW?
IF YOUR HUSBAND IS SERIOUSLY ILL...

Every day, many women face the challenge of caring for a sick husband, and no one has ever said that is easy. But only recently have we learned just how unhealthy family caregiving can be, especially for women caring for their spouses.

When a doctor at Harvard Medical School looked at the heart disease statistics for the more than 54,000 women who participated in the Nurses' Health Study, she found that those who had to care for a sick spouse for more than nine hours a week were almost twice as likely to end up with heart disease.

The study said that the stress from increased financial pressure as well as the stress of juggling work with caregiving may be factors in the increased risk, which is higher than the risk for women who are caregivers of parents or children—where there may be more sharing of the caregiving responsibilities.

If your husband needs your care, please take care of *yourself*, too.

---

who's to say that isn't an appropriate choice for you, to get the benefit of the things you enjoy while accumulating a tiny bit of risk, if any? A little indulgence is part of the enjoyment of life. I say, go for it. Remember, there are no such things as evil foods—just as there are no "miracle" foods. As part of a moderate, varied diet, you can eat whatever you want. The key word here is "moderate."

Q: I've just been diagnosed with high cholesterol—it's 215—and I'm really confused by the "good" and the "bad." I'm sixty-one and considered relatively healthy. Can you give me some general guidelines to get this under control?

A: A high-cholesterol level is one of possibly two hundred fifty to three hundred health factors, all of which contribute to your risk for heart disease. It's just that cholesterol is so easy to measure, and we're so into it, that we make a big deal about it. Thirty percent of people who arrive at the hospital dead from a heart attack have normal or below-normal cholesterol levels, while many people with high-cholesterol levels live very long lives. So, I wouldn't get crazy about the numbers.

If you are taking care of yourself and eating appropriately, the number may not matter. After all, if every person in the universe ate exactly the same diet, we would still not all have the same cholesterol levels or longevity.

It's made more confusing because there are subtypes of cholesterol. There's a good cholesterol, HDL, which should be high, and LDL cholesterol, which should be low. The first line of attack would be to reduce saturated fat intake, eat your fruits and veggies, cross your fingers, and get some exercise. There's a lot we don't understand. For instance, the French eat tons of saturated fat and seem to have better cholesterol levels and fewer heart attacks than we do.

Perhaps it's all the fruits and vegetables they eat, and perhaps it's their attitude. We can't count on anything here. Relax.

Q: My mom is premenopausal, and her cholesterol has gone from 170 last year to 260 this year. She only weighs 125 pounds and sticks to a vegetarian diet. What would make her cholesterol level go up so suddenly?

A: I'd repeat the test. I can't tell you how many times cholesterol tests have been inaccurate. You can take it three times during the week, and it can be different. Sometimes it can be different three times a day.

It is important that your mother find out what's really going on. That is a huge increase in a year's time, and menopause or perimenopause shouldn't change those numbers.

There are many other tests they can perform to predict a risk of heart attack, and if they think that she has a high risk, and her cholesterol level turns out to be the same the next time, then you might consider doing further tests.

But first, I'd repeat the test. You'd be surprised how infrequently that is done. Doctors get one test and automatically put people on medication for the rest of their lives without retesting. If it's something serious like that, we want to make certain that medication is needed.

Q: My mom is seventy-six, 5′5″, and weighs 160 pounds—or is about 35 pounds overweight. Otherwise, she's in good health. Isn't this weight bad for her heart? Does she need to worry?

A: Many people are surprised to find out that almost all the studies show: When you get into your senior years, in general, being overweight is not associated with mortality. If those pounds were going to harm you, you would have died a long time ago. Consequently, we also have no evidence that, if you lose weight, you will do any better. In fact, most of the studies find that when older people try to lose weight, they make themselves less healthy and increase their mortality. That's the opposite of what the diet industry is telling you, but that's the scientific proof so far.

If your mother has any of the diseases associated with being overweight, like high blood pressure or diabetes, her doctor may still advise her to lose some weight.

Q: My father has just been diagnosed with congestive heart failure. Can you help me understand this? I'm not sure what his prognosis is, and his explanation of what his doctor said hasn't been very helpful.

A: First, go with your dad to his next doctor's appointment and don't leave until you understand what's going on.

Congestive heart failure (CHF) has many causes, including coronary artery disease, diabetes, viruses in the heart muscle, and high blood pressure. While there are some genetic relationships to those, CHF is a final end point that means the heart is weak. When whatever disease your father has starts to affect the strength of the heart muscle, less blood is pumped, then fluid pressure backs up, and you get swollen ankles and fluid in the lungs. This can be treated with medication unless the heart is too far gone.

Alzheimer's, Dementia, and General Memory Loss

Q: Is Alzheimer's hereditary? My mom has just been diagnosed with it, and I'm not only worried about her but wondering what my future holds.

A: There is a hereditary component to Alzheimer's disease, especially if your mom is under sixty, but your risk is only slightly increased, and, therefore, the odds are that you won't get it, because most people don't.

There isn't much you can do about it except stay active and keep your mind occupied, which is something you want to do anyway, for your basic happiness in life. People who keep using their minds have lower rates of this disease.

So, I would not fret, and we expect to soon have the ability to diagnose this long before people get the disease. Your much bigger challenge right now will be your mom's care as the disease progresses. Talk with your siblings and your father—if he is still alive and involved in your mother's life—about long-term plans. There are also a ton of books on this subject as well as other resources; see pages 311 and 312 for more information.

Q: My girlfriend's mother has vascular dementia, and the doctor made a point of saying it's not Alzheimer's. What's the difference? When I was a child, my grandfather was diagnosed with hardening of the arteries. Since he forgot who everyone was, and eventually had to be hospitalized, I'm assuming that would now be called Alzheimer's. Am I right?

A: Dementia is the symptom we see in elderly people as they lose their mental functions. While there are many causes, from vitamin deficiency to brain tumors to neurological disease, the two most common causes are Alzheimer's and hardening of the arteries.

Hardening of the arteries happens when less oxygen gets to the brain, and dementia sets in. Alzheimer's is a specific disease, and the cause is still unknown. With Alzheimer's, the deterioration is relatively steady and relentless. Mental function deteriorates, and so does personality; often, once-happy people may become angry or bitter.

With vascular dementia, the changes seem to occur in more defined steps, with personality and insight better preserved than in Alzheimer's cases. Also, strokelike symptoms may eventually appear, such as weakness in an arm, leg, or eye muscle.

Q: How do you know when someone with Alzheimer's needs to go into a nursing home? I am having a horrible struggle making a decision about my husband's care.

A: This is a very difficult decision to face, and there is no clear line to cross over, no crisp and clean medical test that gives an answer.

When a person just can't care for themselves anymore, or becomes hostile, or wanders away and becomes a danger to themselves, then the time for a nursing home may have arrived. I can tell you that the most common reason that elderly people are put in long-term care is loss of bladder control. Their family usually can't deal with that at home. Very often, the care in a nursing home can be better than the care provided by the family. The staff is profes-

---

DEAN'S LIST: ALZHEIMER'S BOOKS

Hundreds of books have been written on Alzheimer's—for people who have Alzheimer's, for their families, for caregivers, and for anyone who wants to do what they can to keep their brain sharp. Here are just a few that provide solid information, insight, and solace.

Alzheimer's Disease: A Guide for Families and Caregivers, by Lenore Powell, Ed.D., with Katie Courtice.

Dancing on Quicksand: A Gift of Friendship in the Age of Alzheimer's, by Marilyn Mitchell

Death in Slow Motion: My Mother's Descent into Alzheimer's, by Eleanor Cooney

The Memory Cure: How to Protect Your Brain Against Memory Loss and Alzheimer's Disease, by Dr. Majid Fotuhi and Peter Rabins

Staying Connected While Letting Go: The Paradox of Alzheimer's Caregiving, by Sandy Braff and Mary Rose Olenik

There's Still a Person in There: The Complete Guide to Treating and Coping With Alzheimer's, by Michael Castleman, Dolores Gallagher-Thompson, Ph.D., and Matthew Naythons, M.D.

The 36-Hour Day: A Family Guide to Caring for Persons with Alzheimer Disease, Related Dementing Illnesses, and Memory Loss in Later Life, by Nancy L. Mace and Peter Rabins

sional, and they can do things that you just can't do, and, very often, the patient is happier.

Caring for a loved one with Alzheimer's is probably the most stressful job in the world. Recently some researchers wanted highly stressed subjects for an experiment on how stress relates to wound healing. They chose people caring for demented patients as the most stressed-out people in the universe.

Beyond the actual work and the time it takes, you're dealing with pain, love, anxiety, and anger. You have thoughts that you feel guilty about; I know the kinds of things that run through a person's mind.

I think you might be asking me the question because you feel the time for the nursing home has come, and maybe you have guilt about that. You are the person who will go on. You need to care for yourself, too. Too often, caregivers lose sight of that.

Q: I'm forty-two, and occasionally I find myself forgetting where I parked the car at the mall. Is this the first sign of Alzheimer's? If not, is there anything that can be done to prevent Alzheimer's?

A: The onset of Alzheimer's occasionally happens to people in their fifties, but that's rare. So your age is the best indicator that you're just distracted when you park.

So far it seems that there are no pills, vitamins, or nutrients that are proven to have a significant impact on your risk for Alzheimer's. Research shows that the best protection seems to be using your brain.

It's possible that the cause of Alzheimer's may go back to our youth. A classic study of nuns when they entered the convent found that in their teenage years those who had poorer vocabularies and less ability to express themselves in writing were the most likely to get Alzheimer's sixty or seventy years later.

The more educated you are the less likely you are to get Alzheimer's, but again, there are no absolutes. The famous English novelist Iris Murdoch is probably the most notable intellectual to suffer from the disease in recent years— and the only one whose story was made into a movie.

Q: I'm a fifty-two-year-old woman in very good health, but my gynecologist has put me on estrogen because of my frustrations with grasping for the right word. Is she overreacting, or am I overreacting to getting "old"?

A: Short-term memory loss and a slight decline in mental abilities are part

DID YOU KNOW?
STAY SMART: HAVE A CUP OF COFFEE

Anyone who has listened to my show knows I *love* coffee. Well, according to a study from the University of California at San Diego, older women who share my passion may have a leg up on those who don't. Unfortunately for me, the results for older men who drink coffee weren't nearly as definitive. In short, researchers tested 890 women, and one of the factors was coffee consumption. In acuity tests, women eighty and older who were lifetime coffee drinkers scored higher on eleven of the twelve tests involving memory, calculation, and categories (for example, how many animals can you name in a minute?). Score one more for a good ol' cuppa joe.

and parcel of growing older. And our expectations of what we should remember are unreasonable. Every time we forget a phone number or lose the keys, we think there's something wrong.

Stress also contributes to short-term memory loss. It happens to all of us.

If we measure short-term memory in a hundred people, who—like you—feel they have abnormal memory loss for their age, we find that very few of them have a deficit; it's all in their head.

Knowing this, if you are still worried, I would want you to take a standard memory test. A simple list of items to memorize and repeat will give you and your doctor objective evidence to use in making a decision. Many people just need to hear they are within the normal range.

If you do have a significant loss, a neurologist should check you out, because that is not a symptom to take lightly.

On another point, I think we've overmedicalized menopause, and we've just learned a hard lesson with estrogen. The common thinking had been that estrogen would prevent some of these problems that naturally occur. We've now learned that estrogen is a bad idea for most women in menopause, because of its side effects—and it doesn't improve memory.

Men have similar changes, but they don't have a menstrual period that stops all of a sudden and tells them they've reached a certain age. Women, unfortunately, have to face this, and I think it creates unnecessary anxiety.

Menopause is not a disease and doesn't seem to be as bothersome in other cultures, where women aren't pummeled with so much scary news. Also, it's important to know that certain side effects of menopause, like hot flashes, vaginitis, and thin bones, are treatable without estrogens.

See related questions in chapter 4.

Strokes, Parkinson's Disease, and Other Neurological Disorders

Q: Occasionally, my husband's right hand shakes when he's holding a glass of wine or a cup of coffee, and I'm beginning to think he has Parkin-

---

The Edell Report
Stroke Checklist

I'm amazed at how many people still don't know the signs of a stroke. If you have one or more of these symptoms, don't fool around. Call 911, because the sooner a stroke is treated, the better your chances of recovery.

Some people fear that having a DNR gives a hospital license to provide substandard care. If you have those fears, get a second opinion from your primary care doctor.

- *Sudden numbness or weakness of the face, arm, or leg, especially on one side of the body*
- *Sudden confusion, trouble speaking or understanding*
- *Sudden trouble seeing in one or both eyes*
- *Sudden trouble walking, or dizziness, loss of balance or coordination*
- *A sudden, severe headache with no known cause*

---

son's disease. Is there anything else it could be? And what kind of doctor should he see? Of course, he'd rather just ignore this.

A: If your hand starts to shake when you do things like reaching for a cup, it's usually a more benign form of tremor. Alcohol temporarily lessens this type of tremor and anxiety aggravates it. It may be inherited, and most physicians would not do much about it.

With Parkinson's, the tremor occurs when you are still and not using your hands. As soon as you try to do something, the tremor will disappear. I once knew a surgeon who had Parkinson's. He would walk into the room shaking like a leaf, certainly not inspiring confidence in the patient. But as soon as he picked up the scalpel, he was as steady as a rock. This, of course, didn't last as his Parkinson's progressed to the later stages.

When in doubt about tremors, the doctor to see is a neurologist, who specializes in all matters related to the nervous system.

Q: Have you ever heard of something called transient global amnesia (TGA)? My father was recently diagnosed with this, but he isn't saying much about what happened.

A: TGA is an attack where a person suddenly becomes confused and loses memory about recent events and even things that happened several years ago. It's caused by a temporary decrease in the flow of blood to the brain, and memory loss can last as briefly as a few minutes to as long as many hours. This almost always goes away, and most people do not have a recurrence of it. A small percentage of folks who have this—around 10 to 15 percent—will eventually have a stroke. This is due to a temporary lack of oxygen to a part of the brain.

TGA should not be confused with transient ischemic attacks (TIA), which are commonly known as "mini-strokes." These need to be addressed immediately, because about 10 percent of the people who experience them go on to have a full-blown stroke within ninety days.

While dramatic memory loss occurs with TGA, people with TIAs suddenly become confused or have trouble speaking or understanding what's being said. Other symptoms include sudden numbness or weakness, usually on one side of the body, sudden and severe headache, dizziness or loss of balance, or trouble seeing out of one or both eyes.

Even if the symptoms pass quickly, you must see a doctor immediately. I mean within twenty-four hours, not a week later.

DID YOU KNOW?
A LITTLE VODKA IN YOUR CAPPUCCINO?

In 2003, an experimental drug that combines caffeine and ethyl alcohol—it's called caffeinol—has shown good results in early-stage testing with a small number of stroke victims, though not with those stroke patients who also had serious heart disease. The drug has reduced brain damage in rats, but still faces extensive research.

Q: When I wake up in the morning, my arm or hand may be numb. Isn't this one of the signs of stroke?

A: Waking up in the morning with a numb arm is usually caused by sleeping in a funny position that pushes on any one of a number of nerves and blocks the nerve impulses, and thus you have the numbness. A stroke, of course, can cause numbness as well as weakness.

It's unfortunate that most people are unaware of the warning signs of a stroke, because we can help people the most in the first few hours after a stroke. As time goes on, it becomes harder and harder to do anything, so we need to be more aware of stroke symptoms (see the list on page 293).

A stroke can be caused by a hemorrhage or a lack of blood flow to parts of the brain because the arteries are blocked. If you get to the hospital quickly enough, clot-dissolving medications can get rid of the clots that are clogging the arteries.

Q: I belong to a board of directors. One gentleman, who has always been an excitable guy, has returned to the board after recovering from a stroke. Now the other members tell me not to disagree with him and risk upsetting him, because I might cause him to have another stroke. Are they right?

A: When I sat on a board, my mandate was to represent the stockholders by doing what's best for the company. If that means arguing, that's what I'm required to do. I don't mean to be cruel, but he shouldn't be on the board if his health is affecting his ability to meet his obligations.

My opinion on this is probably a moot point, however, because although many an angry mother has yelled, "You kids will give me a stroke!," there is no clear evidence that anger induces a stroke. Certainly someone at some time has had an argument and five minutes later had a stroke. But assuming cause and effect would be a mistake.

A stroke is caused by either a hemorrhage or a clot, and chronic stress and chronic agitation could, over a long period of time, lead to physiological events that would lead to a stroke.

We have found that the rates of heart attacks, and strokes to a lesser degree, do increase during panic—an earthquake or a fire, for example.

You can go easy on this guy, of course, but you also need to speak your mind.

Q: Last month my wife, who is seventy-eight, went to the doctor for a monthly blood test. After the nurse and doctor both checked her pulse, they sent her straight to the hospital emergency room. It seems she was on the verge of having a stroke. She feels very lucky, and she now realizes that the shortness of breath she experienced the day before the hospitalization was a warning sign. Is there something more she could have done to keep this from happening?

A: The most likely possibility here is that your wife was experiencing atrial fibrillation. As the atria wiggles at a high frequency, the blood can clot. Then the ventricle pumps out that clot, which can go to the brain and block the blood flow. A risk of stroke is more likely in people who have this type of arrhythmia.

And an irregular pulse is always something you should check with your doctor. The pulse should have a regular beat to it. It's hard to say that shortness of breath is a warning sign for stroke, but it is definitely a serious symptom. Any shortness of breath has to be investigated immediately, because it implies there is something wrong with the breathing mechanism or the heart.

Q: My uncle had a stroke several years ago, and his right arm and hand have been almost useless since then. At sixty-five, he's still a relatively young man; is there any kind of therapy that might help him?

A: A stroke is kind of like a heart attack in the brain, and one result can be that the cells than control certain parts of our body die. It is possible that other cells in the brain can take over some of those functions, but after a few years pass, such changes are less likely.

However, physical therapy can be useful. One relatively new and very interesting technique is called mirror therapy, where a mirror is positioned so that the patient, while trying to move their hands or arms symmetrically, can watch their good arm in the mirror. Somehow the brain, with its unique vision, sends impulses to help stimulate the disabled part of the body. This is not mainstream therapy, and it is not yet widely available, but early research has been positive.

Another option is biofeedback. Encourage your uncle to go back to the doctor who's been treating him—or to find someone new who will take a closer look at this situation. His best bet may be a physiatrist, a medical doctor who specializes in physical medicine and rehabilitation. For information about this specialty, as well as information on doctors in your area, check out *www.aapmr.org*, the Web site for the American Academy of Physical Medicine and Rehabilitation.

Q: I just saw a newspaper story about "silent strokes." Are they any different from regular strokes? Do they have the same warning signs?

A: Silent heart attacks and silent strokes are very frustrating. Many people go to the doctor and the doctor says, "My gosh, you've had a heart attack," and you have no memory of any untoward event. The same can happen with a stroke.

The mechanism in a silent stroke is similar to that of a regular stroke in that it's akin to a heart attack in the brain. There's a lack of blood supply to a part of the brain due to a clot or a hemorrhage. The difference with silent strokes is that you didn't notice any changes to your body at the time it happened. However, silent strokes can cause memory problems, a change in your gait—you suddenly start walking different—or even your mood. Most of the time it's passed off as a sign of aging.

It's very important to recognize that the symptoms of a silent stroke, if they are noticeable, come on rather quickly. If someone has been noticing memory loss gradually over a couple of years, that's not a silent stroke. All strokes have significant and permanent symptoms, such as weakness in one side of the body or a severe change in the ability to speak or think.

Glaucoma, Cataracts, Magnifying Glasses…

Q: My eighty-year-old dad still has 20/20 vision, but he just flunked his driving exam; the examiner said his peripheral vision is bad. Under-

standably, my dad is upset—and scared. He has a doctor's appointment, but I hope you can tell me what's going on. Will he go completely blind?

A: I can't give you concrete answers about blindness without actually examining the eyes, but it is likely your dad has glaucoma.

The routine type of glaucoma does not cause symptoms, which is why we want everyone, once they hit middle age, to have regular glaucoma tests. When the peripheral vision goes, the central vision—which is really more important—is still preserved, but eventually that will go, too, if the disease is not treated. So, in your dad's case, if he were looking down a long table, he would probably see everything down the middle of the table, but nothing along the sides.

A visual acuity exam will not pick up glaucoma, simply because the central vision is not affected in early glaucoma. However, an eye exam that includes checking eye pressure and peripheral vision will pick up early signs and symptoms.

Both optometrists and ophthalmologists can do pressure tests; just make sure to ask if you are being tested for glaucoma.

Q: Can you explain the difference between regular glaucoma and angle-closure glaucoma? My dad has just been diagnosed with the "angle-closure" type, and I had never heard of it.

A: First of all, it's good you are learning more about this disease, because it is more common among people who have a family history of it. This type of glaucoma strikes about 10 percent of all people who have glaucoma, and Eskimos, Asians, women, and the elderly are more likely to have it.

QUIZ

Who is at higher risk of getting glaucoma?
A) Caucasians   B) Hispanics   C) African-Americans
D) Asians
(*C: African-Americans. Glaucoma is treatable but it cannot be cured. Senior citizens and those who have diabetes or a family history of glaucoma are also at higher risk.*)

Its name comes from the fact that it occurs when the iris (the colored part of the eye) gets sucked into the drainage mechanism out toward the white part of the eye. The eye fluid can't get out, and the pressure suddenly rises.

Often there are no signs or symptoms before an attack, but with an attack there are symptoms that include ocular pain—which can be among the most severe pains seen in medicine—and/or redness, blurred or decreased vision, colored halos, headache, nausea, and vomiting. The preferred treatment, laser peripheral iridotomy, makes a hole in the iris to drain the fluid. It's a quick and simple operation that cures the condition for good.

Q: I am going to be seventy-six, and I have macular degeneration. My left eye is much worse than the right. I thought I heard you say that lutein was a good thing, and that it may even reverse the degeneration. Since my doctor hasn't said anything about this, should I bring it up?

A: Lutein and similar supplements are among those rare products found in health food stores that might be beneficial, though there's lots of disagreement among ophthalmologists about their effectiveness and not much proof. Do talk to your doctor.

We have found in surveys of people with macular degeneration that those who consume more fruits and vegetables in their lifetimes seem to have a lower rate of degeneration. But what we don't know is if that means these people also got more exercise and were less likely to smoke. This is hard to pin down.

Lutein is a yellow pigment found in a variety of fruits and vegetables, from broccoli and spinach to all the green veggies, plus tomatoes, oranges, even eggs. These same foods have other nutrients that also have been found to be beneficial in preventing or slowing the progress of macular degeneration.

Q: I'm having trouble reading "close up," but my neighbor told me I'm going to weaken my eyes if I buy a pair of drugstore reading glasses. I really don't have the extra money to go to the eye doctor right now, and this would be a lot cheaper, but I don't want to hurt my eyes. Is she right?

A: One of the great constants in biology is presbyopia, the loss of ability to focus on things close up as we age. This assumes you are not nearsighted. Many people use reading glasses they buy in a drugstore, or magnifying glasses. (In the spirit of full disclosure, I have for many years had my own brand of reading glasses.) It used to be thought that these would weaken the eyes, but that's an old wives' tale. There's no problem using anything you can to see better, because straining when you read can cause muscle fatigue and headaches.

Of course, regular eye exams are very important, and if your distance vision is sliding, you need to see your eye doctor.

Q: I'm fifty-two, and my doctor told me last year that I had small cataracts. I didn't have any symptoms then. Now, I have a lot of blurred vision, and he tells me the cataracts have matured and should be removed. Does this mean that I'm aging prematurely?

A: I would not conclude that the rest of you is falling apart. Some people wrinkle prematurely, but they have healthy hearts and they're not showing other signs of age.

Cataracts can be like that, too. There is such a thing as slow-growing congenital cataracts that you have at birth. Also, ultraviolet light is a contributing factor, so cataract development may accelerate in people who spend a lot of time outdoors without sunglasses.

People who lack phytonutrients—who don't eat enough fruits and vegetables—are vulnerable to early cataracts, as are diabetics.

The good thing about cataract surgery is that you can have it whenever you're ready for it, whenever you decide that your vision loss is affecting your life. There's no harm in waiting. The surgery has a great success rate, and that's true whether you get it tomorrow or wait for years. You'll be very happy with the results.

In the meantime, wear sunglasses and eat your vegetables.

Q: I notice in myself and in other people, too, that, as we age, our pupils aren't as bright, and the whites of the eyes aren't as white. Can this be reversed?

A: Over time, fat deposits accumulate in the eye, and they do dull the white color. The clump of fatty cells in the middle of the white of the eye and next to the nose also gets bigger as we age. A slight yellow cast or a dull color is normal.

You can try over-the-counter vasoconstrictors—eye drops—that are made to erase the redness of irritated eyes. Otherwise, I don't know of anything that will undo this natural process.

Yellow that is more than slight is a sign of liver disease. If the whites of the eyes become yellow, a person should see a doctor right away. That's jaundice. A freckle or mole in the eye can indicate melanoma (cancer), so don't ignore those either.

As for changes to the pupil, those aren't a normal part of aging. A dull or cloudy pupil is a sign of disease, so, if that's the case, see a doctor.

The pupil is the little black round hole in the middle of the iris that opens and closes in reaction to light. Healthy pupils are a deep, rich, reflective, liquidy-black color. If it's cloudy, you should not see well out of that eye and you probably have a cataract.

Q: I've been wearing glasses since I was twelve, and I'm now fifty-four. As the years go by, I need stronger and stronger glasses. I've heard ads on the radio about an eye-exercise method that promises to eliminate or greatly reduce the need for glasses. They are offering a money-back guarantee. Do these work?

A: Throughout my professional career I've seen eye-exercise plans come and go, and you've just stumbled across the plan of the month.

This same plan in various disguises has been around since at least the 1920s, when a doctor named W. H. Bates developed the Bates Method of exercises, claiming you wouldn't need glasses. He represented a sort of anti-glasses "philosophy" that proclaims that glasses don't really get to the source of the problem. It's true; they don't. But what they do is correct your vision and enable you to see.

If your eyeball is too big, you will be nearsighted. If your eyeball is too small, you will be farsighted. It's fairly simple. Glasses can't change the size of your eyeball, but they correct your vision so you can see.

I know of no evidence that eye exercises will alter anyone's eyesight. If they did, do you think you would ever see an eye doctor wearing eyeglasses?

There is a treatment that uses progressively flatter contact lenses to change the shape of your cornea. This works to a certain degree, but it's only a temporary fix. You also have to wear retainer lenses at night.

Anytime a guarantee is given on a health product, you should be suspicious, because any legitimate health product will not guarantee its results. No procedure, no device, is 100 percent risk-free, and the producer of a legitimate product knows that.

Squinting will temporarily alter the shape of your cornea to a small degree and can create a kind of pinhole, which improves your vision while you squint, but in terms of getting rid of your glasses, that's not going to happen in the foreseeable future. Of course, there are newer and better kinds of laser surgery to correct nearsightedness and astigmatism. Talk to a professional.

Miscellaneous: Hearing, Wrinkles, Sleep, and More

Q: My mother is convinced that my dad, who is eighty-one, has a hearing problem, and I think she's right. But he refuses to acknowledge it, and every so often he shocks us by repeating something we said in a low voice,

---

The Edell Report
Health and Driving Risks: Watch Out

Driving a car is inherently dangerous for all of us. But when it comes to denying a driver's license for health reasons, authorities tend to pick on people with certain diseases, and it really isn't fair in most cases.

I've told you about how heart disease is the No. 1 culprit when it comes to older people who have car accidents, and one study says this is true, independent of the medications being used. This is because heart problems can trigger such physical manifestations as diminished coronary or cerebral blood flow, cardiac arrhythmia, or anginal episodes.

Other major risk factors among drivers over the age of sixty-five is a history of stroke, arthritis in women, and a number of drugs, according to a report in the American Journal of Epidemiology.

In the arthritis research, University of Alabama researchers say that older female drivers with the ailment were found to be 1.8 times more likely to be involved in a crash than women without arthritis, regardless of whether they fit into the category of at-fault or not-at-fault drivers. While arthritis can reduce some muscle function, I don't think this is a good enough reason to consider denying driving privileges to all women who suffer from joint pains.

I'm worried that as we start examining all the disorders that could

assuming he wouldn't hear us. Although he isn't a vain man, we know he thinks a hearing aid will make him look old. Any suggestions?

A: This tells me that he has some hearing and, of course, he could have some hearing loss. Many people resist getting this treated because of vanity. But hearing aids have changed a lot over the years, and many of them are quite unnoticeable.

I think it's important to have your dad ask his physician next time he sees him if a hearing test is warranted. There are a couple of simple screening tests that doctors can use to see if a person's hearing is adequate. Some people

---

lead to potentially dangerous drivers being on the road, we're going down a slippery slope. For example, by percentage, teenagers have more accidents than all other age groups, so should we ban all young people from getting behind the wheel? Of course not.

When one person having a diabetic seizure caused a crash on the Golden Gate Bridge in San Francisco, there was an immediate call for keeping driver's licenses out of the hands of certain types of diabetic patients. That's ridiculous. The fact is, there are millions of diabetics in this country who drive, and because they're aware of their condition they have a low risk of having an accident.

If someone snores, they could have sleep apnea. That's a very common cause of daytime sleepiness and vehicular accidents. Should all snorers be denied licenses? How about folks with high cholesterol? We could carry this to such an extreme that we'd have to take everyone's license away.

The issue of whether it is safe for certain people with health conditions to drive is of concern to all of us, but I want to see factual information—resulting from valid studies and not based on assumptions—before we arbitrarily deny driver's licenses.

As a final note on how complicated this subject is, the American Medical Association offers a guide to help patients and doctors deal with the issue of impaired older drivers. It's 226 pages! Find it at www. ama-assn.org.

don't mind some hearing loss, and you'll notice their ability to hear can vary, depending on background noise and different situations.

I think it's your dad's decision as long as he's willing to talk openly about this.

Hearing aids are very expensive, and it's often suggested that the patient borrow one similar to the type that's recommended by the doctor, to try it out and see if it helps. It's not a perfect technology, and not everyone benefits from the same type of hearing aid. You might suggest that gently to him and see if this helps. If he refuses, I think at this particular point, since he does seem to have some hearing, you should drop the subject.

Q: As I grow older—I'm sixty-two and in generally good health—I seem to be sleeping less. Is that a good thing?

A: It depends on how you feel about it. While, in general, you hear that you are supposed to get eight hours of sleep a night, that's as silly as expecting everyone on earth to have the same body weight. Some people do OK on less sleep, some people require more. Super Bowl–winning football coach Jon Gruden is one of the more extreme cases of someone who doesn't seem to need much sleep. Reportedly, he usually goes to sleep around midnight and rises a little after three A.M. But, on average, most of us need at least six to seven hours of sleep.

If you feel OK in the daytime, and you're not excessively sleepy—for instance, when you drive a car or try to concentrate on a task—then I don't think this is a problem. But if you find yourself anxious and lying awake all night, and it's bothering you, then seeking help would be important.

You don't have to just take sleeping pills. There's a whole area of treatment called sleep hygiene, which, unfortunately, many physicians don't participate in. In this particular case, they can teach you the skills necessary to sleep better. Studies have shown that while people who take sleeping pills do better in the beginning, after months of this treatment those learning sleep hygiene do much better than those taking pills. (See more about this on page 533 in chapter 12.)

Q: I'm worried that my mother is too old to drive. As you can imagine, this is not a popular topic; in fact, she refuses to discuss it with me or any of my siblings. She's eighty-three, she sees a doctor regularly, she has not had any accidents, and she just passed another driving test. But she moves

slowly, and I'm afraid her reaction time would be terrible in a difficult situation. Any advice?

A: Whenever I get this question on a show, I'm tempted to move right on
to the next caller, because it's a real can o' worms.

First of all, if she has legally passed the driving test you are facing an
uphill battle if you want the license revoked. There is some question about
whether most driving tests are stringent enough for older drivers. After all, it's
easy to imagine passing the test while in the early stages of Alzheimer's disease or having minimal dysfunctions. But to assume that older drivers are automatically bad drivers is a big mistake.

There are certain types of maneuvers that, research has found, are more difficult for older drivers—such as making a left turn into traffic. On the other
hand, they drive more carefully and slowly, much to the annoyance of others.
Yes, your mom moves more slowly, and the reaction time, if we could measure
it, would be slower. But that's probably the case with every driver out there
who has a cell phone or a cup of coffee in their hand or kids fighting in the
back seat.

The 64 million–dollar question is, at what point should we take away the
driver's licenses of senior citizens.

Right now the statistics tell us that Alzheimer's disease, certain heart diseases, and definable neurological disease should be cause for withdrawal of a
license. But I don't think anyone is willing to tackle the issue of taking
licenses from people who are generally healthy but not as spry as they used to
be. The most important thing is to keep trying to talk to your mom without
seeming threatening. And try to observe her driving whenever possible. After
all, other people's lives could be at stake here, too. See more about this on
page 302.

**Q: Is my seventy-five-year-old mother's youthful, only slightly wrin-
kled face any indication of how my face will age? She has protected her
skin from the sun ever since I can remember, and I wasn't as diligent in my
twenties and thirties about that, though I am now.**

A: You have reason to be hopeful, unless you are also a smoker. Sun exposure and smoking are both major wrinkle factors, though the wrinkles induced
by smoking are usually deeper than those caused by the sun. However, there's a
lot of genetics behind wrinkles, so your mother's good fortune could be yours,
too. (For more on wrinkles, see page 317 chapter 7.)

Q: **A friend—she's in her early sixties—recently asked the doctor who did her laser eye surgery if he could remove a bit of skin from her eyelids with the laser. He did, and she looks great. Will her eyelids stay this way, and was she putting her face at risk by having this doctor do it?**

A: In general, this is fairly minor surgery, and people are very happy with the results. There is often excess skin above and below the eyes, and it is pretty easy to remove, as long as you're dealing with a competent professional. Her eyelids will stay younger-looking for a while, but sooner or later the ravages of time and gravity will cause bags and loose skin to reappear.

She's not putting her face or eyes at risk, as long as the doctor is careful. A laser is an expensive toy in some doctors' hands, but in the hands of others it can do things a scalpel can't. Lasers can make more accurate cuts, and do it relatively bloodlessly. Many doctors, though, still prefer to use a scalpel for this type of surgery, claiming that the laser doesn't offer any major advantage. It's really the doctor, not the tools, that will determine the outcome.

Q: **If there's one thing I hate about my aging face, it's the pucker lines all around my lips. Is there anything that can be done that will have a lasting impact? Or will I just be wasting my money?**

A: Pucker lines—basically, the folding of the skin—develop because of certain shapes and expressions that involve your lips. If you are a smoker, for instance, pucker lines are more common. Take a cigarette and look at yourself in the mirror when you are taking a puff, and you'll see how your mouth forms around the lips. I suppose that if you do a lot of smooching in your life, that also makes pucker lines. How you pronounce certain sounds determines pucker lines; some people, for example, when they pronounce the sound "oooh," purse their lips more than others and may have more defined pucker lines.

What to do about it? While this is a difficult area to treat, many physicians are having success with a variety of laser treatments and peels. Also, you can plump up deeper pucker lines with many injections of collagen or newer supporting materials, which smoothes the area around the lips. These treatments have to be repeated, which is one of the reasons doctors are looking for even better substances. There are newer materials coming on the market, so watch for the latest research. No one is yet using Botox around the lips; it would probably make you drool.

Q: My sixty-one-year-old uncle has lost his sense of smell. He blames the loss on living with a wood stove and burning particleboard and wood that had paint on it. He says that the house was coated with smoke and that wiped out his sense of smell. Does that make sense?

A: Losing the sense of smell can occur as a normal part of aging. There is a test for the sense of smell, and I urge people to have it done if they are experiencing any problems. When our eyes and ears give us trouble, we go to the doctor for testing. We should do the same for our nose.

Not many doctors know how to test the sense of smell, but with some effort you will be able to find someone. The University of Pennsylvania Smell Identification Test is a scratch-and-sniff exam that gives a detailed picture of any problems.

He could be correct that the exposure to smoke and fumes did some damage. We have delicate fibers way up at the top of the nose, which attach to the brain.

He should get it checked out, because it might be a problem that can be fixed. Polyps, allergies, and neurological diseases are some of the possible causes.

Q: A family member is getting vitamin B12 injections for pernicious anemia. I have heard that injectable B12 can make you sick because it contains cyanide. Is that true?

DEAN'S LIST: THE GOOD THINGS FOR LIFE

I'm always on the lookout for research that considers the nonmedical ingredients for a long life. Most are common sense, of course, but that doesn't make them any less significant. Here are my favorites:

1. PETS. Yes, they can be time consuming and expensive to keep, but think about what you can get in return: love and devotion, more physical exercise, improved blood pressure and cholesterol numbers, less anxiety and depression, fewer visits to the doctor, and more family fun. How can anyone argue with that?

2. A GOOD LAUGH. If you've had a difficult day at work or gone through a battery of medical tests, throw a great comedy into the DVD player, make yourself some popcorn, and get ready to feel better. I could watch one just about every night.

3. LOVEMAKING. One study found that a good sex life will make you look younger, and other studies indicate it can help decrease some symptoms of menopause. It's good exercise, too. Any questions?

4. A DAY IN THE COUNTRY. I've spent most of my time living in a city, but I always feel better after just a few hours in the wide-open spaces, surrounded by trees and lots of fresh air. And a study from researchers at the Tokyo Medical and Dental University found that senior citizens who live on tree-lined streets and within walking distance of parks have better odds for a longer life.

5. A GOOD GLASS OF WINE. When I sit down to a simple bowl of spaghetti and a nice zinfandel, life feels good. As I've said many times before, if wine were discovered for the first time today, it would certainly be a prescription drug.

6. DINNER WITH YOUR KIDS. Once your kids become adults, it can get harder and harder to make time for get-togethers with just them. But make sure you do it. Sitting face-to-face with my five sons, who have seen me at my best and worst, and who've given me just a few sleepless nights, is always full of pleasure, because we look to the future, not the past.

7. A WEEKEND GETAWAY WITH MY WIFE. You have to plan

them, otherwise they don't happen as frequently as they should. So, get out your calendars and mark off weekends devoted just to your spouse or partner.

8. A MASSAGE. If you've never had a massage, get one. If you've had a massage, you know why I think they are so beneficial to our well-being. All of us have some level of stress, so find a pair of expert hands to work out the worries that have found their way into your muscles. Even fifteen minutes can do wonders.

9. MUSIC. When I'm listening to Bach's six cello suites, both my brain and my body unload the burdens of the moment.

10. A TRIP IN AN RV. For me, that means hitting the open road in my 1952 bus, disconnected from television, the fax machine, and my e-mail. I don't care where I'm going or when I get there. Fortunately, my wife enjoys this just as much as I do.

A: This is an opportunity to raise awareness about pernicious anemia, which is a decreased amount of red blood cells caused by the body's inability to absorb vitamin B12. No matter how much vitamin B12 the patient takes orally—and we don't need much of it—it has no effect, because the stomach is lacking an enzyme necessary to absorb it. One alternative is B12 by injection, and there are now some nasal sprays that might work, too.

Older people are at risk for pernicious anemia, and, unfortunately, the disease may first manifest with psychiatric symptoms. Every time we test a group of nursing-home patients, we find that a small percentage of people who were thought to be demented actually have pernicious anemia, causing neurological symptoms. We give them a shot of vitamin B12, and they do fine.

Cyanide in vitamin B12 is not a problem. Whenever you hear something like this about a molecular formula, knowing a little basic chemistry can prevent panic.

In a dramatic display, my high school science teacher taught the class how elements behave very differently in their various forms. He took a cube of sodium from its oil bath, and it exploded as soon as it was exposed to air. Chlorine on its own is a fatal green gas that has been used in wars. That's sodium and that's chlorine. Well, the combination of sodium and chlorine is table salt.

So, don't worry about the cyanide in vitamin B12. Vitamin B12 is so harmless that it is often used as a placebo. It's a very popular one, too, because it's red. I can't think of any other injectable medicine that is bright, cherry red. Red placebos work better than blue, green, or yellow ones.

Resource List

The National Institute on Aging offers a variety of free publications on everything from getting a good night's sleep to forgetfulness. Go to the Web site at *www.nia.nih.gov* or call 1-800-222-2225.

For detailed information on Alzheimer's clinic trials that are enrolling participants, go to the Web site for the Alzheimer's Disease Education and Referral Center: *www.alzheimers.org*

If you are living with someone suffering from Alzheimer's, consider registering with the Safe Return program created by the Alzheimer's Association: *www.alz.org*

The American Heart Association Web site is packed with information and resources on all aspects of heart disease in adults and children: *www.americanheart.org*

For the latest stroke research, check out the American Stroke Association Web site: *www.strokeassociation.org*

For information on stroke symptoms in English, Spanish, or French, see the National Stroke Association Web site: *www.stroke.org*

At the Arthritis Foundation Web site, assess your joint health. You'll also find a "pain center," a "disease center," and information about diet and nutrition: *www.arthritis.org*

To find detailed information on services for the elderly, call the Eldercare Locator Service at 1-800-677-1116 or visit the Web site: *www.eldercare.gov*

Learn more about the largest comprehensive centenarian study in the world at the Web site for The New England Centenarian Study: *www.bumc.bu.edu/centenarian*

The American Association for Geriatric Psychiatry tackles a variety of topics, in English and Spanish: ***www.aagponline.org***

The Prevent Blindness America Web site has a macular degeneration test you can take at home to help you know if you need to see an eye doctor: ***www.preventblindness.org***

At the Sight & Hearing Association Web site, you'll find five different do-it-yourself vision tests: ***www.sightandhearing.org***

For information in both English and Spanish on eye diseases, including clinical studies now recruiting participants, check out the National Eye Institute: ***www.nei.nih.gov***

If you suspect that an elderly person is being abused at home or in a facility, the National Center on Elder Abuse Web site has a state-by-state listing of abuse contacts: ***www.elderabusecenter.org***

Subscribe to a free monthly online newsletter from the U.S. Administration on Aging: ***www.aoa.gov***

Take a minute or two to see what the Living to 100 Life Expectancy Calculator says about you: ***www.livingto100.com***

If you want to know which hospitals have the most experience with organ transplants, get up-to-date numbers at the Organ Procurement and Transplantation Network Web site: ***www.optn.org***

The Johns Hopkins Health After 50 Web site has in-depth information on a variety of topics: ***www.hopkinsafter50.com***

The American Federation for Aging Research offers a variety of free publications; sign up at: *www.afar.org* It also supports an aging education Web site: ***www.infoaging.org***

For related questions see chapters 1, 2, 3, 4, 7, 8, 10, and 12.

Chapter 7

Botox, Brava Bras, and the Business of Beauty

I looked through the one-way mirror and prepared myself. It's not often one gets a totally honest view of his physical appeal to others. Today was my day, and the stakes were high. I had just completed a television pilot for the Walt Disney Company, and they had hired a firm to evaluate me and the show. That meant "focus groups," gatherings of everyday folks who are paid a small fee to give their opinions about something they've never seen before, responding to questions from a moderator who is determined to get to their core feelings about the product before them—in this case, me.

A bunch of Disney executives were waiting to devour every word uttered about my performance, and they, too, were sitting behind the one-way mirror. Did I mention how uncomfortable this was?

The first group was every man's fantasy. During the question-and-answer session, when asked about my looks, one woman jumped right in. "Oh yeah, he's cute and sexy. I like him." The other women in the group nodded in assent. The corners of my mouth curled up slightly, as I remembered an aunt who used to tease me as a kid, calling me "ug," short for "ugly." Fortunately, Aunt Frances wasn't here today.

Once the moderator had finished with this group, another was led into the room. The torture was about to begin all over again, eventually leading to the same question, followed by a quick response: "I like the show, but the host of the show is not very good-looking . . . not very sexy." Again heads bobbed in unison. I swallowed hard. Aunt Frances must be here, after all.

Beauty is a topic that both intrigues and saddens me. I struggle most with the subject when I take a call from someone battling anorexia or bulimia, a man or a woman who may die seeking the "perfect" self. The underlying issue is mental illness, of course, but it is hard not to look at the social pressures that face us every day, when magazines, movies, and television perpetuate the idea that if you want to be happy, you need to be beautiful—and thin. The concept of inner beauty seems to have few "made-for-media" qualities—and it's not even in the vocabulary for those who make themselves sick obsessing about weight or facial features.

America's obsession with beauty is anything but new—or purely American. In the sixth century B.C., Pythagoras's mathematical determination of what is harmonious in music inspired many philosophers to attempt mathematical definitions of beauty. Much later on, in the 1500s, it was Albrecht Dürer, a Renaissance artist, who carefully measured people's facial and bodily features so he could develop formulas for beauty. Dürer's standards would be repulsive to some of us today, but beauty "formulas" are still used daily by plastic surgeons to shape the "perfect" face.

Curiously, though, computer technology has shown us that what our culture regards as most beautiful is actually *average*. If you take eight or more random faces off the street and layer them on top of one another in a computer, you will come up with a beautiful face with a fascinating summation of the assorted lips, eyes, noses, eyebrows, and chins. In surveys, these composite faces consistently scored higher than the individual faces used to create the composites.

Of course, not every culture shares the same view we have of the ideal lips, breasts, or hips. And cultures can program themselves to believe that certain ideals represent beauty. For more than a thousand years, in China, women's feet were bound, because the tiniest feet—some less than three inches long—were considered the most beautiful and erotic. In the mid-twentieth century, across Europe and North America, curvy women like Marilyn Monroe and Gina Lollobrigida were considered the ideal. Then came Twiggy in the sixties. Enter decades of female—and male—models so thin that the fashion look was eventually labeled "heroin chic." I've never seen the beauty in that.

But what goes around comes around, fortunately, because today many smart, confident, young women are making the most of their zaftig bodies, and you can see them on stage, on television, and on the street. From Queen Latifah to Camryn Manheim, the attitude says, "Look at me." This is my idea of a healthy attitude.

The same can be said of Jamie Lee Curtis, who stripped down to her underwear for a magazine photo shoot, baring love handles and lumpy thighs in order to challenge the "Hollywood myth of perfection." That tells me there's hope for our society.

But many people would trade bodies with Queen Latifah or Jamie Lee Curtis any day of the week, because they perceive these women as beautiful and they've received the message that they aren't. That message can come in a thousand ways—from job interviews and dating experiences to the subtle suggestions of friends or the cruel comments of other kids as a person is growing up.

My Aunt Frances meant well, but no adult should joke with a kid about being ugly. In my book, that's mental cruelty.

The Danny DeVitos of the world—short, fat, and successful—are the exception, not the norm, and studies show that height and weight are two of the biggest factors when it comes to assessing attractiveness. Many of us can do something about our weight, but medical science can't do anything about height—unless a child has a growth hormone deficiency. Fortunately, being a girl and being tall doesn't seem to be the issue it was when I was a teenager, but I still think it can be a huge hurdle to be short, especially for men. Maybe twenty years from now that will be a nonissue, too.

Strides have been made in helping people deal with everything from skin discoloration to bad acne to imperfect breasts. Often it's expensive, and often not covered by insurance, but I encourage people who can make physical changes to do so, if those changes are really important to them—and their expectations are realistic. We don't always have to live with the bodies we were born with.

Most doctors are careful, though, because the pursuit of beauty can be unhealthy. While eating disorders focus on weight, body dysmorphic disorder is a mental illness that allows people to see themselves as hugely disfigured when, in reality, they are just fine. Teenagers and adults can suffer from it, and its severity varies. One of the more extreme symptoms can be the pursuit of surgical correction, even when a doctor doesn't recommend it.

I remember the first time I ever performed plastic surgery—and lived to regret it—long before I knew about this disease. The woman's eyelids were perfectly OK, but she thought her lids were puffy, and she wanted them fixed. I did the operation, and the next few months were a nightmare, because she wasn't happy. She thought her eyes were different, in a bad way. In the end, I don't think any amount of surgery would have satisfied her, and that experience was enough for me; I never did plastic surgery again.

But more often the response to a modest change is positive. All plastic surgeons will tell you about cases where there was nothing much wrong with people, but they insisted on having surgery; the surgeon fixed the perceived problem, and the before-and-after pictures were almost identical. Yet many of the patients went on to experience significant changes in their self-esteem and accomplishments.

Most standards of beauty revolve around youth. And most of us, as we get older, will experience dissatisfaction and wish we looked younger. On this point, our culture is in dire need of aesthetic adjustments. Haven't you seen people who are middle-aged and older who have a true beauty that has come with age? Wrinkles can accentuate positive facial expressions and reveal the "inner beauty" in a way that makes a profound impression on the viewer. Without making a few concessions to age, I think we condemn ourselves to a life of misery. What a waste.

For those who are hell-bent on looking youthful, a booming crop of less invasive treatments, from Botox to lasers to GORE-TEX threads make that easier to achieve than ever before. But lots of folks are providing these services, and not all are equally competent. Do your research and work with doctors who are more than happy to show you lots of before-and-after photos, including some of their "failures." Just as with all other aspects of medicine, it's your right and responsibility to ask questions, to be an informed patient.

Before contemplating any medical treatment for cosmetic reasons, particularly those that are permanent, think carefully about it. Understand your motivations. Make sure you know that this is not going to change your life. If you are alone and depressed, plastic surgery doesn't automatically deliver the right mate to your doorstep or lighten your mood. In fact, it can have the opposite effect. The last time I checked, most of the beautiful people in Hollywood seem to be struggling to have happy lives. No matter what the movies tell us, beauty does not guarantee anything.

As for me, I'm sticking with what I've got, including my intensely curly hair. One viewer of my TV program sent me a note asking, "What's with those bees on your head?" On the street, I have had little old ladies pull it to see if it's real. My ex-wife hated it so much that she constantly brought straighteners home and made me use them. But she's gone, and the curls are still here. Take that, Aunt Frances.

The Face, from Wrinkles to Nose Jobs

Q: I'm forty-five, and I spent a good bit of time in the sun in my youth, and now my face shows it. Is there any cream that actually works on wrinkles—or should I begin saving for plastic surgery?

A: This is a rapidly changing area of beauty treatment, so I wouldn't rush into anything permanent and expensive at your age. But some creams and injections may give you results that will make you happy for the moment.

Vitamin-enriched creams have been a trend for quite a while now, but legitimate research on many of them is still very thin—and oftentimes it is paid for by the companies that make these creams. That said, prescription-only vitamin A creams, also known as retinoid creams, are the first choice for many dermatologists.

One recent study gave the best marks to Avage, which contains one-tenth of a percent of tazarotene, a drug with vitamin A qualities that is also used to treat acne and psoriasis. Another vitamin A cream is Renova, which is considered effective at improving wrinkles and mottled skin, too, but scored slightly lower than Avage.

A small French study of women between fifty-five and sixty years old found that a five-percent vitamin C cream applied to the skin for six months increased the quantity of collagen—the proteins found in skin, bone, cartilage, and elsewhere throughout your body—and improved the way the collagen was aligned in the skin.

In other words, the random arrangement of collagen as seen under a microscope indeed looked like the pattern of younger skin, as researchers told a meeting of the World Congress in Cosmetic Dermatology in Rio de Janeiro. Of course, this antiwrinkle effect is seen under high magnification and doesn't mean your friends will notice a big difference. Vitamin C is acidic, which means it could act like a mild acid peel. (However, don't even think of applying straight orange juice to your face!) It also has an antioxidant effect, which helps protect the skin from UV damage. Either way, the effects are not permanent.

Botox and collagen treatments aren't, either, but they are more effective. Of course, you pay for that.

As many of you already know, Botox has been a headline maker for the past few years for not only its beauty uses but for other, more medical applications. Botox is the brand name for botulinum toxin Type A, which is produced by the botulism bacterium (see more about it in the next question). Commercial collagen is made from cow's skin and, when injected, it temporarily fills out skin depressions and "erases" wrinkles. The main disadvantage of collagen, besides the fact that a few people are allergic to it, is that treatments need to be repeated.

More products are coming soon, including Restylane, a hyaluronic acid that many plastic surgeons and dermatologists in the United States are already using, although it still awaited FDA approval as of fall 2003. A clear gel used for "repairing" lips, facial wrinkles, and facial folds, it is already on the market in Europe and Canada, and has been shown to reduce wrinkles for up to a year.

Another option is a technique that attacks deeper wrinkles. Your doctor removes a small piece of nice, pure skin from behind your ear and sends it to a lab, where they grow more of your own collagen. They send that to your doctor, and the doctor injects the new collagen underneath your wrinkles. With this method, you don't have to worry about potential allergies, but it's not permanent and it's not cheap.

Finally, you might ask about the newest "wrinkle"—the radio-frequency, nonsurgical facelift, which claims to tighten up sagging skin.

Q: I just met a woman about my age (forty-six) and I was amazed when she mentioned that her mildly bruised eye was the result of Botox injections. Is that a typical reaction? And once the bruising is gone, how long will the Botox still have an impact?

A: Anytime you stick a needle into the skin you have a chance of nicking a tiny blood vessel, which will cause bleeding and, therefore, black-and-blue marks. That is not typical, but to be expected in a treatment like Botox. Once the bruising is gone, the Botox will still be effective in numbing the nerve, but she's going to need this again. All Botox does is paralyze muscles that create wrinkles. It doesn't make wrinkles go away. In addition, Botox, when overused, can create an "expressionless" look that is very obvious and strange. Botox does seem to be benign, but its key ingredient, botulinum, is a purified protein made by the botulism bacteria, which is one of the most powerful toxins known to mankind. Of course, Botox has only a minuscule amount of the toxin. Experts say an ounce of pure Clostridium botulinum toxin could probably destroy the entire human race, and it is considered a potential weapon for bioterrorists.

Q: **Everyone in my office is talking about a facelift that doesn't require major surgery and involves strands of GORE-TEX. Isn't that the stuff they use for expensive mountain-climbing jackets and pants? Can you shed some light on this?**

The Edell Report
Age Before Beauty?

"Beauty" research fascinates me, especially when it relates to the relationships between men and women. I have mixed feelings about what the following study says about guys, but here it is.

Given the choice between a young woman and a beautiful woman, whom will most guys pick?

Well, the common wisdom has always been that men will constantly seek out younger beautiful women, because they may give them more children. Men seek youth, basically. But a study conducted in Great Britain challenges these biological assumptions.

Researchers showed images of different women to a few hundred men who were, on average, thirty years old. A picture of a thirty-six-year-old woman, whom a separate group of men had found attractive, was shown along with eight other photographs of women, ages twenty to forty-five, who had been rated less attractive.

The men were told that the beautiful woman was age either thirty-six, forty-one, or forty-five. When asked to pick one woman as a lifelong partner, all three groups chose the beautiful woman, no matter how old they thought she was.

A: I understand why your office is abuzz. This is an intriguing treatment, but it's not a facelift—at least not like those of our mothers' generation.

Doctors know that long before GORE-TEX was promoted in sporting goods catalogs for its strength and durability, it was being used for hernia repair and other surgeries. It is particularly valuable because it's not known to have ever caused an allergic reaction.

When it comes to your face, slender strings of the material are threaded with a needle under the skin to fill out creases caused by aging. There are no incisions, the treatment requires only a local anesthetic, and it usually is done in the doctor's office.

Of course, before you decide to do something like this, make sure your doctor has lots of experience. And look at the photos of folks he or she has already treated.

Q: When I wake up in the morning and look in the mirror, I can tell that I got new wrinkles on my face during the night. When I sleep, my cheekbone squeezes against my eye. It lifts up and causes circular wrinkles around my eye. Will these become permanent?

A: Don't lose sleep over this, but what you say is absolutely true. Our faces fall into patterns of wrinkles based on how we laugh, frown, talk, and sleep.

Look in the mirror and wiggle your face around. The sleep wrinkles are the ones that squinting and grimacing won't duplicate, because your motions didn't create them. Your sleeping positions did. While we sleep, the pillow can push

---

DID YOU KNOW?
DEFINING A SEXY FACE

Luscious lips, big eyes, and a small nose are appealing to both men and women, according to research from the University of Louisville. As for the lips, voluptuous works better for women than men, and women who purse their lips often send a message that they aren't interested in a sexual advance. Finally, it is possible to have lips that are too big, so think carefully about "improving" yours.

and fold our skin into vertical wrinkles over our eyebrows, on our cheeks, almost anywhere. It's like the way folds develop in a leather shoe—which is, after all, made from cow skin—according to how it bends when you walk.

Talking on the telephone creates another distinct set of wrinkles, the pucker-to-kiss lines around the mouth. No one kisses enough to make those vertical lines around the mouth. If you watch someone talking on the telephone, you will find that their lips are puckering as they speak, like they're giving out kisses.

Most of us like to sleep on our sides or our tummies, which gives the pillows open season to fight with our faces. If you can train yourself to sleep on your back, that might help. But then maybe your skin will start drooping down the sides. Just kidding.

Q: I heard an ad on the radio about a face cream used to remove fine lines. It contains vitamin C, vitamin E, and beta-carotene. Does the skin absorb those things?

A: Even if it does, that isn't going to remove fine lines. Vitamin C is ascorbic acid, and high amounts of it could act like a mini chemical skin peel (see the question on page 317). Glycolic acid is another fruit acid that's all the rage in cosmetics, except cosmetic products are only allowed to contain a small amount of it.

In my experience, small amounts of things like vitamin E and beta-carotene are added to skin care products just to justify the price tag and make them sound healthy. Dermatologists, though, do have products that can relieve that leathery look that comes from too much sun.

Q: I've had an area of dark pigmentation on my face for the past twelve years. It covers 60 percent of my face—my cheeks, my forehead, and my nose. It started a few months after I took antibiotics, beginning as one dark brown spot and eventually spreading during the next several years. I've tried lasers and chemical peels, but they just made it darker. What else can I try?

A: The most important thing, first of all, is to understand the cause. Pigmentation like this can be due to Addison's disease, a hormonal disorder, or even pregnancy.

Sometimes doctors recommend going after the lighter skin and darkening it to match, because sometimes lightening up the darker spots can be very tricky, and getting an accurate match also can be very difficult. There are pre-scription-bleaching creams that you can get from a dermatologist, but I assume you've tried those. They are usually the first line of treatment. As you've said, sometimes we do dermabrasion and acid peels and other similar treatments.

Lasers are changing rapidly, and we're able to do more complicated things with skin pigmentation, so you should keep at this, getting a second opinion if you aren't satisfied with your treatment to date. Whatever you do, make sure you see a dermatologist experienced in this area, and look at before-and-after photos of people who've had whatever procedure is being discussed.

The other answer might be skillful use of good makeup. That might be the best solution, because with any of these procedures it will still be very difficult to blend the areas evenly.

Q: When a product claims it has alpha-hydroxy acids, what does that mean?

A: In a limited concentration, these acids can be used in over-the-counter products although the more potent concentrations are available only from your dermatologist or cosmetologist. The acid acts as a peel, which is not going to take care of deeper wrinkles but it might give you a bit of a glow while smoothing leathery skin and sun damage. The amount of alpha-hydroxy in over-the-counter products is so small that the results are minimal.

Q: My daughter has a very lovely, fair complexion, but she has freckles and she hates them with a passion. We just had a little vacation in the Caribbean, and not only did her skin not tan, it also got more freckles. She's really frustrated. I have told her they're cute, and people love them, but she covers them with some makeup so they're more subdued. Is there anything that will fade or remove them?

A: Any parent knows how ridiculous it is to try to discuss such a sensitive topic with teenagers. They have their own ideas, and there is nothing that will change their minds.

A kid will look you in the eye and say, "I'm ugly," and it doesn't matter if you and everybody else lavishes him or her with compliments. That has no impact on teenage self-esteem.

Now for the good news. There is a new laser treatment that is fairly effec-tive at diminishing freckles. If she wants to give it a try, the dermatologist should work on a few in an out-of-the-way spot, such as the back of her cheek, to see how it goes.

Bleaches are another option, but I don't like them, because the results are uneven.

There's nothing she can do to stop freckles, except for covering up or limiting her time in the sun. Being fair, she does need to be careful in the sun anyway.

Q: I'm a twenty-seven-year-old guy and I've always had dark circles under my eyes. I've heard you say that blood vessels close to the surface can cause this. How do I know if that's my problem, or if I have some other problem, like a vitamin deficiency or an allergy?

A: I don't know of a medical name for dark circles, which tells us that they are not a sign of disease.

Some people are just born with superficial veins or with lots of pigmentation—plain old melanin—around the eyes. Age and sun exposure will deepen the color.

Because the skin around the eyes is the most delicate skin on the body, differences among people are quite noticeable. Since this is how your eyes have always looked, you are not ill.

I haven't seen any evidence to my satisfaction that allergies and fatigue cause dark circles. Tiredness can shift the position of the eyelids a little and create a sense of depth or shadow.

Seriously ill people get dark circles, because the amount of fat around the eyeballs actually decreases and results in shadows. Fluid retention and the accompanying swelling around the eyes are early signs of kidney disease.

Because I do a lot of television work, I've learned about makeup—and it's amazing what a little foundation can do. But if you're like most men, you don't want to go there, so, I'm afraid, you're stuck. I don't know of anything else that will lighten the dark circles.

Q: After several years of ruddiness on her face, my fifteen-year-old daughter was diagnosed with rosacea by a dermatologist. I haven't had any luck getting information on childhood rosacea from the Internet. Is there anything I should be aware of?

A: You are lucky that it was diagnosed, because it often is not. Many people have undiagnosed rosacea for years, and it can get worse without treatment. Plus, when a condition appears to be similar among age groups, most studies will be done on adults, which would explain why you're not finding information specific to teenagers. The full name is "acne rosacea," so searching under "acne" might turn up more hits. Also check out our Resource List on page 361 for helpful Web sites.

Despite its name, rosacea is not a true acne. It first shows up as a flushed face—most often in adults between thirty and fifty—and it becomes a ruddy complexion that doesn't go away. One current theory is that it's caused by the body's reaction to a skin fungus. A flare-up can be set off by a variety of triggers, including sun exposure, stress, hot or cold weather, wind, alcohol, spicy foods, strenuous exercise, hot baths, heated beverages—even certain skin creams and lotions.

At fifteen, your daughter is changing from childhood to womanhood, so I'm not sure that her case of rosacea would require different treatment than that for a grown woman. We have found that a cream used to treat vaginal fungus infections also relieves rosacea, and antibiotics have entered the fight as well. Some insurance companies also cover one of the newest treatments from the "high tech" side of dermatology.

The nonlaser "intense pulse light," or photorejuvenation (your doctor may have another name for it), can remove skin discoloration caused by rosacea, broken capillaries, and sun damage. It works on wrinkles, too. This treatment lasts about fifteen to twenty minutes per session, can be painful, and short-term bruising can occur. Dermatologists usually recommend four to six treatments, depending on how discolored the skin is. As you might suspect, this is expensive, but it does produce results.

Although alcohol triggers flushes in some people, it is not an indicator of alcohol abuse. Former President Clinton has rosacea, and so did W. C. Fields. Fields's bumpy, ruddy nose, a condition called rhinophyma, was the result of long-term untreated rosacea.

Q: Is it safe to use Viagra when you have rosacea? My face gets *really* red after I've taken it.

A: This is a tough one. We think rosacea is caused by an overreaction of the body to a particular organism, a fungus yeast that lives on the face. One result is an abnormal flushing (see previous question).

Viagra on the other hand is a vasodilator (something which causes blood vessels to relax or expand). One very noticeable side effect of Viagra is that it flushes your face and you get all red. Doctors tell rosacea patients not to let any flushing happen, which is why they tell them not to drink alcohol, another vasodilator. I am not aware of any current information on this subject. If you have rosacea, and Viagra seems to make it worse, I would report that to your doctor and tell him or her to report that to the FDA. I doubt they even know that there is a possible effect of Viagra on rosacea.

Lasers, Dermabrasion, and Acne

Q: I'm twenty-nine, and in the last few years I've had cystic acne. I've finally stopped breaking out, so I made some calls about having the scars removed. One office referred me somewhere else, because I have too many red marks for them to handle. Is treatment at one of those laser-surgery centers a viable option? I have an appointment, but I'm nervous about it.

A: You have good reason to be cautious. In general, acne scars do not respond well to lasers. Acne scars vary in type and in depth. Lasers, which are mostly used to smooth skin and to remove wrinkles, may be effective on very shallow scars, but not on those that are steeply edged.

I suggest you visit the surgery center so they can evaluate you and you can evaluate them. Take a look at some before-and-after pictures of people with scarring similar to yours. Also, ask about side effects and for some numbers on success rates.

It's always possible that if you were standing in front of me, I'd tell you, "You look great. Your scars aren't noticeable, and you shouldn't do a thing." Maybe you need to hear that. On the other hand, the scars may be bad enough to warrant some attention.

Be very careful of assembly-line laser businesses. This is your face. Get a few opinions before you decide. Injecting collagen and similar substances to lift the skin depressions may be the best way to treat it, though it's not a permanent solution.

Q: What is the best way to get rid of blackheads on my nose and chin? My mother always said that squeezing them would hurt my skin.

A: First, let's clarify the difference between a whitehead and a blackhead. When bacteria and debris collect and erupt beneath a thin layer of skin, that's a whitehead. When exposure to air oxidizes it and turns it black, that's a blackhead. Either way, the blemish is caused by an infection in the pore. The combination of excess sebum secretion because of hormone production and blocked pores encourages germs to grow and cause pimples.

As for treatment, a lot depends on how extensive the problem is. If you have just a few, see if some of the over-the-counter products at the drugstore work for you. Also, dermatologists use a tool that looks like a little spoon with a hole in the middle, which is effective, and I've seen it in drugstores, too.

If the problem is more significant, or self-treatment doesn't work, a dermatologist can prescribe an antibiotic, which stops the process of infection by killing germs. Retinoids like Accutane, which are related to the vitamin A family, also are an option, though I consider it a last resort. (See more about this in the next question.)

The one treatment that won't work is scrubbing your face too much; in fact, in can make acne worse. When I was a kid, I was told, scrub, scrub, scrub—and don't eat chocolate. Both were bad advice. Other new research suggests that stress and high-carbohydrate diets can make acne worse.

Q: I have girlfriends who have taken Accutane and it totally cleared up their skin. Why does my family doctor balk at giving it to me?

I am sixteen. I have very bad cystic acne on my back, and no treatment I've tried has worked, so I can't even wear a sundress. If I don't do something about it, I will have scars.

A: Accutane does work, but it is a controversial medication. It can cause birth defects, and there is debate about whether it's linked to increased suicide risk among teenagers and young adults. Other side effects include dry skin, cracks in the corner of your nose and lips, and altered cholesterol and liver function, though it's believed that these last two effects are temporary.

Your doctor's opinion may be that your acne is not serious enough to put up with Accutane's risks. I've raised a lot of boys, and when one of them had little zits here and there, no matter how much I told him that his face looked great, he thought it was the end of the world.

That said, family practitioners can't be experts in everything from A to Z—arthritis to zits. I really can't say that your doctor is being overly cautious, because I don't know the details of your case. But I don't want you to be uptight about scars on your back when prom night comes around and you want to wear something low-cut.

I'd strongly recommend that you start with a logical series of topical agents. If they fail, try antibiotics. Keep upping the ante, and, if you haven't done so yet, see a dermatologist.

Doctors come in all stripes, and you need to find one who will meet you halfway as a responsible young lady who knows what she wants. However, do not forget that Accutane does cause birth defects. You must understand all the implications of that.

Q: For the last few years, I've been taking an antibiotic—Doxycycline—to treat my acne. The times I went off it, the acne became worse, and my mother wonders if it's because I have a stressful job. Should I be concerned about long-term use of this drug?

A: We have lots of experience with long-term use of Doxycycline, and it appears to be safe. Pregnant women shouldn't take it, however, because it can discolor the baby's teeth.

Doxycycline does have some side effects. It causes sun sensitivity, so you have to protect yourself from sun exposure or you may end up with some nasty rashes. It also can upset the balance of bacteria in your intestines and sometimes cause unpleasant gastrointestinal symptoms.

A few years ago, a study did find that long-term users of antibiotics had antibiotic-resistant bacteria on their skin. No illnesses were linked to these bacteria at that time.

Since this works for you, I'd stick with it.

And as for your Mom's opinion, she may be on to something.

The first serious look at the link between acne and stress, by Stanford University, found college students' acne got much worse during exams.

Stress can cause the release of testosterone, which can definitely cause acne. This may be why people in their twenties and thirties often see their teenage acne return, even if they aren't stressed.

Q: Do laser or chemical peels done by a dermatologist affect the growth of either basal-cell or squamous-cell carcinoma?

A: The sun is the root cause of most skin cancers, which are usually either the basal-cell or squamous-cell type and which are very rarely fatal. The layers of our skin are like layers of a tree. The part of the tree that is alive and growing is the thin layer right under the rough layer of protective bark.

The skin layer that is disturbed by peels is not the cell layer that will cause cancer—and no laser treatment or peel will cure cancer or remove your risk of it. Most likely the peels don't go down into the dermis layer. And the layer that carries cells that can cause malignant melanoma, which can kill you, is also deeper than the layer disturbed by peels.

There is some evidence that retinoic acid–like compounds used in home mini-peels may increase the risk of cancer, because they can directly juice the DNA and growing skin cells. But I wouldn't expect that from the mechanical laser methods or the pure acid methods.

See related questions on page 477 in chapter 10.

Q: I am thinking of having microdermabrasion to remove liver spots. What are the pros and cons?

A: Microdermabrasion blasts away at the skin with a very fine powder to remove small scars, wrinkles, marks, and discolorations. It has pretty much replaced the old face-sanding method and peels that used heavy chemicals.

It can be used alone or to fine-tune other techniques. For example, following a laser treatment, microdermabrasion will even edges and smooth bumps. The cons are that it doesn't always work perfectly, and pigmentation can vary between treated and untreated areas.

The skin around the eyes is one area where microdermabrasion is helpful, because the original, basic dermabrasion is too coarse for that delicate skin. However, it does not erase deeper folds and crow's feet.

As to your question, it can do a nice job with liver spots, but there are no guarantees. I think you should start by looking at the doctor's portfolio of before-and-after photos and asking the tough questions. Seek an honest opinion on the best outcome you can expect.

See more laser-related questions beginning on page 325.

Plastic Surgery: Go Slowly, Do Your Homework

Q: Our sixteen-year-old daughter is focused on her nose, which is as distinctive as her mother's but not unattractive. She has already begun lobbying for plastic surgery, and my wife and I are somewhat divided on this topic. Do you have any guidelines we might consider for this obviously prickly issue?

A: I think a sixteen-year-old who does not have a major nose deformity is too young to make such a serious and permanent decision. Her face is still changing, which should be reason enough not to do anything now.

She needs to think about how her nose fits into the whole face—and how it makes that face hers alone. Many times, when the nose is altered it just doesn't fit the rest of the face and, once the work is done, you can't go back to what you had.

Keep talking to her about how her focus on a single part of her body is having a major impact on her self-esteem. You might also buy her a copy of the *Bobbi Brown Teenage Beauty* book, which focuses on helping girls bring out their natural beauty and gets raves from many parents. Finally, remind her how many beautiful Hollywood actresses and other performers have distinctive noses.

You and your wife also need to present a cohesive voice on this topic; the two of you should decide in private what you agree on before talking further with your daughter. Don't let your daughter play one parent against the other. If that happens, there are likely to be other issues in the future where a similar game is played, and no one wins when that happens.

Q: I hate my cellulite, and it seems that two of my options are liposuction (more intrusive, more expensive) and massage treatments with

---

DID YOU KNOW?
THE BETTER BELLY BUTTON

The American Society of Aesthetic Plastic Surgery doesn't want to miss a thing when it surveys its membership on surgery and non-surgery trends. So, in 2002 they added six new surgeries to the survey list, including umbilicoplasty (belly button enhancement). Often this surgery is necessary for patients who are having a tummy tuck. But not always. It seems that for some folks, an exposed midriff—or a navel piercing—isn't nearly as memorable if the belly button is ugly. I think I'll stick with what I've got.

lotions and oils. Does either work? Does it actually ever make anyone feel better about themselves?

A: Those are two different questions, aren't they? The answer to the first one is no, liposuction, lotions, and oils don't get rid of cellulite permanently. Your dimpled thighs or buttocks may make you miserable, but, unfortunately, a legitimate treatment has yet to be found, though many aggressive marketers would have you believe otherwise.

However, one treatment you didn't mention, Endermologie, is approved by the FDA and may give temporary results. But it's quite expensive and time-consuming, too. And most medical doctors are skeptical.

The answer to the second question is a definite yes. A classic experiment was done many years ago on a group of people who had had plastic surgery that was undetectable to the patients' acquaintances. Observers couldn't tell that a nose was any smaller or that thighs had been sucked out. And yet, the patients felt great.

In other words, the placebo effect of plastic surgery is very powerful. The doctor who made these observations, Maxwell Maltz, explored how mind-body connections affect human achievement. A person who switches from poor self-image to pleased-as-punch can rise from the mailroom to the board-room.

So whether a cosmetic procedure works or not depends on the definition of "works." If a nose job makes someone feel good enough to go after the brass ring, then I'd say it works.

For people with body dysmorphic disorder, though, nothing works. Rather than getting a boost from a questionably successful cosmetic surgery, those who suffer from this type of compulsion can't get enough surgery to mend their "imagined ugliness." They are so obsessed with slight or even nonexistent physical defects that their ability to hold jobs and have relationships is severely impaired.

Q: Four months ago I had a facelift that healed well, but I am now losing my hair near where the incision was made.

A: You are probably losing hair because the incision cut off some of your blood supply, and reduced blood supply is a common cause of hair loss. Your hair follicles are probably still there, so the hair may grow back.

Four months is not enough time for full recovery from a facelift. I tell people, and I'm sure your plastic surgeon told you as well, that it takes at least

The Edell Report
The Perfect Face?

If you've ever wondered how your face compares to the perfectly proportioned face, according to the American Academy of Facial Plastic and Reconstructive Surgery, grab a straight-on frontal photo of your face, a ruler, and a pen, and follow these steps.

1. *Draw four horizontal lines across your face: one at the tip of the chin, another at the tip of the nose, one through the eyebrows, and the last at the top of the forehead. The "classic" face has an equal space between each of the segments.*

2. *On the same photo, draw five equally spaced vertical lines the length of your face, from ear to ear, so your face is now covered by a grid of fifteen boxes. The "perfect" face is "five eyes" wide, based on each individual's eyes. If your face is perfectly proportioned, each eye will be the width of one of the boxes on the grid, and there will be one eye's width between each eye. The perfect nose also will be the same width as one eye.*

3. *Finally, if you want to check every angle, get a profile photo of your face and draw a line from your lower lip to the bottom of your chin. The chin should be even with the lip or slightly behind it.*

six months from the date of the surgery before you can expect to be completely healed.

Some people say that anyone contemplating facelifts should be shown pictures of the surgery or of horror cases before they decide. But the truth is that most people are very happy with their facelifts.

Q: I still have "baby belly" from giving birth four years ago. It's a floppy piece of skin that just won't tighten up. I'm forty-one. I do exercises. What else can I do?

A: Your best bet may be surgery. Here's why. Doing sit-ups will strengthen your muscles, but your skin—not your abdominal muscles—is the cause of your problem. Around age thirty-five we begin to lose the elasticity in our skin; it no longer snaps back as it does in a twenty-one-year-old.

You would respond beautifully to excising that skin, turning that flap into a short, bikini-line scar. Talk to a plastic surgeon.

Q: I'm a twenty-five-year-old single woman and I have a problem: no butt. Is there anything I can do for a really flat rear end? (I inherited this from my mother.)

A: Yes, there is: implants and micro fat grafting. However, these procedures are relatively rare, not every plastic surgeon does them, and you're talking about a part of your body that gets a lot of activity (sitting), so I want you to do your research before taking the leap. Don't go to a doctor who's only done a couple of patients.

The implants are silicone, the procedure is expensive, and recovery, as you might expect, isn't instantaneous. This is not something you do on a Friday, so you can be back at work on Monday. Implants are still a relatively new, and rare, procedure, so we don't yet know much about long-term satisfaction or side effects.

A little more is known about micro fat grafting. According to a report in the *Aesthetic Surgery Journal*, a study based on 566 cases of buttock augmentation found that 50 to 75 percent of the grafted fat remains in place long-term. The authors of this study reported high satisfaction on the part of patients—about 10 percent of the patients requested further augmentation.

Where does the fat come from? Well, it is taken from another part of the

---

QUIZ

Which age group has the most cosmetic surgery, according to the American Academy of Cosmetic Surgery?
A) thirty-five to fifty years old   B) twenty-six to thirty-four
C) twenty-five and under   D) over fifty-one
(A: thirty-five to fifty years old, who had 33 percent of all surgeries. People over fifty-one accounted for 27 percent.)

body with a syringe or a liposuction pump. Then the surgeon makes two tiny incisions in each buttock to inject the fat.

A compression garment is worn for about six weeks (this is normal for liposuction procedures, too). Patients are able to resume most normal activities in two to five days. Mild discomfort may persist for one to two weeks after the surgery. Time will tell with this one.

Q: My thirty-year-old sister is at the point in her life where she can afford breast implants, and she's seriously thinking of getting them. What's my best argument to convince her otherwise? I'm not sure she'll listen, but I think this is such a stupid idea that I have to try and talk her out of it.

A: When people want to improve their appearance, there's almost no argument you can make against it. As far as breast implants go, I remember a study where students looked at airbrushed photos of models. It was actually the same model with different-size breasts in each photo. The students chose the larger-breasted model to be less trustworthy, less moral, and less intelligent.

Please, before you fire off an angry e-mail, I'm not suggesting there aren't decent and smart women with D cups out there; it's just that society has some very skewed views of female breasts. Women tell me that if men wore their penises in the middle of their chests, where everyone could see them, men would be as avid about penis enlargement as some women are about implants.

As for your sister, unfortunately you can't raise the disease argument anymore, because silicone implants don't cause diseases, and saline implants, which are all that's on the market, don't either. But there are surgical mishaps, and the results don't always satisfy the patient. While the vast majority of women are very happy with implants, there are many who are not. Yes, they can be removed, but sometimes you cannot restore the original look of your breasts.

On the flip side, women tell me again and again that they feel better about themselves when they have it done. Will someone please tell me how breasts became such a giant symbol of many women's validity? Breast implants also can create unrealistic expectations. Someone who thinks that new breasts will bring her the perfect mate is setting herself up for disappointment.

Maybe you can convince your sister to at least talk to some women who weren't happy with the investment, before she makes hers.

Q: What sort of an effect does a breast implant placed under the muscle have? I have noticed that my own under-the-muscle implants look weird whenever I pull anything toward me, especially when my arms are chest-high.

A: Probably the No. 1 complaint you'll hear from women who have saline implants under the muscle is that it looks funny in certain positions. And I don't mean just sexual positions. A variety of muscle actions can distort the implant. Such positions or actions can make wrinkles or make it move, and it's different for every woman.

It isn't critical that the muscle attaches itself along the entire surface of the chest wall. The muscle, after all, comes from just the side of your breastbone and sweeps across up to your humerus and helps move the upper arm. You can tense all your chest muscles and see what it does by making different motions with your arm. But with under-the-muscle implants, there seems to be less migration, less capsular contraction, and, in women who are very thin, better cosmetic results. The surgeon goes in through the armpit when it's put under the muscle, so there are no scars on the chest.

Your plastic surgeon should have told you about the unusual appearance of the implant in certain positions. But, as I said, it's variable, and women who are bothered by this just learn not to do those kinds of motions with a bathing suit on or when they're undressed. The silicone implant gives better cosmetic results overall, and perhaps you can switch when they're back on the market, if yours still bug you.

Q: I've been diagnosed with gynecomastia. The doctor says the only solution is surgery. Is that true? Also, what causes gynecomastia?

A: Gynecomastia is enlarged breast tissue in a male. Before I answer your question about treatment and cause, I want to comment on the diagnosis, because some men just have a lot of fat tissue on their chest and that can be mistaken for gynecomastia. In that case, nothing needs to be done. The feel of the tissue should clue the doctor in. Glandular tissue—breast tissue—has a firmer feel than does mushy fat tissue.

Gynecomastia can be harmless. If your doctor rules out breast cancer, which he must do, because it does occur in men, then I think fat sucking is a nifty, simple solution. But because surgery gives them more control, and there is less chance of ending up with ripples, lumps, and bumps, many plastic surgeons would rather remove the tissue surgically.

Medical causes of gynecomastia can be drugs, or hormonal or liver disorders. Common stomach medications, spironolactone (a high blood pressure medication), digitalis (a heart medication), and estrogens prescribed for prostate cancer can all cause breast growth in men. And, possibly, so can marijuana, because of its effects on hormone receptors.

Disorders of the testicles or pituitary gland will create hormone imbalances that can lead to gynecomastia, as can alcoholism and liver disease by impairing the body's ability to break down a man's natural estrogens.

These are, of course, more serious disorders that your doctor should test you for. Other signs of hormonal imbalance would be decreased facial hair and erectile dysfunction.

Q: This is a very sensitive subject with my husband, and I don't know if he would do anything about it, but I'm curious: Will any kind of surgery eliminate his love handles and beer gut?

A: As you seem to realize, people who want to see physical changes in their spouses or partners need to be very careful about how they approach this subject. And, in general, I don't think it's a good idea to pursue such issues bluntly unless the other person brings up the topic first.

Some men undergo liposuction to remove the fat around their waist, but it's not always satisfactory surgery, because a man's fat distribution is different from that of a woman.

While liposuction will remove excess fat just under the skin, men have a higher ratio than women of intra-abdominal, or visceral, fat that lies deep in the abdomen. Because this deeper fat can't be sucked out, you could still come out of the procedure with a protruding gut.

It would take major surgery to reach the abdominal cavity to remove the

---

QUIZ

Which treatment is best for erasing stretch marks?
A) vitamin E   B) any moisturizer   C) abdominoplasty
D) progesterone cream   E) none of the above
(C: "tummy tucks" may remove some marks but not necessarily all of them.)

inner fat layer that helps push the gut out, which is something I'd never recommend. However, some men have trimmed their paunch by using liposuction along with an open surgical procedure designed to remove excess skin and tighten abdominal muscles.

One study of male runners showed that even if you have a consistent diet and exercise regularly, you'll gain 3.3 pounds and add three-fourths of an inch around your waistline every ten years. In other words, you'll naturally put on a little flab as you age.

So, bottom line: If it's your husband's general health that you are worried about, talk to him about your fears and see if the two of you can make some adjustments in your diet and exercise regimens. But, if he's fit, accept your husband's body for what it is.

All This Stuff Called "Body Modification"

Q: I pierced my ears about twenty-five years ago, and the other day one of my earlobes split apart. It seemed to just kind of erode. I've now got two lobes where I had one. How should I fix this?

A: Once the edges of the split start to heal, they won't stick together well. So, you will want a doctor—probably a plastic surgeon—to clean up the edges. Your lobe will probably require a stitch or two, or the doctor may use a medical "super glue."

Of course, if the lobe is infected, that should be treated and allowed to heal before the edges are joined.

Q: I got a belly-button ring about three months ago, and it's not healing properly. It's raw, and gunk is always coming out of it and it hurts. Do you know why this could be? I had it pierced professionally.

A: Belly button piercings usually take the longest to heal of all piercings and have the highest rate of problems. In general, it takes three to six months to completely heal, because it's a very fleshy part of the body.

When you get your ears pierced, the hole heals up quickly. Other parts of the body don't heal as easily. It really depends on the blood supply to the area and exactly what you're piercing. Piercing cartilage, for instance, is notoriously difficult. Piercings that are up higher on the ear that go through cartilage take longer to heal. And the belly button is the worst of them.

Once any piercing becomes infected, which about 25 percent do, the treatment can be tricky. Sometimes doctors advise you to take out the piercing and just let it heal up. And it's possible that the area around your belly button may be so sensitive that it cannot tolerate a foreign body.

If the infection was just setting in, I'd recommend leaving in the ring and using Neosporin, or something like that, though you run the risk of having a reaction to that, too. I would rotate the ring, so that some of the antibiotic goes to the flesh, and I would also put a wet washcloth that's warm or hot on the infection every few hours for several minutes. The idea is to keep it moist; if a scab forms, the infection can be sealed inside.

However, since this has been a problem for a while, see a dermatologist.

Q: My seventeen-year-old daughter hit me up with one of my own techniques. She gave me a choice. She said, "Dad, I'm going to do something next month. Would you rather I got a tattoo or had my tongue pierced?" I picked tongue piercing, because at least it's more temporary, and the thought of a Jimi Hendrix tattoo on my daughter's butt is unappealing.

But I've heard horror stories about kids bleeding to death from botched piercings. Do you have some compelling argument that I can use against piercing?

A: Your daughter is far from alone in her interests of the moment. A 2003 survey by the University of Michigan Health System showed that more than one half of the students questioned had piercings, and 23 percent had tattoos. So, as parents, we aren't alone either—and, by the way, piercings and tattoos are now clumped under the title of "body modifications." Yeow.

Jimi Hendrix was a great guitarist, but I can understand why you wouldn't want him tattooed on your daughter's butt. Boy, is it payback time for the baby boomers or what?

If compelling arguments worked, we wouldn't have kids smoking, using drugs, having sex, or driving drunk. And I've lost some battles in my own home, so I am not an expert. When my boys wanted to pierce something, I screamed and hollered. They did it anyway, but as soon as they started looking for jobs the scrap metal was history, because they learned that people are judgmental about these things.

An argument against the tattoo is that it's permanent. Dermatologists can tell you that most young people who get tattoos live to regret it. All these fads change, and whatever is "in" now will be "out" some day, and then what do you do?

A tongue piercing is temporary, but the crack it can make in your teeth isn't. Dentists can tell you about that side effect. If the hole doesn't heal, she may need a little surgery, and piercings can get infected.

The truth is that most of the time tongue piercings are harmless. Excessive bleeding from one would be very rare, but it has happened. The tongue is vascular, so a professional piercer should know where the major arteries are.

Of course, if it's done without sterile equipment, or by someone unskilled, she is definitely at risk for potentially serious problems like hepatitis C and HIV. Sorry, nobody keeps statistics on these things, so I can't arm you with any.

You can say, "I'm your father and I pay the rent. I don't want anybody with a piece of metal hanging from her tongue at my dinner table." You have that right as a parent—but is this the war you want to have with your kid?

I think the key is to talk to her about why the piercing is important to her. Find out what she hopes to gain from it, and find out what she thinks she will lose by not doing it.

Most likely she wants her friends to think she's cool. This is a sign that she is still a kid. She is emotionally attached to her peers and eager to fit in. That's absolutely normal, but it is a sign of youth.

Let her know that being independent, being mature means being herself and ignoring the fads. Tell her that you will respect her more for not being a sheep and just doing what all her friends are doing. Every once in a while, a kid will get it.

If you can get to the emotional reasons that kids do these things, if you can get them to understand it themselves, then you are well on your way.

Q: My twenty-one-year-old son now has four tattoos on his arms, and I keep wondering what he'll do once he reaches an age where these seem ridiculous. What's the latest on removal techniques?

A: This is still a very dicey area, though lasers seem to be the treatment of choice among dermatologists. Before your son makes any decisions, though, he should be sure the doctor who will be doing the work has a lot of experience removing tattoos; having the right doctor is worth the search.

The next step is to take a look at the doctor's collection of before-and-after pictures. Beyond giving your son a preview of his or her work, this will give him a dose of realism about the results. He can choose a doctor to do just one tattoo and see how it goes before he decides to forge ahead.

Also, some small tattoos can just be cut out with a scalpel, and the skin is then sewn together, leaving a little scar.

If your son doesn't choose to remove his tattoos, he may want to consider what profession is best suited to his body marks. A recent study found that people are much more likely to respond positively to people with tattoos if their attire seems to match the stereotype of a tattooed person. If the tattoo owner is wearing a tie and slacks, the average person is less receptive than if the tattooed individual is wearing jeans and a sweatshirt.

That makes you feel a lot better, right?

See more about tattoos on page 406 in chapter 9.

The Tanning Salon Is Now Open

Q: What have you heard, good or bad, about tanning beds? I am recovering from an accident and don't have an interest in being outdoors, but I'd like to get some color.

A: Tanning beds don't seem to be any safer or any more dangerous than the sun. But they are devices of the modern age, so we just don't have that much evidence on them yet. However, the British Medical Association is concerned enough about their use to recommend government regulation of them. One British survey found that some folks have more than a hundred tanning sessions a year.

Tanning beds use UVA rays, which we used to think were safer than UVB rays, the kind that burn. It turns out that UVA is not completely benign either; there is the risk of premature aging of the skin as well as cornea damage, if you don't wear protective eyewear. Some evidence shows that exposure to rays at a young age may be even more dangerous.

Obviously, the level of risk depends on the amount of exposure. But accepting the risk in what we enjoy can make for a fuller life. The trick is to know how significant the risk is and how many limits we want to place on ourselves. You sound like you enjoy the look and experience of tanning. So the benefit of that pleasure might be worth the risk to you. Of course, a little natural sunshine could have additional benefits, like vitamin D.

DID YOU KNOW?
DON'T FOOL WITH MOTHER NATURE

I harp and harp about the dangers of the sun, but if you still have any doubts about the issue of skin cancer, consider this: About 1.3 million cases of skin cancer are diagnosed in the United States each year, more than all other forms of cancer combined. And while most skin cancer is treatable, there are still 7,800 melanoma deaths every year. If you are ever in doubt about whether you can burn, consider the "summer shadow rule": If your shadow is shorter than your height, you can be burned. If you want to make skin care even simpler, just be sure you have sunblock on between ten A.M. and four P.M.

Q: I wear a foundation makeup that is SPF 15, and when I go outside, I add a sunscreen that is also SPF 15. Does one cancel the other, or do I have SPF 30, double protection?

A: Here's a topic that just seems to confound most of us, and I can see why, when there are several SPF (sun protection factor) grades that really are overkill—yet lots of folks buy them.

First, two layers of SPF 15 do not add up to SPF 30, but you do get a benefit of having a thicker-than-usual application of sunscreen. Laboratories test SPF with a smear that's a standard thickness of two milligrams per square centimeter of skin, but one study found that the average person applies just about one-fourth of that amount. And even after being instructed in applying sunscreen, people still boosted the quantity to just about one milligram per centimeter of skin, which is half as thick as the manufacturer's intended use.

Second, most folks are buying a lotion or cream with much more SPF than any of us need. When enough sunscreen is applied, SPF 15 is the maximum strength you need. There isn't enough sunlight in the day to justify using SPF 30. You'll still find SPF 30 at the store, but the FDA stopped allowing higher SPFs—though sunscreen makers can put a plus sign behind the 30 if they want to suggest something more potent. Don't buy it!

There's more than a bit of irony in all the progress made in the last ten years to educate folks about the dangers of the sun. Statistics show that people who use sunscreen have a higher rate of skin cancer, because the people who use sunscreen seem to think it's a license to bake in the sun. Sunscreen blocks out UVB rays, but most types do not block the UVA rays as well, and these may be linked to skin cancer, too.

So, Dr. Edell says: Use ample sunscreen, put it on 30 minutes before you go out, enjoy that long walk along the beach, but put a hat on—and keep it on. Finally, don't assume that your clothing is protecting you. A typical white t-shirt has an SPF of only 5! And if it's wet—or a loose weave—the SPF is even weaker.

Q: Is the sunscreen I bought last year still good, or should I buy a new bottle?

A: You can use the old sunscreen, although it may have degraded a little, especially if it has been stored in light or heat. In general, the FDA says that sunscreens without expiration dates are good for about three years. When in doubt you can first put it through a limited trial. If it works, go ahead and use it. Any sunscreen is better than no sunscreen.

Q: I have a question regarding those sunless tanning lotions. They keep telling us to stay out of the sun, but we still want suntans. I wonder if there is any data or study on the active ingredients in these products?

A: There are two types of products on the market, one you rub or spray on your skin and the other you take as a pill. I don't like the pill, and it's not legal in the United States anyway. You've got to be out of your mind to take something orally just for the sake of looking like the color of cheddar.

QUIZ

Which of the following can cause dermatitis if you go out in the sun?
A) fig tree sap   B) aftershave lotion   C) lime juice
D) tetracycline   E) all of the above
(E: all of the above. Dermatitis, also known as eczema, comes in several forms. This is called "contact dermatitis." Best bet: Once you know you have a reaction to any of these, make sure to wash them off before going outdoors.)

As for self-tanning lotions, they are safe and, aesthetically, they have gotten one heck of a lot better. There's even the option, available now in some cities, of jet-spray booths. You can get an all-over tan in less than a minute, and this treatment uses the same ingredients found in the do-it-yourself products.

The only danger found in these lotions is that you may assume you are protected from the sun, but you're not. This stuff just dyes your skin, it doesn't block the sun's rays. One study of women who use these lotions found that they are more likely to use regular sunscreen, which sounds good, but they also were more likely to get burned.

By the way, the reason a suntan looks good is a great example of how we self-program ourselves aesthetically and how our standards of beauty change. Victorian women carried parasols to protect themselves from the sun, and at the beginning of the twentieth century, the only people with tans were men and women who worked outside as laborers. Then, in the twenties, fashion designer Coco Chanel went to the French Riviera for a vacation and came back with a tan, beginning the trend of tanning for health and beauty.

The potential for skin cancer is hard to ignore, but I don't think a nice tan will ever go out of fashion entirely.

The Bald Facts About Hair

Q: I want to have laser treatments to remove my beard, because I hate shaving and I don't like whiskers either. I was told that I'm not a good candidate for beard removal by laser, because I have a psoriasis-like condition on my face. I was told that the laser would make the psoriasis weep, and I'd get an oozing rash. Does that sound right to you?

QUIZ

True or False: Any pair of sunglasses will provide your eyes with adequate protection from the sun.
False: Not all sunglasses are created equal. Look for a pair that blocks at least 98% of the sun's rays.

A: First of all, I don't think a laser is an effective tool for removing any man's beard, no matter what the condition of the man's skin. A laser easily covers a large area, so it does a great job removing the patches of finer hair that most women have. But the thick, dense hair on a man's beard is a tall order for a laser. It would take many, many treatments.

Even under a lesser challenge than a beard, laser treatments have to be repeated, because hairs grow back. You would have to be dedicated to the time and expense of follow-up. I think you'd find this to be a far greater inconvenience than shaving.

As for your skin condition, it doesn't sound like psoriasis to me. First of all, psoriasis is not common on the face. Also, psoriasis causes flakiness, not moisture or oozing.

You might want to get this diagnosed and treated. You should definitely have it treated if you do decide to investigate laser treatments. I wouldn't want you going at your skin with a laser until you know what ails it.

Q: Is it true that gray facial hair cannot be removed with a laser?

A: Color contrast between skin color and hair color does make for the most successful laser hair-removal treatments. The laser zooms in on the dark hair against the pale skin, vaporizing the hair and damaging the follicle.

New lasers with broader capabilities are being introduced all the time, and some promise to do a better job on people whose hair and skin color are similar: dark-skinned people with dark hair and pale people with blond or gray hair.

Another technique involves rubbing a black cream on the skin. It accumulates in the pores and attracts the laser to the follicle.

If you do some digging, you will probably find someone who can remove gray hair with a laser, but be sure to ask directly about the person's skill specific to your needs and look at some before-and-after photos.

Q: I was thinking about hair removal from my back. Is electrolysis or laser the best?

A: Your back is a large area, so electrolysis would take a LONG time, no matter how much hair there is. And a laser can do many hairs at one time.

I have not seen a lot of literature on laser hair removal for men's backs, but I would encourage you to talk to at least a couple of different laser practitioners before you make a decision. This field is changing rapidly, and new treatments are emerging all the time.

I just hope you're not going crazy. The issue is: Are you self-conscious about the hair, or is the hair bothering you? If the latter, then you should take care of it. Otherwise, why waste your money?

The laser won't get everything in one visit, and it's more expensive, but it will certainly take care of the problem more quickly than electrolysis can. However, electrolysis may have a higher rate of permanent removal. It depends on who is doing it and what type of hair you have. Curly hair is more difficult to remove with electrolysis, because of the spiral shape of the follicle.

There is also waxing. It hurts, but it is a quick way of getting rid of a lot of hair, but you have to do this on a regular basis.

Now, are you sure you can't live with what you've got?

QUIZ

What's the long-term result of plucking or shaving facial hair?
A) thicker hair   B) darker hair   C) more hair
D) faster-growing hair   E) no change
(E: In case you were wondering, men who shave throughout their lifetime will remove almost 27 feet of hair.)

DID YOU KNOW?
IF IT CURLS . . .

When Swedish researchers used computer-aided reconstructions of hair from Caucasian, black, and Asian subjects, they determined that it's the follicle, not the shape of the hair shaft, that determines whether you have straight or curly hair. Curly hair grows from spiral follicles, which is why electrolysis doesn't always work when curls are involved. The straight needle going into the follicle won't hit its target the way a straight needle in a straight follicle will.

Q: I asked my doctor about taking a drug to fight hair loss. He told me about Proscar. I also have problems with my prostate. Isn't Proscar used for that, too?

A: Yes, Proscar is used to treat an enlarged prostate, and Propecia, the exact same drug as Proscar, works for some bald men. These medications work because they block testosterone, which is an important part of both problems. The difference in the two pills is that the prostate version (Proscar) contains five times as much of the active ingredient as the hair pill (Propecia).

Q: My roommate recently lost a lot of weight, and she is also losing a lot of hair. Are the two related? Should she take a specific vitamin?

A: Usually people lose weight without losing their hair, but there can be a relationship between the two.

QUIZ

How many hairs do you have on your head?
A) 25,000   B) 125,000   C) 750,000   D) 1 million
(B: 125,000.)

Of course, the basis of weight loss is to burn more calories than you consume, and in some people that seems to affect the hair follicle. The hair loss is almost always reversible. I've known women to lose a lot of hair that then grows right back in.

Hair is so important in our culture that I always advise a woman who is suffering from hair loss to visit a dermatologist. The doctor will pluck out a few hairs and, by looking at the roots, will immediately know if a condition other than the weight loss is the cause of the problem. Other nondisease causes of hair loss are stress and heavy exercise.

I know of no specific vitamin or nutrient that your friend should take.

Q: My nineteen-year-old son is very image-conscious and insists on bleaching his hair every few months. Is this going to have any long-term effects on his hair or his general health?

A: Well, it could be worse—say, neon orange or purple. Or he could be sporting a two-tone Mohawk.

Seriously, you may have heard reports claiming that beauticians and people who dye their hair have higher rates of assorted diseases. This has never been confirmed, but if there is a danger it would involve people who are around these dyes every day. I don't know of any health effect that happens with bleaching other than damage to your hair.

Q: I'm desperate to deal with my baldness, which is getting worse by the day. How do you feel about hair transplants?

A: The main risk is that you could end up with a bad hair day—forever. And that's a pretty big risk in my book. As for the medical and surgical risks, they are fairly small.

QUIZ

The color of our eyes and hair may tell us more than we want to know. Who ages faster?

A) blue-eyed blondes   B) brown-eyed blondes

C) blue-eyed brunettes   D) brown-eyed brunettes

(A: blue-eyed blondes.)

Early on, the most common error surgeons made was putting the hair plugs in rows, so your head looked like an orchard. When you look at someone who has a bad hair job, the transplants are obvious and unsightly.

Another very important aspect is the hairline; good surgeons create a natural hairline using much smaller grafts, sometimes down to two or three hairs. This gives a more natural appearance. You should also recognize that this is a time-consuming, expensive and sometimes frustrating procedure. You need to be committed and you want to look at lots of before-and-after pictures before you pick the surgeon.

Of course, most doctors don't offer photos of their disasters, and most people who have transplants are satisfied. But you need to be patient, and you need enough hair elsewhere on your head that you can spare.

The Hype and the Facts Behind Creams, Lotions, and Oils

Q: My friend says that my body cream, which has a lot of nut oils in it, will be absorbed through my skin and make me fat. I told her this is nonsense. But she did scare me a bit when she pointed out that estrogen cream is put on the skin to be absorbed into the body. Is the same true with fat?

A: This is preposterous, of course, but if you want to keep her as a friend I wouldn't respond quite that way.

The body is not capable of absorbing fat into the bloodstream from the skin. It is the body's digestive system that breaks down fat, protein, and any other substances that we put in our mouths, turning it into smaller, absorbable components that will be metabolized as nutrition or waste, or stored as fat.

Skin can absorb some medications, like estrogen, especially when combined with certain chemicals that the pharmaceutical companies know will allow the best absorption. Fat is a large molecule, however, and any piece that got through the skin would be so tiny it would have no influence whatsoever.

Oils and other substances in moisturizers seal in moisture, but they don't actually do the moisturizing. When you wash yourself, your skin soaks up the water, and the lotion you rub on afterward prevents that moisture from evaporating quickly.

Your friend is a lucky gal to have time to worry about the fat in lotion when

The Edell Report
Don't Waste Your Money

Given women's—and some men's—passion for moisturizers, and their constant pursuit of something even better, you would never know that this beauty aid is really very simple. It's not the jojoba or the aloe that makes it work; all moisturizers break down into two ingredients—an occlusive (petroleum jelly and/or an oil) and a humectant (something that allows your skin to retain moisture, such as glycerine). That's it.

Moisture does not come from moisturizers. Moisture comes from water. After you bathe or shower, the way to moisturize yourself is to seal in the water on your skin with an oil-based product.

If you don't believe me, here's what the Berkeley Wellness Letter *had to say about it: "You may think that skin absorbs moisture or oil from a moisturizer, but it doesn't work that way. The skin absorbs little from a moisturizer. The moisturizing effect comes from the protective factor (usually some form of petroleum jelly or oil) and from the humectant. Thus, the product keeps your skin's own moisture from evaporating."*

All those other ingredients—vitamins, liposomes, hormones, and collagen—are useless.

One Consumer Reports *comparison of thirty moisturizers found that Vaseline Intensive Care Dry Skin formula, at about 30 cents an ounce, worked best. The most expensive product tested was $16 per ounce, and it did less moisturizing than the cheap stuff.*

in other places people worry about death, war, and starvation. Has our obsession with fat gone off the deep end or what?

Q: I have severely dry skin. Is there any correlation between that and the amount of water I drink? Also, some body oils are made to be put on after a shower. Does that mean I should apply them while my skin is still wet?

A: Skin is dead, so, to tell you the truth, I don't think drinking lots of water makes a lick of difference in keeping it moist, although that is certainly the common advice. How you hydrate your skin externally and the dryness it is exposed to environmentally are what does make a difference.

Of course, adequate hydration is necessary for bodily functions, but the blood regulates the concentration of water in our system. The result of drinking an excessive amount of water is not increased moisture in the skin, but a full bladder.

Trapping moisture on your skin is the way to treat dry skin. A moisturizer seals in moisture, so the trick is to put on a moisturizer after a bath or shower when your skin is fully hydrated. It seals in the dampness in your skin. Pouring moisturizer on dry skin does no good and may keep out environmental moisture.

So I recommend that you apply body oil before you are entirely dry, although I think you can towel off a little.

The shinbone is the driest place on the body. For many of us, this site is not a happy sight. It's the spot dermatologists use to assess the dryness of skin, and it's a good spot for you to do a test of moisturizers.

Manufacturers aren't doing head-to-toe clinical tests on moisturizers, because most products don't do the job. The most effective one we have— petroleum jelly—is esthetically displeasing. But it's the best at creating a barrier that prevents water from evaporating from skin.

Q: I've heard you say that petroleum jelly is a great moisturizer, but I have semi-oily skin. Will the jelly clog my pores? Also, whenever I use a toner, I get this supertight feeling. Is that how toners work?

DID YOU KNOW?
THE INJECTABLES: WHAT'S WHAT AT A GLANCE

If you're confused about the various wrinkle treatments currently on the market, check out the chart from The American Society for Aesthetic Plastic Surgery on the following pages.

	HYALURONIC ACID	BOTULINUM TOXIN	FAT INJECTIONS	BOVINE-BASED COLLAGEN	HUMAN-BASED COLLAGEN
Name	Restylane, Perlane, and Restylane Fine Lines	Botox and Myobloc	Fat Injection	Zyderm and Zyplast	CosmoDerm and CosmoPlast
What it is	A substance found in all living organisms	Botulinum toxin type A—produced by Clostridia Botulinum bacteria	Fat transfer from one part of the body to another	Derived from purified bovine (cow) collagen	Derived from human collagen
How it works	Adds volume	Temporarily relaxes the muscle	Adds volume	Adds volume	Adds volume
Injection Areas	Nasolabial folds, forehead wrinkles, smile lines and lips	Forehead, frown lines, crow's feet and vertical neck bands	Nasolabial folds, crow's feet, lips, frown lines, and facial recontouring	Nasolabial folds, crow's feet, frown lines, and lips	Nasolabial folds, frown lines, crow's feet, feet, and lips
Results	Up to 12 months	Up to 6 months	Highly variable: months to years	Up to 6 months	Up to 6 months

Average cost*	Unknown	$399 per procedure	$1,282 per procedure	$399 per procedure	Unknown
US availability	No—FDA approval pending for cosmetic use	Yes—FDA approved for frown lines; other uses are "off-label"	Yes—Does not require FDA approval	Yes—FDA approved	Yes—FDA approved
Back To Work	No downtime	No downtime	Minor: 1–4 days Extensive: 7–14 days	No downtime	No downtime
Possible Reactions	Swelling, redness, and tenderness	Bruising, redness, droopy eyelid, flu-like symptoms, headache	Swelling, bruising and lumpiness	Slight bruising and allergic reactions	Swelling, redness and bruising
Other Considerations	Does not require allergy skin test	None identified at this time	Requires a donor site (i.e., thighs, abdomen, or buttocks)	Requires allergy skin test—at least one month wait	Does not require allergy skin test

*According to American Society For Aesthetic Plastic Surgery 2002 statistics

A: I don't think you need anything at all on your skin. If you have naturally oily skin, you don't need a moisturizer, because your skin oils will replenish on their own. The oils that are removed when you wash your face are probably replaced within hours.

As for toners, most of them contain alcohol, which evaporates rapidly and dries your skin. Skin does not need toners. Dermatologists will tell you to avoid them, and so do I.

Let's face it, there are no rules for the cosmetic industry. They can sell you anything: Wrinkle creams that are bull, toners that dry your skin, and moisturizers to take care of the dry skin caused by the toners. And all for a pretty penny.

The two best things you can do for your skin are to stay out of the sun and don't smoke.

Q: I want to get rid of a scar that I've had on my wrist for forty years. What faith do you have in the scar-fading creams that are advertised?

A: None at all. You'll get the same results that you would rubbing your own saliva into that scar. In fact, nothing will fade a forty-year-old scar. Studies of aloe vera and vitamin E show them to be useless, too, even on a scar that's a week old.

The best thing to do for a fresh scar is to disturb the tissue as little as possible. In other words, leave it alone to heal.

If this scar has really become a problem for you aesthetically, talk to a plastic surgeon, who may be able to disguise it, remove it, or hide it. Generally that is done by making an incision along the body's natural lines and wrinkles. The wrist wrinkles where you fold your palm up, so it's possible to hide a scar in that wrinkly fold. But there's nowhere to hide an incision that runs the length of the arm.

Q: I have chapped lips, and someone told me that Campho-Phenique is a good over-the-counter medication for that. Its package doesn't list treating chapped lips as one of its uses though. Is it OK for this use?

A: Campho-Phenique is an old-time remedy for cold sores, but I think it could be irritating for chapped lips. I recommend you use a good-quality lip balm instead.

Let's look at what might be causing or aggravating your dry lips. Licking them will exacerbate the chapping, so you've got to avoid that. Sometimes older folks get vitamin deficiencies that can cause chapped lips. Chapping, especially in the corners of the mouth, can be a sign of infection, too. And dentures can cause trouble by stimulating too much saliva.

The one treatment pitfall you should know about is that people actually get addicted to lip balm. Their lips feel dry without lip balm, and they end up getting hooked on it. It's like getting hooked on nose drops. There are no halfway houses or Lip Balm Anonymous groups for people with these habits, but they are real. Also, lip balm can make matters worse by sealing in a fungus that needs treatment with antifungal medications.

If your lips stay chapped, even if you're using a reasonable amount of lip balm, check with your doctor to see if one of these other problems is the source of your trouble.

The Finer Points About Fingernails and Toenails

Q: I've got brittle and cracking toenails as the result of a fungal infection. I was advised to take an oral antifungal medication. What is your opinion of these drugs?

A: Unless you're a foot model and your livelihood depends on close-ups of your feet, I'm not sure any medication is worth fooling with.

Oral antifungals, such as Lamisil, are better than their predecessors, but they are still a potentially toxic group of drugs. You have to take them for eight months to a year, and often they don't work. In the meantime, they get into your bloodstream and go everywhere in your body, from your eyeballs to your knees, and eventually where you want it, your toes.

You have to take a dose that's strong enough to do battle with a disease that's growing on the underside of the toenail, a spot that is not within easy reach of the bloodstream. Delivering the medication where it will be most effective is difficult.

A topical product called Penlac also takes eight months to a year to get rid of the fungus, but at least you're not dosing your entire body with it. You paint it on like toenail polish. It works for slightly more than half of those who use it. See what your doctor has to say about it.

The folk remedies recommended for toenail fungus are soaking your feet in tea or in hot water and vinegar, but I have no idea how effective this is. The most important thing is to keep your feet dry to prevent the growth of the fungus, and it might even go away. But nothing will deliver a quick fix.

Q: I have been getting acrylic or silk wrap on my nails every week for years. Is there anything I need to worry about? I chipped the fake nails off last night, and my real ones are paper-thin.

A: I'm not surprised. There are a couple of problems that fake nails encourage, and brittle nails are one of them. Just as your skin becomes dry without proper moisturizing, so do your nails.

The stuff used to create the fake nails dries them out. Most nail-care products contain alcohol and solvents, which are the worst things for your nails. Dry, split nails are a common problem that I'm asked about all the time.

Fake nails don't breathe like your regular nails do, and this creates another problem. A recent study found that hospital nurses who wear fake nails have more germs and fungal infections under their nails than do nurses with real nails. Also, fake nails can harbor infections that aren't detected, because the wraps hide them.

During a thorough physical exam, a doctor looks at the patient's fingernails, because the fingernails tell a lot about a person's health. For example, fingernails can alert a doctor to thyroid disease, anorexia, or vitamin deficiency. Among the details a doctor might pick up are ridges that run across the nail. They tell a doctor that you had a major illness when those ridges formed. Vertical ridges are simply a part of aging and mean nothing. White spots are usually a sign of trauma to the nail, and are nothing to worry about either.

Clubbing, which is an outward bulging of the nail, can indicate heart or lung disease. And the opposite condition, where the nail is concave, can mean anemia or thyroid problems.

Of course, the doctor can't study your nails if they are smothered by fakes.

I really do recommend that you let your nails breathe sometimes. And be sure your manicurist is a licensed cosmetologist or esthetician.

QUIZ

Which grow faster, fingernails or toenails?
(Fingernails; the index fingernail grows fastest, nails grow faster during daylight, and illness can slow nail growth.)

Q: This is pretty insignificant, but I'm bothered by it. For the past couple of years my nails have not grown. They're thin, they crack, they snag. What can I do?

A: The growth of fingernails changes with the weather, and it varies from finger to finger. Nails grow faster on your right hand, on the longer fingers, in daylight and in summertime. Pregnancy can influence the way your nails grow, too.

In my experience, the one thing that can slow the growth of fingernails and toenails is vascular supply. If you have any kind of arterial or vascular insufficiency, that's a possibility, but it is fairly unusual unless you're a smoker or you have heart disease.

The other things you described are mostly due to the fact that as we age, our nails become brittler and thinner, just like our skin does. But most of us don't care for our nails the way we care for our skin. Nails need to be moisturized, like skin does.

And we put our hands in all kinds of detergents and all kinds of drying agents, and then we buy a bunch of products for our nails, which are the worst thing, because all of them contain organic solvents that will evaporate any moisture that happens to be left in our fingernails.

Whenever you put your hands in water, I would moisturize them. I'd avoid nail polish for a while and consider wearing gloves. You also can do detective work: When you're using detergents or have your hands in water, wear a glove on only one hand. After a few weeks, see if there's a difference between your hands.

Mention your concerns the next time you see your doctor. But I think you'd know if you had pulmonary or heart disease or something like that.

Q: I have very weak nails, and my friend, who loves health-food stores, told me about a silica-gel pill that would make my nails stronger. She was right. I have been taking it for a month, and my nails have really improved. But my concern is that the carton says it comes from silicon, "which gives structure to all living things throughout the plant and animal world." Have I been swallowing the stuff that breast implants are made of?

A: Silicon is an element, the second most common one in the earth's crust. The material used in breast implants is silicone—put an "e" on the end—which is a polymer. Silica is a mineral, a granular form of silicon.

I cannot imagine that silica gel is responsible for improving your nails, because it has nothing to do with nails. Weak nails are almost always caused by dryness or other problems. And it takes a long time for nails to respond to treatment; it takes the amount of time needed for the nail to grow completely out before you can expect a new, healthy, strong nail. It's like expecting that something you take internally would cure your hair's split ends. That doesn't make sense, does it?

I'm glad your nails seem to be improved, but that gel has nothing to do with it.

Q: I have a friend who claims that a visit to a manicurist could expose me to an infectious disease. She says the tools usually aren't sterilized correctly, and she's very picky about where she goes. This is one of the most relaxing parts of my week. Do I have to start worrying about this, too?

A: I'm afraid your friend is right. But if you select your salon carefully, and you are sure they are doing the right things with their implements, you can relax again.

Here's the situation. Regulation of salons in many states varies from mediocre to nonexistent. A study by a team at Baylor College of Medicine in Texas—which got twenty-four states to respond to its survey—found that none of those states require salons to sterilize implements. Many states do require salons to disinfect their tools, but the research team said that isn't enough to protect people from disease.

As you know, when a manicurist is cutting cuticles—or scraping the tough skin from the bottom of your feet—she might draw blood. Yet only two states of those surveyed require workers to be screened for HIV or hepatitis B and C. And only one state required technicians to wear gloves.

Footbaths are another dicey area of treatment, because a person can pick up fungal and bacterial infections. A salon should clean the tubs after each use, first with a bleach solution for ten minutes, then with a disinfectant for ten minutes. Of course, the problem is, how are you really going to know that is happening?

Ask your friend what salon she uses and go from there. Also, don't hesitate to ask questions at the salon. You may have to pay more for your manicure and pedicure, but you will have peace of mind.

Miscellaneous: From Bigger Breasts to Spider Veins

Q: I read about something called a Brava bra in a fashion magazine. Is this legit?

A: The one medical study I've seen on this product does indicate the potential for developing larger breasts, but the size increase is modest, at best. And the product is new enough that there are no studies yet about the staying power of such "growth."

The Brava "breast enhancement and shaping system" is also quite costly (about $2,500–$3,000) and requires a major time commitment for the user, so check it out thoroughly before you make the leap. You need to ask yourself: Do I want to be wearing suction cups for ten hours a day for six to eight weeks, so that I can possibly increase my breasts by one cup size? That sounds like a lot of work to me!

However, if you are looking for more symmetry with your breasts—rather than larger breasts—this appears to be a viable option. You have to have a prescription for the bra, so talk to your doctor about whether this is the product for you. Or you can start at the company Web site, *www.brava.com*.

Q: I'm thinking about having sclerotherapy to remove spider veins. Something called Sotradecol would be injected into my veins. Since this is cosmetic surgery, I don't want to take any unnecessary risks. Do you know anything about the safety of this procedure?

A: I can't say that any medical technique is 100 percent safe, but I've never heard of any problems with sclerotherapy. It is possible for the needle to go in the wrong place, which would cause inflammation, but I've not heard of that happening a lot.

The best way to weigh the risk is to ask the doctor what complications or side effects he or she has seen. The doctor will say, "Well, one in fifty patients get this; one in one hundred get that, and one in two thousand get the other." You will then be able to decide if these are chances you're willing to take.

The American Society for Dermatological Surgery has called sclerotherapy the "gold standard" for treatment of leg veins. With sclerotherapy, very high concentrations of salt or other chemicals are injected into the vein, causing inflammation. Then, the vein is collapsed with a compression bandage for a time, so no blood flows through, and the veins scar shut. The first day or two of recovery can be quite painful.

A San Diego, California, vascular surgeon has also introduced a treatment involving glycerin-foam injections that he claims will produce the same results as sclerotherapy but without the side effects. That's very new, so stay tuned.

Finally, there's a clever process called a radio frequency—closure technique, in which a catheter delivers radio-frequency energy to the vein, which causes the vein to shrink and to seal shut.

After hundreds of thousands of these procedures have been done, we will have a lot more statistical data. Based on what we know so far, I have seen nothing but encouraging results.

So, find a dermatologist who does all these procedures, and he or she should be able to recommend the one that is best for you.

Q: I'm a fifty-three-year-old man, and my wife says my yellow teeth

DID YOU KNOW?
FORGET ABOUT THOSE DIMPLED THIGHS!

You know the male cliché about guys not noticing "stuff"—like a new haircut or even a new hair color? Well, add cellulite—the accumulation of subcutaneous fat, usually in the hips and thighs—to the list.

According to one French study, most men say they don't really notice it, and others are clueless about its existence. One in five guys thought it was a type of battery, and one in three men said they had no idea what it was.

Of course, most women know what it is—about 80 percent of all women have some—and said it was their biggest cause of misery. Four out of five women said they feel negative about themselves because of cellulite.

Folks, we need to shift our worry meters toward something a bit more substantial—and controllable.

make me look older. Should I buy one of those drugstore treatments or should I talk to my dentist? Does anything really work?

A: Most dentists are against the do-it-yourself method simply because if the bleach gets near your gum line it can increase your chances for periodontal disease. The one-hour Brite Smile method, which is done at a dentist's office (or at a Brite Smile office), is very effective but expensive, and the results after any of these techniques are not permanent. Your teeth usually look great the day after—or when you reach your peak whiteness—but then quickly yellow again. How fast, depends on your eating habits. Remember, even green and orange vegetables with a lot of beta-carotene and other pigments can stain your teeth, as do tea, coffee, and cigarettes. Money aside, I think the Brite Smile method is the best technique at the moment.

Q: I'm considering having permanent makeup applied to my lips. I want a natural color and an outline, just for enhancement. The color would be light—it hardly looks like lipstick. What's the downside to something like this?

A: I have to warn you that as we age, things sag. And permanent makeup is attached to the skin and next to impossible to remove.

When your skin sags, your lips will, too, and your outline and color might fall down like clown lips. When you apply makeup every day yourself, you have the freedom to cheat a little bit and reshape your mouth.

Sometimes I've seen a woman put on lipstick and say, "Oh, that looks horrible" and wipe it right off. Well, you can't wipe this off and start again. Obviously, you want to work with an experienced (and licensed, if your state requires it) technician. Test the dye first, too, to be sure you're not allergic to it.

I'm not sure what the gain will be. Unless you have arthritis or a visual

QUIZ

Where is the thinnest skin on your body?
A) lips   B) ears   C) between your fingers   D) eyelids
(D: eyelids; the skin is one five-hundredths of an inch thick; the rest of our skin averages one-twentieth of an inch in thickness.)

impairment, putting on lipstick isn't that tough. Now, I could never accurately put eyeliner on my own eyes, so I certainly understand wanting that as permanent makeup. But again, if something goes wrong on the eyelid, repair would be next to impossible. And trends do change. Remember the sixties, when makeup was taboo?

Q: I'm thirty-seven years old, and over the last couple of years, I've been developing what my wife calls skin tags on my back, shoulders, side of my neck, and armpits. Should I be concerned about them?

A: My mother used to tell me to take a hair and tie a knot around the skin tags and choke the little suckers until they turned black and fell off. However, I didn't listen to my mother and neither should you.

Skin tags are benign skin growths that typically appear in the areas you named. We think that some people have a gene that predisposes them to these tags.

Some researchers are exploring a possible relationship between skin tags and an increased risk of polyps in the colon, and while there's nothing conclusive that I know of, ask your dermatologist what he or she knows about this topic. When you reach your late forties or early fifties, you might want to have someone take a peek inside your colon just to be sure everything's OK.

And, if you want, the doctor can zap them off in two seconds.

Resource List

For details about everything from a facelift to a breast lift, plus a surgeon directory, check out the Web site of the American Society of Plastic Surgeons: *www.plasticsurgery.org*

Go to the patient/procedures section of the American Academy of Facial Plastic and Reconstructive Surgery Web site for before-and-after pictures, a "physician finder," as well as extensive information on all types of facial surgery: *www.facial-plastic-surgery.org*

The American Society for Aesthetic Plastic Surgery Web site will help you find a surgeon: *www.surgery.org*

The American Academy of Dermatology has tons of information on acne, aging skin, eczema, and more: *www.aad.org/*

For the latest info related to Botox, go to MedLine Plus, the Web site produced by the National Institutes of Health and the U.S. National Library of Medicine: *www.nlm.nih.gov/medlineplus/botox.html*

Current information from the Food and Drug Administration on breast implants can be found at *www.fda.gov/cdrh/breastimplants*

For the latest research on rosacea, visit the Web site of the National Rosacea Society: *www.rosacea.org*

Get the full picture on hair transplants for men and women, as well as a directory of transplant doctors, at *www.hairtransplantmedical.com*

Chapter 8

Healthy Minds, Healthy Lives

A healthy body is a great thing, but why are so many of us reluctant to include the mind when we think about good health?

I know about this because I've been there.

I was very unhappy as a young man in medical school. Early in my life I had wanted to be an artist, but practicality gave way, and I started college studying architecture. I didn't enjoy that or several other majors that I considered ever so briefly, and ultimately reality presented itself. I had to commit to something that would stick.

I decided to go to medical school because a friend of mine was going to be a doctor and I figured I was at least as smart as he was. Good, rational thinking, huh? But there were lots of folks just like me out there every day—kind of lost and confused. Some of us eventually got lucky—or got help—and some of us didn't. In my case, I was caught in the throes of depression and didn't even realize it.

The process of getting a degree nearly finished me. I had never made my peace with my decision, and I was a very unhappy person. When the clinical years came around, then the end of medical school, and the internship and training, it only got worse. The responsibility, the stress, and the hordes of sick people made going to the clinic a dreadful experience. When you are depressed, the practice of medicine can be very depressing. After all, people don't go to doctors because they want to have a good time.

Prozac wasn't making headlines in that era, and even though I was a physician, I couldn't identify my problem. Being a male only compounded it. Men are much less likely to recognize the symptoms of depression and even less likely to seek treatment. A man is also four times more likely than a woman to kill himself.

Depression is more common in women, but women have the ability to spontaneously talk about their issues and they are less embarrassed about getting help. Most men can't talk about, and they don't even recognize the warning signs: sleep problems, withdrawal, irritability, loss of interest in hobbies and work. They just plop down in front of the TV for endless hours of ESPN's *SportsCenter.*

Of course, I blamed all my problems on medicine, but it wasn't that simple. During medical school I continued painting and tried to sell my paintings through a gallery. But even when I sold one, I got depressed, because the woman who bought it was going to put it in the guest bathroom. Of course, I had an ego, and I thought it should be front and center in someone's living room. Nothing was working the way I had expected it to.

When I eventually sought out a therapist, I realized it was the best thing I had ever done for myself and those close to me. I knew it wasn't weakness but strength that made me drop the guy stuff and get help. Plus, my therapist taught me new skills to help combat the thinking errors depressed people make, like blaming themselves and linking negative thought patterns. In the years since this time in my life, I have encouraged many men and women in similar situations to pursue talk and drug therapy. I wish I could feel more confident that most folks take my advice.

Let's face it: The stigma of mental illness still exists, and the cost to our society is huge, not only because of suicides, divorce, family abuse, job loss, and homelessness among so many people who could be so easily helped.

Depression seems to be more common today than ever before, perhaps because we are doing a better job of tracking it and other mental illnesses—and because we know more, though not a lot. Anxiety seems to be emerging, along with stress, as a powerful inducer of depression, but by the same token, many of us seem to learn or inherit a way of thinking that keeps our mood down.

We know even less about happiness, though there do seem to be people who are born happy. Doctors call it hyperthymia, and while it doesn't look like an illness, doctors aren't quite sure why some people seem to cruise through life in a euphoric state. Because these people don't go to psychiatrists complaining that they are too happy, there are very few studies of it.

Once upon a time, we defined happiness as optimism. If you were optimistic about the immediate future, we didn't think there was much more you needed to enjoy your life. However, it would seem that a little pessimism can be a good thing. People who are overly optimistic seem to have a harder time dealing with life's bumps, which inevitably come along.

In fact, some people who are hyperthymic eventually develop bipolar disorder (once called manic depression) or deep depressions. Nevertheless, there are people who maintain this high state of being, and scientists are beginning to explore this side of mental health.

Often when I talk to people about depression, one of the reasons they don't see a doctor is because they are afraid of being put on antidepressant medications. We live in a funny society, one where many of us turn to illegal drugs or alcohol because of depression but would refuse to take drugs prescribed for depression. This is crazy thinking, and it hurts not only the depressed individual but everyone close to him or her. I know this won't be the last time I say this, but depression is an illness—not a weakness—and it is highly treatable.

So are many other mental disorders, and this is the best time yet in modern society for doctors, therapists, and patients, because a record number of psychopharmaceutical medications have been approved or are in the research and development pipeline, with the biggest advances coming in the area of antidepressants with fewer side effects. But don't wait for the next hot drug. The current crop of medications is highly successful, especially when used in conjunction with talk therapy to help folks navigate their way through life at a higher level.

While you are on medication is often the best time to learn how you became depressed and how to deal with depression in the future.

Unfortunately, that treatment combo is not the norm. Psychotherapeutic drugs, I believe, are often overprescribed by doctors who don't have the time or the training to give you the appropriate combination of talk therapy *and* medication. And, of course, managed health care programs encourage inexpensive solutions—and talk therapy ain't cheap.

While depression is a hot topic, anxiety and stress are getting their share of attention. Our lives are full of stress, because there is, indeed, a lot of pressure on us. We are expected to do so much more than our forebears. We have e-mail and voice mail, plus telephone calls and faxes and snail mail. We now have so many ways of giving and receiving information that it can easily become overwhelming, whether we're focused on the world situation or the problems of our children or friends. Women are expected to be stellar parents and wage earners, and men are expected to fill both roles, too.

Like mood changes, a certain amount of anxiety and stress is healthy. Depriving animals in a laboratory of either element shortens their life span. Yet we are now learning about the profound effects on our health that depression, anxiety and stress can have. We already know that what's stressful for you may not be stressful for me, but we don't know why. We each have to understand and accept our differences; while fishing may have a calming effect on you, it would drive me nuts. So I don't do it.

How you cope is what's critical, and recent research shows that most of us do a mediocre job with this. Going to a yoga class once a week or taking the occasional long, restful weekend is probably not enough. It's more important to handle the stress as it's happening, and whatever you use to relax—a dog, tennis, hiking—needs to be woven into the tapestry of your day-to-day existence on an ongoing basis.

Our inborn skills at dealing with life make us all different, and sometimes it's less a matter of changing who we are than learning how to handle our mental environment in a way that works better for us. For instance, sitting in traffic drives some people crazy. It's kind of funny, isn't it, because you aren't really doing much, and most of us have all the comforts and technological advancements available in our cars, from CDs to cell phones—yet being "stuck" or not getting where you want to be as fast as you want to get there can put some people over the edge.

The point of all of this is that most people do not have a handle on what's going on inside their heads. We hardly recognize our depressions, and we refuse to admit our stress and anxiety, so we do nothing about them until we get very strong signs—a meltdown at work or a crumbling relationship.

These are very important parts of our lives—and where we spend the majority of our time. After all, you are what you think. When we find ourselves not doing well with work or family, it's time for a mental inventory.

I know a marital counselor who calls his job divorce counseling, because by the time people come to see him it's often too late. No one teaches us about how to have successful relationships; we don't have to take a test to get a marriage license. And yet psychologists tell us that they can give us surveys before we get married and predict which relationships will make it. Perhaps some day couples will have to complete that survey before getting a license—just so they know what they're getting into.

When we do find real happiness and contentment, there's a dividend. Duke University Medical Center looked at people with heart disease and found that being happy and cheerful gave you a 20 percent better survival rate. That's a lot more than your treadmill will give you. Even after taking into account how sick the patients were initially, as well as major factors like smoking and other bad habits, cheerful people still had a significant advantage.

But please don't think you have to be happy—or content or anxiety-free— every minute of every day. That's not reality and that's not my message. We all have bad days, down days, stressful days. It's swinging too high or too low that needs to be fixed. When bad weeks at work turn into bad months at work, something's wrong. If your spouse notices a change in your personality, you need to pay attention. Talk to your doctor, because there is so much that modern medicine and good therapists can do to make you feel better.

If Tipper Gore, Charley Pride, Frances Ford Coppola, Ben Stiller, and Kitty Dukakis can be open about their mental health problems, why can't you?

Depression and Bipolar Disorder

Q: My middle-aged daughter is a successful businesswoman whose life is now going very well, following some stressful years. She has healthy kids and a good marriage. But, for the past month, she has been constantly tired. She sleeps six to eight hours a day, after being in bed all night. She says she isn't in pain and she doesn't feel sick, but she has no energy. She is very often cold, too. She is reluctant to see a doctor, but her husband and I are worried. What should we say to her?

A: You have a right to be concerned, because this is not healthy behavior. However, my big fear is she will see a doctor who will immediately diagnose her illness as chronic fatigue syndrome. That's the worst label in the world, because chronic fatigue syndrome is a supposed disease that has no known cause, no means of diagnosis, and no cure. This is a last-resort diagnosis, and other things should be considered first.

Fatigue can be correctly diagnosed if the doctor starts from scratch with a full battery of tests, including those for thyroid disease and iron deficiency, which are often accompanied by a sensation of coldness.

Another possibility is a sleep disorder called apnea (see more about this in chapter 12), which causes the afflicted person to unknowingly and frequently snore and stop breathing during the night. And a few patients who are labeled with chronic fatigue syndrome turn out to have rare parasitic infections.

But far and away the most common cause of abundant sleepiness is depression. There's a dangerous myth that a successful job and family life preclude depression. Well, depression is a disease, and we can get depressed when life is good, just like we can get the measles when life is good.

The point at which we achieve success is the point at which many of us question our lives. A person who has spent years pinning their happiness on a great job, money, and security can be scared into depression when that day finally arrives, because they realize that belief was totally flawed.

As for how to approach the subject, I think it's best if her husband tackle this head-on with her, since her continued unwillingness to acknowledge an ill-ness—no matter what it is—is not healthy for her family. After that conversation, you can let her know that you are concerned, too.

Q: Do you think I am better off seeing a psychologist or a psychiatrist to talk about some minor issues in my life? I am a mildly depressed single guy in my thirties.

A: Regardless of professional degree, you will get the most from finding a person with whom you feel simpatico. Is the doctor easy to talk to? Do you feel comfortable with the way they talk to you? And consider how important gender is before you get recommendations. Some women like talking to other women, some don't, and the same goes for guys. You might want to talk to two or three different doctors before making a commitment to one.

As for the difference between psychiatrists and psychologists, and which is best for you, here's where you'll see a bit of my bias.

Psychiatrists have medical training that includes a residency in psychiatry. They are M.D.s and they treat serious mental illnesses like schizophrenia, manic depression, and obsessive-compulsive disorders. Many of these doctors are very skilled in talk therapy, too.

Because they are medical doctors, psychiatrists can prescribe antidepres-

The Edell Report
Workday Blues?

If your job gets you down, you're not alone. According to one study of 900 workers, jobs with high demands and low decision authority can cause you to become excessively depressed. And another study of six major companies found that unmanaged stress and depression are the two most costly factors when it comes to company medical expenses.

The Johns Hopkins University researchers looked at 905 full-time employees in Baltimore, Maryland, and concluded that those with high job strain had a greater prevalence of major depressive episodes. They also had more depressive symptoms.

Women generally suffer more depression from this job strain than men, according to an American Journal of Public Health *report on the study. However, unmarried men are also at a higher risk of depression from the work environment than their married counterparts.*

Another study, analyzing the behavior of more than 46,000 workers, found stress and depression to be more expensive for the companies than smoking and obesity.

The bottom line is that heavy demands in your occupation can give you a bad case of the blues, especially if you don't have much to say about the situation.

If you see yourself in this picture, start looking at your life outside of work. Your personal interests and hobbies—especially if they include some kind of exercise—may make the difference in how you feel.

---

sants and other medications. Of course, this is helpful for patients who will benefit from drugs. Sometimes, though, psychiatrists can rely on drugs too much and too soon.

In general, as a group, I think psychologists (those with Ph.D.s, that is), are more skilled in talking with you about the lumps and bumps of daily life—family, marriage, and career—than psychiatrists, perhaps because they can't prescribe drugs by law and therefore are more focused on talk therapy. They also are less expensive than psychiatrists.

A good psychologist knows which patients will benefit from talk therapy and which patients should be referred for psychopharmacology. In some medical practices, psychiatrists and psychologists work as a team, one focused on the talk, the other focused on medications.

Rather that getting a name out of the Yellow Pages, see if any of your friends or a family member already has a good doctor they can recommend. Or, ask your primary care physician for names. Getting recommendations from trustworthy sources almost always makes this process more successful.

Finally, you said you are "mildly depressed," but, because you're a guy, you might not be admitting, even to yourself, how you really feel. Guys can be ripped apart with the deepest, darkest, death-defying depression and not even know it, or not want to say it. Make sure you are completely open with whomever you choose to see. You've already taken a big step by deciding to see a doctor, so make sure you collect the payoff. Congratulations.

Q: Two years ago, I had strange feelings that lasted maybe four months. I thought it might be depression, so I took some St. John's Wort, and they finally went away. But then I had all this energy—I was up at four A.M., accomplishing all kinds of things.

DID YOU KNOW?
WE NEED HELP!

In 1999, there were 1.7 times as many suicides as homicides. And among Caucasians and blacks, single black mothers have the lowest suicide rate, while white males account for more than 70 percent of all suicides. This is scary, folks, and it should tell you just how much of a stigma remains when the subject is mental health. Guys, when are we going to acknowledge that a mind is just like the rest of a body—and sometimes it gets sick and needs treatment?

A few months ago, the tiredness set in again. I didn't feel suicidal, but didn't have any energy. This time I went to the doctor, and he recommended Prozac, but I didn't want to take that, so I decided to do talk therapy. The therapist also suggested medication and gave me some samples of Paxil. I put them away, but my husband finally got disgusted with me and convinced me to try them. I took 10 milligrams—I refused to take 20 milligrams—every day for about a month and I didn't feel it was having any effect, so I just stopped taking it.

Now my question: Is there a way to know if I have manic depression?

A: I can see where you're going with this. You're one of those do-it-yourselfers. The symptoms you described are classic for manic depression—which is also known as bipolar disorder—and most people don't understand that a person can spend a lot of time in the "up" or manic phase of the illness. You may feel grandiose and delusional, and you'll accomplish all kinds of things, but then again, sometimes you get yourself in trouble and don't accomplish much, and then you go down.

In your case, the highest priority should be committing to one doctor you trust and following that doctor's advice. If he or she prescribes medications, please remember that psychiatric drugs take time to work.

Paxil is an SSRI (selective serotonin reuptake inhibitor), and they can be tricky for treatment of manic depression, especially since there are other drugs that specifically address the disorder. So, go back to your doctor, be very specific about how you feel, then stick with one regimen and see if it helps you. You're bouncing around and that's worrisome.

I don't really understand your reluctance to take these medications. They can help; they save lives and they can improve your life. At this point, don't set limits on dosage; that's silly. Who cares if you are on 10 milligrams or 30 milligrams, as long as it helps you? I am confident you will get results with a combination of medication and talk therapy.

Q: I have been on anti-depression and anti-anxiety medications for two years, and now my family doctor, who has handled all my treatment so far, wants me to see a psychiatrist for medications management. Is this necessary?

A: I would encourage you to do this sooner rather than later, and I just wish your doctor had made this suggestion a while back. Too many patients are treated for complicated mental illnesses by general practitioners and other doc-

The Edell Report
The Hot Button Called Chronic Fatigue

When I talk about chronic fatigue syndrome, I get angry calls. That's because, to date, the evidence supports a diagnosis of this as a mental disorder rather than a physical illness. I find one study particularly compelling.

In searching for the possible genetic and environmental causes of chronic fatigue syndrome, researchers at the Department of Medicine at the University of Washington reviewed the health problems of 127 pairs of twins. One twin had had chronic fatigue syndrome for at least six months, and the other was not fatigued.

The evaluation found that the twins with chronic fatigue syndrome had high rates of other conditions—fibromyalgia (widespread pain in muscles and tendons), irritable bowel syndrome, chronic pelvic pain, multiple chemical sensitivity, and TMJ (jaw pain)—and that their twins rarely had any of these other illnesses. For example, 70 percent of the twins with chronic fatigue syndrome also had fibromyalgia, compared with 10 percent of their twins.

There's a pattern here that's impossible to ignore. These other illnesses have causes that are not fully understood, but we feel there are strong links to stress, anxiety, depression, or somatization. The symptoms of chronic fatigue syndrome, fibromyalgia, and multiple chemical sensitivity are all similar. That's suspicious. It is also suspicious that none of them can be diagnosed by any known test that finds any physical cause. Of course, some cases of TMJ and irritable bowel syndrome can be linked to a bad diet, or disease. But people can become physically ill by the power of their brain, and that doesn't mean they suffer from mental illness. The symptoms are real to them but not based on physical changes. Cognitive and behavioral therapies can be very effective in treating these problems.

The evidence keeps stacking up on this issue, but I'll change my mind as soon as solid, contrary proof comes along.

DID YOU KNOW?
THE PINK SLIP SYNDROME

Thanks to downsizing, bankruptcy, and corrupt practices, lots of companies are cutting their payrolls—or going out of business—and that means lots of folks are losing their jobs, sometimes for the first time in their lives. Well, if you are one of those people, give yourself a good, long time to recover. A recent study by the University of Michigan shows that the negative consequences of unemployment can last up to two years, even for those people who found new jobs. Financial strain and loss of health care benefits are two of the most stressful factors that can lead to depression and loss of self-esteem. Is this you? If so, please find a support group or a therapist to help you through this tough spell.

tors with limited training in this field. It is as inappropriate for your gynecologist to prescribe Prozac as it is for a psychiatrist to do a Pap smear. Depression is highly treatable, but not all medications work the same in all patients—and some people who are depressed don't need them. Mental health is not as straightforward as, "You're depressed, here's a pill."

Nowadays, some psychiatrists who specialize in medications are finding success with "cocktails" that combine two or more drugs. But it can take months to figure out which cocktail works best for a patient.

A lot has changed in the field of psychiatric medicines in the past few years, and it will continue to change. This means good things for almost everyone dealing with mental illness.

Q: I've taken several different antidepressants over the last few years. After beginning the first one, Prozac, I was in marvelous shape mentally; but after a month, I developed a side effect, sexual dysfunction. Now, I'm on trazodone and I still have trouble getting an erection. Do all antidepressants come with this issue? This is not what I had in mind as I face forty.

A: Sexual problems are a very common side effect of antidepressants—but erectile failure is not a common one. However it can be the first sign of heart disease, diabetes, and some other conditions. And it can have psychological origins.

I want you to start by making an appointment with a urologist. Tell the doctor about your particular problem. As you know, we live in the era of the little blue pill, Viagra; maybe that will help you.

What's curious about your case is that trazodone is being used to treat erectile failure. One of its side effects is a prolonged, unwanted erection.

Some antidepressants are less likely to cause sexual problems—Wellbutrin and Serzone, for example—so, after you see the urologist, talk to your psychologist/psychiatrist about trying something else.

Q: I will be taking a drug test for a military job. They're going to test my overall fitness, and take urine and blood samples. My life is on a bit of a bumpy road right now, so I'm taking 40 milligrams of Paxil each day. This is something I don't want the military to know about. If I skip my medication for a few days, will it clear from my system and not show up on the test?

A: To my knowledge, antidepressants leave your system within twenty-four hours, so a few days of abstinence might help you avoid detection. But the military may not be looking for signs of this type of drug; antidepressants are not part of a typical screening. However, if someone wanted to look for evidence of them and was willing to spend the money, there are tests that can detect them.

QUIZ

In 2000, the No. 1 reason for hospitalization of women between the ages of eighteen and forty-four was the delivery of a baby. The No. 2 reason was:

A) plastic surgery   B) depression   C) asthma   D) fibroids
E) back problems

(B: 205,000 women were hospitalized for depression; 139,000 women were hospitalized for fibroids.)

You might want to think more about what this job means to you. Would you have to stop taking a medication that's important to you? If the job application asked whether you are taking prescription medications, and you lied, that's not a promising start. Are you sure this is what you want?

Q: My husband suffers from depression. None of the medications he's tried have helped, but he has had a lot of success with cognitive therapy. However, he still gets depressed every day around noon. What else can he do?

A: Our bodies do respond to circadian rhythms. Hormones and neurochemicals fluctuate in the course of a day and do alter our moods. Timing medication with his rhythms may prove to be very helpful.

For depression, I wholeheartedly support the combination of medication and cognitive therapy, which usually focuses on a person's current problems rather than rehashing his or her entire life from childhood. Your husband should be very specific with his psychiatrist about how he feels at various times of the day, so his doctor can experiment with different medication times.

We are finding that even the effect of chemotherapy varies depending on the time of day that it is given. In addition, diseases from arthritis to chronic pain syndromes seem to have cycles.

I wonder what hour of the day your husband would feel his low point if he took a trip to a dramatically different time zone. What happens at noon in his daily life at the moment? And does the depression happen on weekends? Perhaps there are hints in the answers to these questions.

Q: Is there really a kind of depression that only happens in the winter? My sister says that's what she has, but I'm skeptical, because she tends to be a hypochondriac.

A: Well, your sister may be a hypochondriac, but you need to be more supportive, because it's very possible she has been diagnosed with seasonal affective disorder (SAD). It's a real ailment and very treatable.

With SAD, the onset of depression-like symptoms is probably linked to sunlight—or lack of it. As the seasons change, some folks' biological clocks are thrown out of sync. Melatonin fluctuation may trigger symptoms of depression, and it is produced at increased levels in the dark. The worse months are usually January and February, and women are at higher risk. These same people usually have no signs of depression in spring and summer.

One treatment is called "bright-light therapy," but some patients respond to just being outdoors during daylight for more time in the winter than they might be on a normal summer day. Antidepressants are also used to treat SAD.

Of course, there are people who hear about this illness and convince themselves they have it. I'm not saying that's the case with your sister, but it is possible.

Diagnoses in Children

Q: My friend's seven-year-old boy is a very angry child. After ruling out attention deficit disorder, his doctor diagnosed him with bipolar disorder. My child has bipolar disorder, too, but he was an easygoing kid, never angry, and he wasn't diagnosed until age eighteen.

How does a doctor determine that a child has bipolar disorder? Is there some kind of brain-wave test?

A: This is a diagnosis to be cautious about, and your friend should get a few more opinions. There is a disturbing trend toward diagnosing younger and younger kids with psychiatric disorders. These are difficult enough to diagnose in adults who are at least able to talk accurately about their symptoms, but a seven-year-old is not going to have that capability.

We don't have a brain test for bipolar disorder, and no manual has a checklist saying that three out of four of certain behaviors, persisting for six months or a year, are the signs of bipolar disorder.

QUIZ

What behavior may have links to depression?
A) teen smoking   B) childhood obesity   C) drug usage
D) all of the above
(D: all of the above; one study found that nondepressed teens who smoke have a higher risk of developing depression, and separate research involving almost a thousand children found that chronic obesity is linked to psychiatric disorders in both children and teenagers. Many studies have linked drug usage to depression in both teens and adults.)

It is possible that the boy has been diagnosed correctly, but certainly there has to be more to go on than his anger. Maybe it's appropriate anger? Has the child suffered a loss, or is there a family dynamic at the source of his anger? At age seven, the boy's personality is still developing, and kids seem to be almost naturally bipolar. They go up and down very easily.

I think the overall motive, to diagnose these disorders as early as possible in hopes of successful drug treatment, is a good one. But we don't yet have hard evidence to back up the diagnosis and treatment of many mental disorders in kids.

Bipolar disorder used to be called manic depression, and bipolar personalities are depressed most of the time. But they do have bouts of mania, during which they are emotionally high, they can't sleep, and they become delusional. In this phase, you feel invincible and your behavior can be extreme. You might spend every cent you have on ridiculous business ventures, or get involved in destructive sexual situations.

Many famous, highly productive, creative artists have been bipolar, including Virginia Woolf, Ernest Hemingway, and William Faulkner. Some stayed manic most of the time—that's a rare form—and were depressed less frequently. Effective bipolar medications are a relatively new phenomenon, and not that long ago many people with this illness could not be effectively treated and either committed suicide or spent much of their lives in asylums and psychiatric hospitals.

Q: We have a sixteen-year-old boy who is seriously struggling with depression. So far, he has responded only slightly to medications, and the psychiatrist we are working with says it may take months to find the right medications formula. In the meantime, he has been briefly hospitalized because of his suicidal tendencies. We can't find any intensive outpatient treatment programs for teenagers in our community, and our doctor has suggested the possibility of a therapeutic boarding school. What do you know about these programs?

A: Most parents find it a very scary prospect to consider letting their child out of their sight, especially when that child is struggling. So, recognize that you are in an emotional state and be careful in doing your research.

I am very familiar with these schools, and I think legitimate programs can play a significant role in helping troubled kids, especially in programs where talk therapy—both individual and group sessions—is a strong, frequent component of the curriculum.

The Edell Report
Is Your Teenager Depressed?

I don't want to scare every parent with a child between age twelve and eighteen, but this recent report should be a wake-up call.

Researchers at Columbia University surveyed nine hundred parents of children eighteen and younger, and 89 percent said they were confident they could tell if their teenager were depressed, and 90 percent said they would be able to tell if their child were suicidal. However, 88 percent did not think most parents would recognize a child's depressed behavior. And 69 percent did not think other parents would recognize a child's suicidal behavior. In other words, we believe we know how to read our kids, but that most other parents don't know how to read their kids.

The survey also found that 65 percent of the parents did not know about reliable tests for teen depression and suicide. These tests aren't perfect, but they do identify many troubled kids who can be helped.

Of course, raising teens is always a challenge, and knowing when teen behavior crosses the line from just difficult to dangerous is never easy. But a lot of parents are fooling themselves when it comes to their knowledge of teen depression, because suicide is the No. 3 killer of teenagers in the United States, coming right behind accidents and homicides.

If you have concerns about your child, insist that he or she see a therapist or your family physician. Teaching youngsters how to deal with their problems through talk therapy, either one-on-one with a doctor or in peer groups, is underutilized. They will probably fight you on this, but tell them you won't take no for an answer. Then follow through.

One caveat: The use of antidepressant medications has never been subjected to rigorous, long-term studies, and many experts feel we are overmedicating many kids. And there is a suspicion, not yet proven, that some of the medications—for instance, Paxil—may increase the risk for deeper depression and suicide.

The best way to find the right program for your child is to use an educational consultant; see if your child's psychiatrist can recommend someone in your region. Good consultants are familiar with programs across the country and will interview you and your child before recommending the best programs for you. Please don't go school-hunting on your own. There are bad programs out there that aren't helping kids, but their marketing materials make them sound pretty appealing to desperate parents.

Unfortunately, all these programs can be very expensive and are not covered by insurance (though the specific psychiatric expenses may be covered), and most of them do not offer financial aid.

Finally, be prepared to do battle with your teenager about this treatment plan. Your son probably won't buy into this idea and may claim that his treatment should be his decision. However, it isn't. You are still the parent and he is still the child until he is eighteen. Once he turns eighteen, you will have a lot less control over this situation. Try to help him while you can.

Adult ADD and Wellbutrin

Q: I'm forty, and I have been diagnosed with ADHD (attention deficit hyperactivity disorder). I'm reading _Driven to Distraction_ and boy, it's the story of my life. I change jobs every few years, I am a little impulsive, and I don't focus very well. Because I'm a regular listener to your show, I know this is a controversial issue. What do you think about an ADHD person taking Wellbutrin? And what can I tell my wife, because she is freaking out about this?

A: I always ask myself if the type of behavior that you describe is a symptom of a disease or is it just who we are? I say "we" because I, too, am an energetic, impulsive, and easily distracted person. I've had lots of jobs, and I've never done well with the corporate scene. I walked out of my surgical practice in a snit, a very impulsive move that eventually led to a radio career. Change can be good.

I like the theory that some of us are natural hunters, some of us are farmers, and society needs us all. The problems come up when we are shoved into boxes. Rather than conforming to the box by drugging and labeling ourselves, I think we need to make intelligent, healthy choices about how we live.

Energy and impulsiveness can be used to our advantage as we mature and understand ourselves.

Answering your question about Wellbutrin is easy. If it helps you, good. And if it doesn't, you can stop taking it. I have no objection to an adult making a choice to take a drug that is being monitored by a physician.

My main concern with ADHD is that kids, especially kids under five years old, are being diagnosed with it and put on drugs. Right now, this is happening way too often to kids who've barely begun to take shape emotionally. And we have no proof it helps them in the long run.

Q: I graduated from high school with a 4.0 grade point average and was accepted to the University of California. In my freshman year, I began having immense problems studying. I can't concentrate, and I don't retain as much as other students do. Someone suggested I might have ADHD, so I went for testing. The examiner decided I probably don't have ADHD, because I didn't show any signs of it until college.

I never had to study in high school like I do now. I was able to get great grades without sitting and concentrating for a long stretch. Is it possible that I was misdiagnosed, and I do have ADHD?

A: As you may have noticed in the previous question, I have a bias, and a lot of research supports my bias. ADHD is diagnosed much too often, and a large number of people are being labeled with ADHD because they fall at the skimpy end of the bell-shaped curve rather than in the crowded middle.

All people have strengths and weaknesses. Distractibility seems to be part of the nature of people who are labeled as having ADHD. This can be an advantage. Distracted people are attracted to and quickly notice changes in their environment. If you were on a safari in Africa, you'd be the first in your group to spot the wild animals, because your attention would be darting all over the savannah.

Let's look at your situation from a slightly different angle. You are attending what many consider the best public university in America. You are in classes with kids from all over the country who were tops in their classes. For the first time in your life, you are being challenged. I think you're being too hard on yourself. No one I know believes he concentrates as well as he should or remembers as much as he wants to. And, of course, given the choice between studying and not studying, most of us would just as soon go to a movie, right?

You seem to have a fixed idea about the right way to study. If you allow yourself to find your own style, without trying to fit into a mold that doesn't work for you, I think you will be successful. There is nothing wrong with studying for a few minutes, getting up and walking around for a bit, and then returning to your books. Many people learn more effectively like this than by slogging through material for two hours straight.

The question of whether someone can develop ADHD as an adult is very controversial. Some experts say yes, others say no. If you were diagnosed with ADHD, what would that mean to you? That you would take drugs for it? I would really hate to see you go that route because it just doesn't seem necessary.

See more ADHD questions on page 218 in chapter 5.

Anorexia and Bulimia

Q: I'm twenty-one and I'm anorexic. I know I have a problem, because I've been in inpatient care and I currently see a therapist. I've taken a lot of diet pills, but they don't help me lose weight. Is Metabolife safe for me to take? How about laxatives? I'm five-foot-two and weigh seventy pounds. I want to weigh sixty pounds.

A: Eating-disorder questions are some of the saddest, scariest, and most frustrating questions I get on my show. And, in your case, your weight goal is not compatible with life.

Diet pills are not working for you because your body is fighting further weight loss. You are saying to me that you want to kill yourself. At seventy pounds, your heart muscle is on the verge of giving out right at this moment. What will kill you is losing protein from your heart. As for laxatives, Metabolife, or any other weight-loss product—NO!

If you want to live, you have to acknowledge to yourself that you cannot trust your perceptions. When you look in a mirror, you don't see your real body. You see a distortion. Your eyes and brain are lying to you.

Anorexia is a terrible disease that's rooted in desperation about having power and being in control. Young women who are anorexic don't ovulate or have periods. They are attempting to hold back the future, to delay maturity.

Research has found that an anorexic distorts the image of her own body size as well as portions of food. To a person with anorexia, a hamburger is as large as a human head. A person with anorexia might recognize that a model at a one hundred twenty pounds is way too skinny, but still consider herself fat at seventy pounds.

Since you've been in therapy, you understand enough to know that you can't trust what you see. You have to let go of that and trust that other people are telling you the truth. I know that this is very difficult, but it's not impossible.

Your own beliefs will do you harm. You have to accept as truth what other people tell you. Please tell your therapist exactly what you told me, because your life depends on it.

Q: My sixteen-year-old daughter has been in the ballet for the past eleven years. She's a vegetarian and would like to tone and reshape her upper thighs, buttocks, and midsection. She's concerned about her weight as well.

She's dancing thirteen hours a week. She eats many carbs, but not enough fruits and vegetables. You know how that goes. Are there any products or videos on the market you would endorse?

A: I don't understand what type of products you want to know about, but what she truly needs is help with her denial. I cannot imagine that a sixteen-year-old who has been dancing for eleven years needs to tone her thighs, buttocks, and midsection. My guess is that she doesn't need to lose even a pound, yet she's obsessed with her weight.

Your child is on her way to an eating disorder. Young girls who are ballet dancers and gymnasts have the highest rate of eating disorders of any segment in our society. Please have her talk to a therapist about how she sees her body before this situation becomes more serious.

Schizophrenia

Q: I have a friend in her late forties who is becoming increasingly paranoid and hostile. She hears voices, and she believes that her neighbors are attacking her with lasers. She has put foil on her windows and she won't sleep at home anymore. She sleeps in her car or at a friend's house.

Do you have any ideas about how I might help her? Her family lives out-of-state and can't care for her. I have talked to her about seeing a doctor, and sometimes she says she will, but she never acts on it.

A: You are in a tough position, especially because she could easily become paranoid about you, and if so, your ability to help her will decline. It's tricky.

Encourage her to see a doctor, because the proper diagnosis can lead to effective treatment. While her symptoms—hearing voices and suspiciousness—are the classic symptoms of paranoid schizophrenia, some physical conditions can cause symptoms of mental disease. Also, schizophrenia usually manifests before age forty.

Pernicious anemia, which is caused by malabsorption of vitamin B12, can manifest as dementia. There is also a form of early vascular dementia. Both of these conditions are treatable.

If your friend is in communication with a primary care physician, you might try alerting that doctor and getting your friend to go in for an exam. The doctor can make arrangements for a psychiatrist to talk to her during the visit.

It would be unfortunate for her to avoid help until her paranoia hurts her or others. But if it does come to that, she might then get the medical help and medication that will control her symptoms.

She needs a psychiatric, and perhaps a neurological, workup.

Q: I've been diagnosed with schizophrenia. I'm taking Risperdal and I'm feeling OK now, but what am I up against?

A: What a schizophrenic is up against is that he can't tell what's real from what's not real. Your brain fools you. Schizophrenia is a type of mental illness known as psychosis. Psychotic people experience breaks with reality.

The reality distortion may be in the form of a delusion or a hallucination. A delusional person doesn't know who he is; if someone thinks he is Jesus Christ, he is delusional. Hallucinations are seeing things that aren't there or hearing voices that aren't speaking.

These imagined experiences are only real to the person with schizophrenia, which causes isolation from other people and can lead to antisocial behavior. The patient might hear frightening voices that make threats or give commands that are dangerous to the patient or to other people.

You should be very encouraged by the fact that you're feeling OK on the medication. Modern psychopharmacology shows promise in keeping the symptoms of schizophrenia under control, and in your case they seem to be doing the job. Recent research also has raised hopes about identifying a certain gene or genes that may be an indicator of schizophrenia. If a single cause can be found, that's a big step toward finding a treatment.

Also keep in mind that something as simple as exercise, even taking a walk, may calm the anxiety that can overwhelm a schizophrenic person.

Grief and Anger

Q: I've been going downhill since my husband passed away not long ago. I cry all the time and I just can't seem to function right. I feel horribly down and at a dead end. Should I see a psychoanalyst or a psychiatrist?

A: Losing a spouse can be devastating. Your loved one has passed away, so you really have to expect to feel a lot of pain and grief for a while.

A psychoanalyst provides more long-term treatment and tries to find the root causes of behavior, sometimes retracing the phases of a person's life. Such extensive treatment is probably not necessary in your case, but a lot of evidence shows that talk therapy in combination with antidepressants is beneficial in relieving this type of crisis.

Either a psychologist or a psychiatrist will be able to help you. If the psychologist thinks that drugs will help you, he or she will have access to a physician who can prescribe them. Psychiatrists are physicians, so they can prescribe medications. What's more important than the therapist's specific training is that you find relief and comfort in your sessions with whomever you choose.

Q: Can you please explain the term "anger management"? I have a husband who seems to spend a good part of his waking moments angry—at me, his job, and his kids. Would this help him?

A: Anger is one of the more negative psychological manifestations, and it can play a significant role in overall health, according to recent research. Many people, for instance, can be depressed or anxious, but when you add anger, it seems to accelerate the likelihood of heart attacks, strokes, and other health problems.

Just as important, it is no fun to live with or around anger. There are two schools of thought about what to do. Many psychologists and psychiatrists would say that you need to get at the core issues: Why is he angry? Who is he angry at? And why does this spill over to you and his children?

Other experts take a more cognitive approach. They say it doesn't matter what's going on, it's a matter of learning how to manage it. And, yes, anger-management techniques can be very helpful. When they feel anger building up, folks are taught how to respond with specific exercises, from deep breathing to meditative-type methods.

Personally, I can't help but feel that someone who is angry all the time has deeper, core issues that could be managed or sorted out with psychotherapy. Many men are very reluctant to admit that psychotherapy is needed; they see this as a sign of weakness. Yet I would turn it around and say it is a very strong and centered individual who has the guts to do something for himself and his family. Who will benefit the most? He will, of course.

Will this situation get better on its own? Not likely. And if it isn't addressed, it could have a long-term impact on your children. You need to have a private talk with your husband about your concerns, and if he isn't willing to address this, you may face some hard decisions about your marriage.

Anxiety and Stress

Q: For almost a month I've had headaches all day long. I also have been exhausted, nauseous, and lightheaded. Then, a few days ago, I felt tingling in my left arm. That went away, but I have continued to have headaches and nausea. My doctor says that stress is causing these symptoms, and he gave me medication.

I have been through much greater stress than I'm under right now, and it did not affect me physically. What's my doctor talking about? Should I get another doctor?

A: These are very tough symptoms to nail down, and your doctor is a gutsy guy for calling it stress and sending you away with sedatives. Your symptoms could be the symptoms of somatization, which means there is no physical explanation for them. And, believe it or not, this is the most common reason for all doctor visits. In fact, one study reports that 60 to 80 percent of people who go to doctors' offices have symptoms that are not caused by physical illness.

This doesn't mean that the patient doesn't feel physically ill, but that disease is not the cause of the illness. Rather, the body is coping with whatever is coming at it, very often stress, by feeling physically ill.

Nonetheless, before throwing pills at a patient, it is prudent for a doctor to rule out a heart attack, a gallbladder problem, or a brain tumor as causes of the symptoms. But doctors are in a tough position, because in the current climate, nobody—not the consumer and not the insurance company—wants to pay for lots of expensive tests for rogue symptoms.

Nausea that persists for weeks is more likely to be psychosomatic than to be a sign of a serious illness. And nausea that precedes a headache is very likely to signify a migraine. If you do have that kind of temporal association, see a neurologist, because he or she will be able to diagnose this and treat you appropriately.

Fatigue is a very common complaint, and most often the cause of it is no mystery—too much running around and not enough sleep. We put unreasonable expectations on ourselves. And if you are depressed, that will certainly tire you out.

The Edell Report
Women and Worry

I've spent my life telling my Mom, "Don't worry," and, finally, I know why.

Recently, scientists at the National Institute on Alcohol Abuse and Alcoholism (NIAAA) found that women with one particular variation of a single gene scored high in tests measuring anxiety levels. The researchers combined DNA analysis, recordings of brain activity, and psychological tests to reach their conclusion. Scans of electrical activity in the brain also showed signs of an anxious temperament.

Everybody inherits two copies of a gene—one from each parent—that affects the production of an enzyme called COMT. Women who inherited two copies of the Val 158Met variant of the gene scored highest on the worry meter, because that gene produces significantly less COMT. However, guys with a similar genetic makeup didn't score as high on anxiety.

Previous studies have shown that women generally have lower COMT levels, and another recent study at the same lab found that the variant gene can be linked to a higher level of brain response to pain and stress.

So, if you're a woman who worries, blame it on your mother and father—and learn some relaxation exercises.

In some rare cases, lightheadedness, nausea, and tingling in the left arm turn out to be heart disease. However, because your symptoms have been going on for so long, I don't think that's what's ailing you. Another possibility is a low-grade virus, which could cause a group of symptoms like these.

If you don't begin to feel better in a week or two, get another opinion.

Q: Can you help me understand why I am so uncomfortable going out with friends? I'm single and in my twenties and I know it's not healthy to be nervous about something as easy and casual as getting together for dinner on a Saturday night. And I absolutely freeze at a party where I don't know most of the people.

A: This sounds like a straightforward case of what's called social anxiety disorder or social phobia. People who suffer from this have a fear of being scrutinized, embarrassed, or humiliated when they are in public. Of course, none of us particularly like that, but people with this disorder react in the extreme, and research indicates that it may be caused by a deficiency of serotonin or norepinephrine, which are both brain chemicals.

But you don't have to stay home forever. Two medications—Effexor XR and Zoloft—were recently approved by the FDA for treatment of this problem. If those drugs sound familiar, that's because they are also used to treat depression and general anxiety. Subsequent testing showed that they can work for social anxiety as well.

Q: I thought I was having a heart attack, but after I had all of the stress tests, the blood work, the chest X rays, and the EKGs, the doctor determined it was anxiety. Now, several months later, I'm starting to lose my hair. When I wash my hair in the morning and check my hands, there is hair all over my hands. Is that normal for a 43-year-old woman? I'm even wondering if some of these anxiety things are hormonal.

A: Hair loss can happen after major stress or anxiety, and there usually is a delay of three or four months, just as you are experiencing. As you have noticed, the hair loss can be severe; I've seen women lose almost all their hair. The good news is it grows back.

However, I don't want to assume your hair problems are due to anxiety; I'd hate to see you miss a case of alopecia or male-pattern baldness. All kinds of things can happen in a woman that can cause hair loss, so you should see a

The Edell Report
What Do We Fear, What Should We Fear?

Those of you who listen to my show on a regular basis know that I have a few health-related hot buttons, and "misplaced fears" is a big one. Too often we worry about the wrong things!

That's the same message you'll find in a book called Risk. *According to authors David Ropeik and George Gray, our fears far outweigh the risks associated with hazardous waste, silicone breast implants, artificial sweeteners, nuclear radiation, mammograms and pesticides on food.*

But that doesn't mean there isn't serious stuff that we should put on our "worry radar." Ropeik and Gray say that many of us don't worry enough about the sun, indoor air pollution, accidents in the home (falls, poisoning, drowning, fire and choking), medical errors and antibiotic resistance.

So, fix that broken front step, put all your dangerous house cleaners on a shelf where kids can't reach them and when you worry, worry about the right stuff.

---

dermatologist. The doctor will pluck some hairs out of your head, look at them under a magnifying glass, and then he can tell you what's going on.

Q: I'm feeling more anxious every time I see a TV commercial about anxiety. What signs should tell me if I'm a candidate for these medicines? And do they really work? And what are my other options?

A: One way to treat this is to stop watching those television commercials. You also need to know that everyone has anxious moments—anxiety is a normal and healthy part of life. A life without it would not only be dull but animal research has found that a lack of any anxiety or challenges can actually shorten your life.

In terms of when and how you should consider treating anxiety, start by knowing that there are many ways to go after anxiety that do not involve drugs. If you are anxious, try something simple first, like relaxation. You can do this formally by learning meditation, yoga, deep breathing, or other exercises.

Another approach is to aggressively and regularly do things that are not only fun but also relaxing. Anything from rigorous daily walks to gardening, cooking, tennis, or some other hobby that involves physical exertion and stimulation may do the trick. I always recommend this as a first step, because it can be rewarding, allowing you to grow as a person.

This is an obvious component to a healthy life, yet many people do not schedule relaxation and antianxiety time for themselves. We schedule everything else in our lives, but somehow, when it comes to this, we seem reluctant to acknowledge its importance for our overall well-being. Of course, identifying those things that cause you anxiety may be fruitful, too.

When anxiety starts to interfere with your home and work life, when you don't feel you can enjoy life, it's time to take stock. Antianxiety medications are an effective treatment, but the best ones often have a side effect of sedation, which may not be desirable to you. Talk to your physician.

Q: Ever since kindergarten, my brother throws up when he gets stressed out. He's now twenty-eight and was diagnosed with psychosomatic vomiting several years ago. He has been taking Prilosec. His esophagus is ulcerated, and that has him worried. Is there anything else doctors could do for him?

A: Since he's getting medical care, I'm going to assume that his doctor has taken the important first step of ruling out all physiological causes of the vom-

QUIZ

What's the most stressful month of the year, if you consider such life-affecting activities as marriage, death, divorce, job changes, hospitalizations, and house purchases?

A) June   B) December   C) January   D) September

(A: June is No. 1, according to a study by a sociologist at Whitman College in Washington. September ranked second, and December was among the lowest scoring months. Maybe we enjoy holiday dinners more than we think?)

iting. When there is no medical or physical cause, then the diagnosis is psycho-somatic vomiting, and your brother needs to know that he's not alone and it is treatable. A good psychologist familiar with this condition can help him gain control and get off the medication.

Stomach acid needs to be kept in its proper place—the stomach—where it aids in digestion. Outside of the stomach, where it doesn't belong, it can rot teeth and, as your brother is experiencing, burn the esophagus.

Q: I went to my doctor because I'm extremely nervous. I shake all over, especially when I'm driving, and sometimes I have to pull over and stop the car. My doctor sent me to a psychiatrist, because he couldn't find anything wrong. The psychiatrist prescribed Librium. I took it for about four months, and the shaking did go away. But whenever I go off the pills, I start shaking again. Do I need to be on medicine for the rest of my life to keep this under control?

A: I want you to get a second opinion—or go back to your current doctor—because I think the diagnosis and the drug are slightly off base. Librium is an old-time sedative, and what you are describing sounds more like phobia or panic attacks.

You may have agoraphobia, which is a fear of public places. For someone with agoraphobia, driving around—being out and about—can bring on panic attacks. People with severe agoraphobia don't even go out; their anxiety forces them to stay home.

Librium is a drug that we don't hear much about anymore; Valium replaced it, and we now have drugs that are far superior to either of them. But too often in these days of managed care, people who walk in to see psychiatrists walk out with prescriptions for sedatives and not much else.

There are clinics that specialize in phobias and panic attacks that I believe will be more on target for you. If you decide to stick with your current doctor, tell him or her that you suspect you might be agoraphobic and that you want to see someone who knows how to diagnose and treat you.

Trauma, Phobias, Fears, and OCD

Q: I witnessed a murder five years ago, and it has taken a terrible toll on my life. I used to be a very independent person and a workaholic. But

for a long time after the incident, I was on a lot of medication and I couldn't focus, so eventually I lost my job.

I still feel like someone is after me, and I have nightmares. I had counseling for a while, and I was told I have obsessive-compulsive disorder (OCD). I have been taking Prozac, but whenever I try to wean myself, I begin having anxiety attacks and nightmares again. Is this what the rest of my life will be like? I really want to work again.

A: Going off the medication and returning to work are admirable, worthwhile goals. But I think they are too demanding for you to accomplish without getting more help. You could be suffering from posttraumatic stress disorder and need specific medications for that.

You are coping with fears and anxiety that seem to be akin to phobias or OCD. Seeing a murder doesn't cause phobias or OCD, but if someone was on the verge of having one of those syndromes, something traumatic could push them over the edge. Don't make it harder by beating up on yourself because you can't work this out on your own or wean yourself off the medications. You might want to give cognitive or behavioral therapy a try, or you can return to your original doctor if you felt you had a good connection with that person.

The best way I know of for gaining control of a phobia is desensitization. A therapist will be able to slowly acclimate you to facing the work world again. By taking tiny risks that will make success easy to come by, you will gradually rebuild your confidence.

It may be hard work, and there may be more bumps in the road, but you can have a better life. Good luck.

Q: When I was younger, I had no fear of flying, but now that I've hit my thirties, I am deathly afraid to get on a plane. My heart jumps, and my palms sweat, and I have to clutch my wife's hand to get through it. Is there anything I can do about this?

A: There is a lot you can do about it, but one thing that won't help, as you know, is logic. I could tell you the truth, that your life is so much more at risk when you're in a car, and I could rattle off the statistics that prove that per mile and per hour air travel is the safest way to go, but logic is no weapon against phobia.

To top it off, human nature is such that we focus on major negative events, like plane crashes. Thousands of planes take off and land safely each day, but that doesn't make headlines. However, the extremely rare crash is big news. It's tragic, of course, but it is extremely rare.

What you can do about your fear for the short term is to see your doctor for a light sedative, like Valium, before your next flight. Take a Valium and you'll be OK. But you don't need drugs to deal with this for the rest of your life. Fear-of-flying clinics can be found in almost every city, and the cure rate is spectacularly high.

Virtual reality is one of the techniques used to treat this phobia and a multitude of others, from the fear of spiders—arachnophobia—to the fear of germs. For example: If someone has a fear of heights, the subject puts on virtual-reality goggles, which simulate the experience of climbing a long, steep staircase. Once he is comfortable with that, the images gradually become more and more challenging. Eventually the person acclimates to each one and is able to face his fears in the real world. Most fear-of-flying programs have access to empty planes that you practice in on the ground, until you are ready to take off.

So sign yourself up, because who wants to sit at home when you can be traveling around the Greek Islands or visiting a small town in Italy?

Q: I am concerned that my boyfriend has obsessive-compulsive disorder. If I make an idle comment about mailing a bill after dinner, he brings it up all through the meal and while we're cleaning up. "We've got to go to

---

QUIZ

People who suffer from obsessive-compulsive disorder (OCD) may engage in which of the following activities:

A) "cleaning" (excessive hand-washing)

B) "checking" (always looking to see if the doors are locked)

C) "repeating" (saying the same thing over and over)

D) expressing distasteful thoughts and impulses

E) all of the above

(E: all of the above; OCD afflicts more than 3 million people in the United States.)

the mailbox." "We've got to get that bill mailed." "We've got to do this; we've got to do that." I sometimes think that he is afraid of doing something wrong, so he says it over and over again. Do you think this is OCD, and is it connected to anxiety?

A: OCD and anxiety are definitely connected. I once did a story on a fellow with such severe OCD that he stopped his car every quarter of a mile so he could look underneath, just to be sure he hadn't run over someone. This was one very anxious man.

As the name indicates, the disorder has two parts, obsession and compulsion. Obsession is an invasion of recurrent and persistent thoughts, ideas or images. Compulsion is a behavior, usually a senseless, repetitive one, that an individual feels compelled to perform because of the obsession. A classic OCD behavior is compulsive hand-washing, which is triggered by obsessive thoughts about germs.

Of course, I can't be sure that your boyfriend has OCD—it can be tricky to diagnose. We always have to ask at what point does anxiety or compulsion cross the line from personal persnicketiness to a psychological disorder? For many of us, a little obsession is what gets the job done.

It is generally agreed that the line is crossed when the anxiety and action seriously impair a person's ability to function on the job or in personal relationships. Obviously, this behavior is a problem in your relationship, from your point of view. I don't know that I would define "Let's go to the mailbox; let's go to the mailbox" as full-blown OCD, but I would say your boyfriend is behaving in an obsessive-compulsive manner. However, snap diagnoses are dangerous, and your boyfriend deserves to get an opinion from someone who can spend some time with him.

Many psychologists think that people who suffer from OCD can be taught certain little mental mechanisms to give them some control. Other patients may be helped by medication. Have an honest discussion with your guy and ask him to talk to a psychologist, for the sake of your relationship and his long-term good health.

Q: I have a compulsion to pull out my eyelashes. I've taken a number of drugs, but none of them helped for very long. Prozac worked for about three months and, during that time, I completely stopped pulling my eyelashes without even realizing it. My shyness also disappeared while I was on Prozac, because I stopped caring about what people think of me.

I have chatted about this with some people on the Internet, and it seems like none of the drugs work permanently. Is there anything new on the market?

A: You have an obsessive-compulsive disorder called trichotillomania. It's not terribly rare, but it is more common in women than in men. If you yank out your brows and lashes so severely that they don't grow back, you can end up in serious trouble. Otherwise, compared to other bad habits, this is not that harmful physically.

Fortunately, trichotillomania is no longer the "secret" disorder that it once was, and there are support groups. And, as you know, you can find a lot of contacts and information online.

As for new drugs, it seems that a new SSRI—selective serotonin reuptake inhibitor, which is what Prozac is—comes out every week. And they all have different profiles and side effects. My advice on medication is to keep trying them, under a doctor's care, of course. Raising the dosage on the Prozac might also help—but your doctor needs to decide that. In addition, you should explore behavioral therapy, where you can learn appropriate exercises and substitute behaviors.

But keep in mind that even professionals who are experts in the field of obsessive-compulsive disorder cannot agree on treatment, and they have a hard time identifying when compulsive behaviors cross the line from normal to abnormal. I think the patient is usually in the best position to determine that.

Q: My forty-two-year-old sister has been diagnosed with multiple chemical sensitivity (MCS). I want to understand her illness, which often seems to get in the way of her daily living, but so far, everything I've read about this raises concerns about her mental health. Can you explain this illness to me?

A: I have been accused of being insensitive—and much more—for my stand on this question. But the truth is that there is no proof that such a disease exists. And I am hardly alone in my belief: The American Medical Association, the American Academy of Allergy and Immunology, the California Medical Association, the American College of Physicians and the International Society of Regulatory Toxicology and Pharmacology have all said the same thing. Still, it is a hot topic among lawyers, politicians, researchers, and regulatory agencies, and people have been awarded workman's comp because of MCS.

The basic claim is that patients with MCS—it's also called "environmental illness"—are supersensitive to artificial elements in our environment, everything from deodorant to hair spray to floor cleaners. Because of that, many folks make major changes in their lives, from getting rid of all the furniture in their home to stopping all activities outside the house. It sounds like that's what you're seeing in your sister's behavior.

The problem is that when you surreptitiously expose such patients, unbeknownst to them, to the substances they claim they are sensitive to, they don't react. And, as you found, there is a very high rate of various psychological problems in such patients—often depression and anxiety.

The vast majority of patients are women, usually between the ages of thirty and fifty, and frequently they have determined the diagnosis by the time they see their doctor. Unfortunately, there are doctors—some call their field "clinical ecology"—who almost encourage the delusion and do a great disservice to their patients.

I think this disease is actually something like a phobia. Some folks are phobic about germs, others unseen chemicals. When suggestible people watch a television story that tells them that a few molecules of some chemical in the air can make people fatigued and forgetful, well, some folks start feeling fatigued and forgetful. Technically, we call this mass sociogenic illness (MSI).

The good news is, a lot of research indicates that cognitive behavioral therapy helps. But first the patient needs to be convinced that this could be a psychological illness—and, often, that's nearly impossible.

Of course, there are toxic substances in some environments. This is why we always investigate such possibilities before concluding that it's all in your head.

See page 397 for more on MSI and page 545 for more on MCS.

Q: Someone in my family is burying us under clutter. The house, the garage, and the yard are stuffed with junk. Of course, the person saving it doesn't see it that way. Right now, there's not enough room on the kitchen counter to put two pieces of bread side by side to make a sandwich. When does a "pack rat" need help, and what can we do about this?

A: When a person's behavior interferes with his or her self-esteem or family, social or business life, it stops being a quirk and starts being an abnormality that needs professional help.

If the clutter is a constant source of battling and distress, your family should get help from a psychologist or psychiatrist. Psychology considers pack-rat behavior to be a form of obsessive-compulsive disorder. Psychological profiles of pack rats show that they have weak boundaries between their belongings and their selves. We all find ways to cope with a world that is not under our control. For the pack rats, security and control are tied to keeping stuff.

However, we do have to allow for different styles of living. When I walk through the newsroom where I work, I see desks piled with junk and other desks that are neat as a pin. Working side by side with our differences is healthy, as long as the operation—be it a newsroom or a family—is functioning.

It sounds like your family is struggling. If the family member who is doing all the "packing" won't acknowledge the need for help, then maybe all the family members who share the house should sit down and discuss personal boundaries for each person, as far as where they can store stuff in the house, with the kitchen and living room off-limits to all but essential items for that room.

Q: I used to work in an oncologist's office, and the job had a terrible emotional effect on me. I now have an overwhelming fear of cancer. My doctor thinks that medication might help me. Some of the research I've seen says that medication is effective, and other reports say it's just a Band-Aid and that the patient should get to the root of the problem. Do you have any guidance for me?

A: In order to work in the medical field, we have to build emotional barriers. If we aren't able to do that, the suffering that comes knocking on the door will freak us out. Successful medical staffs develop the ability to be caring and compassionate and at the same time stay emotionally removed.

You could be bordering on a phobic reaction, and the latest thinking is to treat phobias with desensitization. This process of losing fear through gradual exposure is used to treat all types of phobias, and it's possible a desensitization program could be designed to deal with this issue.

Of course, a certain amount of fear about cancer is healthy and normal. Fear can motivate us to take care of ourselves, and it certainly is what gets most women in for a mammogram.

I don't think there's anything wrong with taking advantage of medication while looking for a desensitization program. Yes, it's a Band-Aid, but when I cut myself, I want a Band-Aid, because it does the trick. When I take it off, the wound has healed.

Another important thing about Band-Aids is that they are temporary aids, and that's what you want in your medication, too. No one is suggesting that you handle your phobia by taking drugs for the rest of your life.

Life is precious. You must have gotten that message by being around death as much as you were. It's time to enjoy your life again.

Q: I have a panic disorder, and my OB-GYN nurse practitioner put me on an antidepressant. She started me at a very low dosage, but I'm only taking a half tablet instead of the whole one she prescribed, and it's doing wonders.

But when I went to my follow-up appointment and told my nurse prac-titioner that I was only taking a half tablet and had started seeing a thera-pist, she was unhappy with me. She said the panic disorder is completely biochemical and can't be treated with therapy, and she wants to raise the dosage. Should I follow her advice?

A: I would slam a doctor for such an absolute position, so I'll do the same to a nurse practitioner who shouldn't be treating a complicated psychological disorder.

The basic goal in using pharmaceutical medicine is to take the smallest dose that gets the desired effect. I'm willing to agree — and literature sup-ports the opinion — that panic disorder has a physiological component, but, like depression, environment plays a role, too. These disorders stem from a complicated combination of biochemical, genetic, and environmental causes.

By seeking therapy you are taking charge and taking care of yourself. It's a wonderful, positive thing to do. I suggest you tell your therapist the whole story and get his or her opinion. This is the therapist's area of expertise, and it is not the expertise of someone in the OB-GYN field.

I support the movement for ancillary medical personnel like nurse practi-tioners and paramedics when they are in appropriate roles. But any health prac-titioner working outside of his or her league is dangerous.

With panic disorder there are a lot of other things you can learn to do to mitigate the symptoms. We find that breathing exercises, yogic breathing, and similar activities may be helpful. This is because the first thing that happens in a panic disorder may be a carbon dioxide shift in the blood. You get a little anxious and then you start to increase your breathing. Carbon dioxide levels drop, and this causes certain pH and chemical changes in the blood that can trigger the panic attack.

Teaching people something as simple as breathing exercises is helpful. Even though medication can help, I always think it's worth going off medication now and then to see how you do on your own. That's common sense to me.

Miscellaneous

Q: I recently read a story about how a bunch of children at one school came down with a rash, and in the end the rash was blamed on "hysteria." It sounds to me like the school isn't taking responsibility for something in the building that's causing an allergic reaction. Does this make sense?

A: "Mass hysteria" sounds like a dirty word, and many people resent it when it's applied to them, yet it's one of the most important concepts that any health consumer can understand. In medicine we call it mass sociogenic illness (MSI), and it's responsible for enormous amounts of sickness in America that often go undiagnosed.

The typical case will be people in a single building who all of a sudden get sick in a very short period of time. Nausea, headaches, fatigue, and rashes are common symptoms. This is all due to the powers of suggestion. Another way of looking at it is explained by the concept called "nocebo." What's that? Well, If I give you a medicine that is a phony medicine but I tell you it will cure you, many of you will get better, and that's a placebo. Well, the opposite is also true, too. If I give you something and tell you it will make you sick, many of you will get sick. That's a nocebo.

MSI has several typical characteristics. One of them is that the illness occurs only in people who can see other people getting sick or hear them getting sick. In other words, if there is something legitimately bad in the ventilation system, then people will get sick according to the pattern of ventilation. But if a bunch of people in one classroom get sick, it's difficult to understand why everyone in the school wouldn't get sick. What always happens is that one or two people get sick first, and then another bunch of people who are near them, and, before you know it, everyone is claiming illness.

Toxicology reports never find anything toxic in the environment. There have been recent cases of rashes in schools, all of them due to MSI, even though parents don't want to accept that and accuse the school managers of not doing their jobs.

I'd much rather be told that my child is psychologically normal and reacting the way most humans would in a situation like that, instead of knowing he or she had been exposed to some mysterious toxin.

MSI is an important concept, and yet there are times when people are being exposed to bad things that are making them ill. You can't immediately say that any outbreak is due to MSI; you have to do the standard tests for toxins in the

DEAN'S LIST: WANT TO KNOW MORE ABOUT DEPRES-
SION AND BIPOLAR DISORDER?

Many excellent books have explored the experience of battling
depression and manic depression.

The Beast: A Journey Through Depression, by Tracy Thompson
An Unquiet Mind, by Kay Redfield Jamison
Darkness Visible: A Memoir of Madness, by William Styron
*I Don't Want to Talk About It: Overcoming the Secret Legacy of Male
    Depression,* by Terrence Real
More Than Moody, Recognizing and Treating Adolescent Depression, by
    Dr. Harold S. Koplewicz
The Noonday Demon, an Atlas of Depression, by Andrew Solomon

environment and make sure that's not the cause.

**Q: I did a lot of LSD in the sixties and seventies. It's been a long time
since I've done drugs of any kind, but I'm still getting flashbacks. The doctor gave me Prozac and put me in group therapy. Is there anything else I
can do?**

A: LSD is a drug that was initially called a psychotomimetic, which means
it mimics psychosis—by inducing delusions and hallucinations—which is why
people took it.

Psychosis, by definition, is the loss of reality. If you hallucinate or are seeing things that aren't there, or are hearing voices that aren't there, that, by
definition, is psychosis.

But what we have found is that for people who were borderline psychotics,
or would develop psychosis later on, LSD was particularly treacherous in its
effects. In fact, the drug may have precipitated a psychotic state in any number of people.

Your situation also depends on what else you took, because who took just
one drug in those days? The thought is, what you may be experiencing now is
the beginning of some mental difficulty that needs to be treated independ-
ently, whether you took these drugs twenty or thirty years ago.

What is done is done, and you need to look forward. If you're experiencing hallucinations, which is what people often describe when they describe "the flashback," then that needs to be treated. And treated more powerfully than with Prozac or another antidepressant; you may need antipsychotic drugs.

So when you go to your psychiatrist, make sure that you tell him or her exactly what's going on. Now's not the time to be secretive. You may be developing a mental problem that needs serious treatment.

Q: Can you please help me understand why my daughter is cutting herself? This wasn't a suicide attempt, according to her doctor. She just started seeing a psychiatrist about this, and I'm very scared about her future.

A: I can understand why you are scared. It is almost impossible not to be terrified whenever our children do anything to hurt themselves.

As you probably know, your daughter's "cutting," or self-mutilation, is not a one-time incident, and there may be a variety of reasons that she is doing this to herself. It can be a mental disorder—and it can raise your daughter's risk of suicide—but that's not always the case. Sometimes it can occur because the cutter wants attention, is involved in drugs, or is simply doing it because of peer pressure. The behavior is more prevalent among teenage girls than boys, it usually starts in the early teens, and it may last as long as ten years. Some cutters describe a sense of control over and distraction from the psychological pain they feel in their lives.

In some cases, cutting is also linked to a personality disorder or an eating disorder, and young adults who were sexually or physically abused as children may become self-mutilators. As you can see, this is not an ailment that comes with simple, straightforward explanations.

You have already taken a good first step by getting your daughter into therapy. Antidepressants or mood stabilizers also may be part of the treatment. Don't assume that your daughter can just "stop" this behavior if she wants to. Sometimes the cutter is suffering from an impulse-control disorder. With time, the psychiatrist should be able to figure out the best way to help your child.

Resource List

For information on a variety of topics, click on the "public" box on the home page of the Help Center at the American Psychological Association Web site. It can help you determine whether you need to see a psychologist. It also provides information on a variety of topics, from stepfamilies to eldercare to marriage: *www.helping.apa.org/*

The National Institute of Mental Health Web site has information on clinical trials and the latest research, as well as specific information, in English and Spanish, on major disorders: *www.nimh.nih.gov*

The Web site for the Anxiety Disorders Association of America includes a "self test" as well as guidance on finding a therapist: *www.adaa.org/*

At the National Strategy for Suicide Prevention Web site, find state-by-state lists of prevention programs as well as the latest information on suicide research: *www.mentalhealth.org/suicideprevention/*

The Web site for the National Center for Post-Traumatic Stress Disorder has information for military veterans and others who suffer from PTSD: *www.ncptsd.org*

The National Mental Health Association has more than three hundred affiliates around the country where you can get information on services and support groups. Find the affiliate directory at *www.nmha.org*

For detailed information about OCD, go to the Web site for the Obsessive-Compulsive Foundation: *www.ocfoundation.org/*

For information on mood disorders and to find a Depression and Bipolar Support Alliance support group in your area, go to *www.dbsalliance.org*

If you are interested in starting a self-help group, find more information at the National Mental Health Consumers' Self-Help Clearinghouse: *www.mhselfhelp.org*

The National Child Traumatic Stress Network provides guidance on how to help a child who has experienced physical or domestic abuse or some other traumatic event: *www.nctsnet.org*

For extensive information on all aspects of mental illness go to the National Alliance for the Mentally Ill Web site, *www.nami.org*, or call the NAMI Information and Service Center at 1-800-950-NAMI (1-800-950-6264).

Some psychologists and psychiatrists are certified by the Academy of Cognitive Therapy. You'll find the list of certified members at *www.academyofct.org*

For related questions see chapters 2, 3, 4, 5, 6, 7, 9, and 11.

Chapter 9

The Dirt on Infectious Diseases

OK, so I admit it. For a significant portion of my life, I have been a little finicky about germs. First, I must blame that most convenient of scapegoats: Mom. From her I learned that just about everything in the universe was covered in filth. Medical school didn't help. You are taught that Mom, indeed, was right, that the world is awash in germs, not to mention all the gross infectious diseases you come in contact with.

I'm lucky, though, because after decades of avoiding suspicious doorknobs and pushing the flush handles of public toilets with my foot, I was cured with something akin to shock treatment. My mother-in-law had purchased a trailer that we were using while waiting to move into a new house. The holding tank for the trailer's toilet was full, and we had pulled the trailer to a dumping facility at a local gas station. Just for the record, I had no experience emptying a holding tank.

I couldn't figure out why, after I slid back the three-inch gate valve at the bottom of the tank, nothing was happening. I grabbed a clothes hanger to poke at the opening of the valve, where a thin layer of settled waste was tenuously holding back the onslaught. But not for much longer.

Thirty-five gallons of human waste burst onto my face, and when I finally stopped screaming, I was cured. I had seen the worst and I had survived.

I'm not as judgmental of my mother's germ-crazed generation as I once was. They remember when infectious disease was truly worthy of the paranoia. In 1900, the top three killers in the United States were pneumonia, tuberculosis, and diarrhea/enteritis. Today those diseases don't show up on any American Top Ten list.

Other countries are not so fortunate. While we tote around expensive water in plastic bottles and whine about the safety of our public water supply, each day six thousand children around the world die from easily preventable waterborne diseases. Yet we, with the safest water and food supply in the world, complain the loudest. Sorry, but you won't get much sympathy from me.

One of the most difficult aspects of dealing with infectious diseases is the fear factor, as well demonstrated during the 2003 SARS panic. I'm not saying it's unreasonable to have some fear of things we barely understand and which can cause seemingly sudden death. On the other hand, there are a lot of folks who just worry too damned much, or they worry about the wrong diseases and do nothing to prevent the more common ones worthy of our respect.

A couple of years ago, a resort area in Italy banned bikini-clad patrons from sitting in outside bars and coffee shops for fear that the scantily dressed customers would leave the potential for diseases on the plastic chairs. Sarongs and other cover-ups sold well that year. Talk about theater of the absurd.

Then there's influenza, which kills 20,000 to 30,000 Americans in an average year, yet many who should get flu shots do not. And even though we have the safest food in the world, 76 million of us annually suffer food-borne gastroenteritis, with 325,000 hospitalizations and 5,000 deaths. Most of that would be preventable with the simplest upgrade in our food-handling practices. We resist reasonable solutions like radiating meat to kill infectious organisms. Sorry folks, but that makes no sense.

Our day-to-day behavior is full of contradictions, too. Many women admit they hover over toilet seats in public rest rooms, suspending their buttocks in the air to avoid contact with the dreaded toilet seat. Yet, if no one else is in the rest room, many will leave without washing their hands.

Mothers try to protect their kids from germs by purchasing antiseptic cleaners but refuse to get them vaccinated. I get angry phone calls almost every week on this topic—because of fear and misinformation. For the record, one more time: Vaccinations protect your children from horrendous diseases; they don't cause autism.

While most of us don't truly fear the common cold, we have abandoned common sense when it comes to this illness. How else to explain the millions of unnecessary visits to doctors and emergency rooms every year for an illness that does not require medical care.

Colds now cost $40 billion a year in the United States alone—more than asthma, heart failure and emphysema—even though they will go away by themselves. We spend almost $3 billion annually just on over-the-counter medications and we push doctors for antibiotics that not only are useless against the cold but increase the development of antibiotic-resistant bacteria. Colds are caused by viruses, and antibiotics only help with bacteria. Save your money.

So, what should you worry about? When should you go to the doctor?

Well, polio, plague, smallpox, diphtheria, and a long list of scary diseases are hardly heard from anymore, but others have taken their place. Germs continue to be a formidable foe for medicine, and their tactics keep changing. Flesh-eating germs, SARS, and the West Nile virus make headlines, and they have killed people, but the overall risk is still very, very small.

Your best and only weapon is to stay in touch with the facts—not with people who are panicking—and learn as much as possible. Learn what the real threats are and how to effectively deal with them. And throw out the old wives' tales and just plain nonsense. Colds are not caused by cold weather. The drain of your kitchen sink is the dirtiest place in the house, not the toilet. Undercooked poultry can cause salmonella, and so can the knife you just used on the chicken—if you use it, unwashed, to slice the tomatoes. AIDS is a preventable disease. Ebola will not reach you. Wash your hands. Don't touch your face a lot. Bio warfare is scary but it's not as easy to pull off as it sounds.

Finally, don't forget that germs can be good for you—in your intestines, germs help with digestion and make vitamins for you—and you have lots of them. Benign germs (five hundred to one thousand species!) live in and on your body and help keep out the pathogenic ones. Unbelievable as it may sound, you have ten times as many bacteria cells as regular cells. Bad germs can't invade you if good germs are taking up space. Even exposure to germs in early life seems to toughen up the immune system and protect against allergies later on. Kids raised in clean environments have more asthma and allergic diseases.

If we all took a blood test to find antibodies to different infectious diseases, which means that at some time in our lives we were infected, those tests would show that most of us have been infected with herpes, cytomegalovirus, Epstein-Barr virus, and other intimidating stuff. We just didn't know it, because we didn't get very sick. Don't believe me? Go get tested.

Pick and choose wisely what you worry about in life, especially when it comes to the scariest stuff. Life's too short, and you can't control the roulette wheel. When SARS contaminated one floor in a Hong Kong hotel, do you really think there was anything those unlucky folks could have done differently to protect themselves? No way.

Hepatitis A, B, and C

Q: My close friend was diagnosed with hepatitis C when she was nineteen. We're both now thirty-two. What are my risks of contracting it from her? We shared cigarettes when we were younger, though we don't do those things now. Are there any risks involved?

A: A lot of unanswered questions remain about hepatitis C. We do believe it's becoming semiepidemic, because the disease can remain dormant in someone's body for decades with no hints, no symptoms that it's there. Then, many decades after the person did something that infected them, they come down with liver disease, maybe even needing a liver transplant, and the cause was this festering hepatitis C virus.

It was originally called non-A/non-B, and we thought it was transmitted by transfusions and that was that. Then we found it could be transmitted with needle and drug use. Now we're finding other ways that it could have gotten into the body. Risks include sharing toothbrushes, razors, or other personal care articles that might have blood on them. And tattooing and piercing can introduce hepatitis, if the practitioner does not follow good health practices.

In addition, we have discovered that snorting cocaine through any type of tube could transmit it. Cocaine is a very intense vasoconstrictor; it constricts your blood vessels and can cause little patches of tissue to die, so you can get a little bit of blood in your nose that gets on whatever instrument you used to inhale it. If the tube or hundred-dollar bill is passed around, and there is blood left on it, infection is possible. We believe it may be strictly the blood contact that's doing it and not contact with mucus or saliva.

We do not think it can be transmitted by kissing, sharing saliva or by casual means. Although people with multiple sex partners do have higher rates of Hepatitis C, sexual transmission seems to be uncommon.

If you had called me and said this was your husband, and you wondered if you should use a barrier method of birth control to protect yourself during sex, I wouldn't know how to answer you. Sexual transmission *seems to be* one of the least likely ways of contracting it, but I don't know with certainty if that is true. It's very difficult to do research on human beings when it comes to sex. But the official word from the Centers for Disease Control is that if you have sex with an infected steady partner, the risk of infection is low.

But I've digressed from your question. You probably don't have hepatitis C, but a simple blood test should give you peace of mind. Since our knowledge about this virus is still evolving, it's better to be a bit conservative. We don't want to find out down the road that we gave people bad advice.

Hepatitis C is a disease against which we are making progress, but there is still a lot of work to be done.

Q: I have just been diagnosed with hepatitis C. I went to my doctor, because I had dark urine and blood in my stool. I also had fatigue, muscle aches, and a high fever. How contagious am I to my two small children, ages four and eight? And could I pass it on to my baby if I have another child?

A: From what is known at the moment, you're not likely to be a risk to your kids, but you could pass it on to a baby if the hepatitis is active at the time of the delivery.

See the previous questions for more on this topic and talk to your doctor before you get pregnant again.

Q: My twenty-one-year-old son has gone tattoo crazy, and he now has four on his arms. Is there a health reason I can use to talk him out of getting any more?

QUIZ

True or False? Hepatitis B is much more infectious than HIV.
(True: Hepatitis B is one hundred times more infectious than HIV.)

A: Try this: In the United States, 10,000 people die each year from hepatitis C, 4 million Americans are chronically infected, and there are 36,000 new infections each year. If you have a tattoo, you need to be tested.

According to one study, people who received tattoos in a commercial tattoo parlor were nine times more likely to be infected. In this study, 18 percent of people had a tattoo. Of those with a tattoo, 22 percent were infected with hepatitis C.

That's one in five of you with tattoos. However, folks with tattoos may take other risks, so just because someone gets hepatitis C doesn't mean it came from a tattoo. Anyone considering their first tattoo—or yet another statement of love, outrage, or art—should be very careful about who does the work. There are no laws about tattooing ink; it's the only substance I know of that you can legally inject into the human body that does not require FDA approval. And the chemicals in tattoo ink are the same as those in auto paints. A disposable needle is a must.

Q: A friend of mine was recently diagnosed with hepatitis C and is taking interferon. Isn't interferon an experimental drug? I'm worried about my friend.

A: No. Interferon, which is usually combined with an antiviral drug, has been used successfully with hepatitis C for some time. Unfortunately, it doesn't work for everyone. The treatment can last from six months to a couple of years, and depression, fatigue, moodiness, and flulike symptoms are possible.

Your friend will need your support, because this is a serious illness, and the treatment is not an easy one for many people.

Q: In 1990 and 1991, I had hepatitis B. Since then, I have felt fine and my tests have been negative. Could I still transmit hepatitis B through sexual intercourse?

A: Feeling good and getting negative test results does mean that you are not likely to be secreting the virus any longer, but that's something only a doctor can determine. Ten years is a long time, so check in with a physician about your health status.

Hepatitis B is transmissible through body fluids and blood, and also through sex, although we're having difficulty nailing down exactly how that happens.

We now vaccinate youngsters for hepatitis B as a part of routine childhood immunizations.

The Edell Report
Hepatitis Clarified

The word hepatitis simply means inflammation of the liver, and it can be caused by alcohol, drugs, or a variety of infections. Hepatitis A, B, and C are the most common strains, and they have both similarities and strong differences. Hepatitis carriers don't always have symptoms, but the common signs for all three strains, if they occur, include jaundice, fatigue, abdominal pain, and loss of appetite. One thing to remember: If you have ever had any hepatitis you cannot donate blood and you should not drink alcohol.

Hepatitis A

- *Spread from person to person through fecal-oral contamination of food. This is why restaurant hygiene is critical to everyone's good health.*
- *Casual and sexual contact can both be transmitters.*
- *Once you've had it, you cannot get it again.*
- *A vaccine exists, but your best protection is regular hand-washing.*

Q: My sister-in-law's blood tested positive for hepatitis A. She doesn't remember having it, but many years ago she was exposed to it, so she got the vaccine at that time. Is it possible that the vaccine caused her to test positive? Or could she have had hepatitis A without knowing it?

A: Hepatitis A is definitely a disease that you can have without knowing it. Many viruses are like that. We call these subclinical infections.

Hepatitis A is often mistaken for the flu because it has flulike symptoms: aches and pains, fever, and a generally crummy feeling. It's highly contagious and accounts for about 65 percent of all viral hepatitis cases, including C. The most distinctive hepatitis A symptom is jaundice—yellowing of the skin—but that doesn't happen to everyone.

Her blood test showed hepatitis A antibodies, which means that at some point she was infected by that virus. The shot she got years ago when she was

- *Can occur in epidemics.*
- *One-third of Americans have had it.*

Hepatitis B

- *Spread by bodily fluids, sexual contact, and intravenous drug use.*
- *Symptoms may be nonexistent or slow to surface, and are less common in children. They can include jaundice.*
- *Can become chronic infection.*
- *Vaccination recommended for all children.*

Hepatitis C

- *Most people have no symptoms and carry the infection their entire life.*
- *Transmission occurs when blood from an infected person enters the body of an uninfected person, often through intravenous drug use.*
- *No vaccine exists, but the disease can be treated in many people with interferon/ribavirin.*
- *Four million Americans have it.*
- *It's the No. 1 reason for liver transplants.*

initially exposed was probably a gamma globulin shot, which is given to ward off the infection. Gamma globulin contains the antibodies from someone who had the disease. If she had been tested right after getting the shot, she'd show the antibodies, but its effects are very short-term, so it is not the cause of the antibodies she has now. She had hepatitis A at some point.

Hepatitis A is passed along in food that is contaminated with the feces of an infected person. Which is just one reason why it's always critical for food handlers to wash their hands well after using the bathroom.

Q: We got a notice in the mail from the school saying that my twelve-year-old seventh-grader needs one of those hepatitis B shots. That sounds scary. Should I be worried about this?

A: You shouldn't worry about the vaccine, but you should worry about hepatitis B. While hepatitis B can be sexually transmitted, and it can kill you, I haven't heard of anyone being hurt by the vaccine. You need to protect your child.

We're starting to vaccinate small children against it, and at the same time we're playing catch-up with the teenagers through their schools.

I vaccinate my kids, and I've never had a moment's doubt about doing that.

Colds and Influenza

Q: You've talked before about having colds and washing your hands and keeping clean, but no one has ever spoken about the toothbrush. Can you recatch your cold from using a toothbrush that you used during a cold?

A: There is research claiming you can recatch strep throat from reusing your own toothbrush, but I have seen nothing about colds, and I would assume that is unlikely.

First of all, when you get a cold, you should become immune forever to that particular virus. So the next time you get a cold, you have a different virus.

You might think that's good. If you knock them off as you move through life, you're not going to get a cold again. But it doesn't work that way, because there are hundreds of cold viruses.

I also doubt that a virus would survive too long on a toothbrush after it dries, but, if it did, you would already be immune to that particular virus, so it wouldn't be a problem.

However, if you have some time on your hands and you want to be really careful about keeping other members of your family from being exposed to this virus, you could put the toothbrush in the microwave briefly. Microwaves work by heating water molecules, which vibrate the hydrogen and create heat. Just put the damp brush in until it gets hot.

Germs can jump around among toothbrushes that share a holder, so your toothbrush can spread your cold if there are other brushes in the cup. When you are ill, a thoughtful gesture would be to throw your toothbrush in the microwave, or dry it well and put a cover on it.

Q: I'm forty-eight and in good health, and I've never had a flu shot, mostly because I'm kind of afraid of them. When do I really need to deal with this?

A: You can relax a bit, because you have two years before you should bite the bullet.

The Centers for Disease Control recommends that everyone over fifty get a shot every year, though the biggest concern in the fifty-through-sixty-four age range is those who are at high risk—people in long-term care facilities; adults and children over six with preexisting heart and lung conditions, including asthma; and adults and children over six who go to the hospital regularly because of diabetes, kidney disease, AIDS, or other immune-system problems. Women who will be more than three months pregnant during flu season also should be inoculated.

There is nothing to be afraid of, and this is nothing to take lightly. The flu can be a killer—twenty thousand to thirty thousand people die from it in the United States each year. Some day, if we have enough vaccine, the shots will be recommended for everyone, because the flu takes a terrible toll on our nation's health.

The vaccine itself is completely safe, as far as we know, though there have been some bad batches in the past. The other thing to keep in mind is that it's manufactured in the late summer, when we're just beginning to take a wild guess as to what particular viruses will cause influenza in the next year. It's different every year, and the vaccine can only handle three or four flu viruses, when there may be hundreds and hundreds of them out there.

So, the shot doesn't necessarily protect you against every flu strain. But it's a big leap from no protection at all.

Q: It seems like my daughter takes her five-year-old to the doctor every time she has even the tiniest cold. I've tried to explain what you've

---

QUIZ

Which virus causes the common cold?
A) coronavirus   B) equivirus   C) ratovirus   D) rhinovirus
E) unknown
(A, D, and E: the coronavirus is the cause of most adults' colds in winter and early spring; the rhinovirus— "Rhin" is Greek for nose—often causes colds that occur in spring, summer, and fall. But many other viruses can cause colds, and some have yet to be identified.)

said on your show—about this being a waste of her money and her doctor's time—but she won't listen. What else can I say?

A: As you have heard me say many times, most colds are caused by viruses, and most get better on their own without the need for medical care. Despite this, one study found that 66 percent of parents surveyed believed that bacteria could sometimes cause colds, and more than half reported feeling that antibiotics—which target bacteria—could cure colds. So your daughter is not alone when she goes to the doctor's office.

Amazingly, almost one quarter of the parents surveyed said they would bring their children to the emergency room if they developed a cold. And you wonder why people working in emergency rooms are stressed out? Can you imagine trying to be patient with overprotective parents when you have people with gunshot wounds and heart attacks waiting for medical attention?

You may not win this battle with your daughter, but please tell her that there just isn't much doctors can do for a child with a runny nose and a cough. The best thing she can do for your granddaughter is to see that she gets rest and fluids and, if necessary, nose drops for comfort.

If the symptoms are more serious, of course, such as a high fever or ear pain, or if the child has difficulty breathing, then it is time to call the doctor to see if you should go in, just to make sure the child does not have anything else in addition to her cold.

Each year in the United States, 1.6 million adults and children visit the emergency room for simple colds, and 25 million get harmless colds checked out in a doctor's office.

Finally, there is research showing that people who are given antibiotics by a doctor to treat a cold once are, understandably, more likely to return to a doctor's office for their next cold. This is not a good thing for a child, because when he or she really needs antibiotics, they may not be as effective.

Q: My husband and I are battling over our toddler, and we need your help. He thinks our toddler caught a cold and then an ear infection because I washed his hair at night, and he went to bed with his hair a little damp. My husband says the cold goes into the pores of the head. I say this is a myth. Can you settle this, please?

A: I have this same argument with my mother, who still believes that going outside with a wet head will cause a cold. I wonder how many other mothers and fathers still yell about this to their children every morning as they race off to school?

But you are right, and your husband is wrong. Dampness or exposure to cold air isn't going to do it. Research has found that throwing people naked into snowbanks does not cause them to catch colds. We also know that colds are not transmitted by touch, although that's what most people believe. That's what I was taught in medical school and what I told people for the first ten years of my radio program.

But in doing research for my first book, *Eat, Drink, and Be Merry*, I found out that's not it at all. As disgusting as this may sound, researchers had people play poker with snot-laced cards, and that did not transmit colds.

Colds are transmitted through the air. Breathing in as few as fifteen to thirty virus particles will do it. The problem with a cold is that it's called a "cold," which suggests temperature. But try using the medical word for cold, coryza, and see how far that will get you.

So why do people seem to get more colds in winter? Because we spend more time indoors, where virus transmission is more likely. But our cold immunity can vary throughout the year, and stress can be a big factor in how many colds each of us will have.

Q: When I get a fever or flulike symptoms, my impulse is to get into a

DEAN'S LIST: IS IT A COLD OR THE FLU?

The following symptoms should guide you to a self-diagnosis:

	COLD	FLU
fever	rare	usual (can be high)
headache	rare	usual
general aches, pains	slight	usual (often severe)
fatigue, weakness	quite mild	usual (often severe)
stuffy nose	common	occasionally
sneezing	usual	occasionally
sore throat	common	occasionally
chest discomfort	mild to moderate hacking cough	common (can be severe)

bath as hot as I can stand it, over 110 degrees. I do this about three or four times a day until I feel better. Since you've said the body uses a fever to fight infection, do you think raising my heat is curing me?

A: You are talking about what's called fever therapy. For the first half of the last century, we raised people's temperature on purpose, because we thought it might help. The research has not been conclusive, though, and, to my knowledge, we are not sure that heating the body reproduces a fever's infection-fighting abilities.

When I get the flu, I have awful chills, and I have been very tempted to jump into a hot tub or spa. But being in 110-degree water can be flirting with disaster. There is a lag period between the time when your internal body temperature starts to rise and the time when you register the change. So your temperature may be dangerously high without your knowing it. People have died this way from being in a hot tub. Respiration becomes very rapid as the body goes into overtime to cool off.

So, to be on the safe side, when I get a flu with chills, I get under a pile of blankets until I sweat. I can't recommend your approach.

Q: I have what I suspect is the flu, and I've been locked up in my room since Saturday. I haven't kissed my wife or my son, and my father is coming for a visit. Is there a way to know if I really have the flu, and how do I avoid giving it to my child or my father? When am I free from giving it to anyone?

A: A lot of progress has been made in the past few years, so no one needs to go into hiding without first taking a test at the doctor's office. The results are available in about thirty minutes, and the two tests now being used are considered moderate to reasonably accurate.

Also, the FDA has approved two drugs that shorten the duration of flu symptoms if taken no later than forty-eight hours after the symptoms appear.

As with many infectious diseases, including the common cold, your flu may have been the most infectious to your loved ones before your symptoms began, before you even knew you were sick. You are probably still contagious, but you're less of a menace than you were at the start.

The flu can be deadly to old people, so, if your father is elderly, take care not to expose him. Don't cough and sneeze and slobber on anyone. There may be viruses in your saliva, and we think the flu is mostly spread through droplets. By the way, has your dad been vaccinated?

Q: I'm seventy-eight years old, and I had a flu shot two days ago. Yesterday I felt bad, and today I feel like I've been hit by a Mack truck. I don't even want to stand up. I've got aches and pains in my muscles. Did the flu shot make me sick?

A: No. The belief that the flu shot will give you the flu is a myth. However, the shot does cause some people to feel a bit crummy and achy, and it may cause pain at the site of the injection.

It takes a day or two for the shot to become effective, and I have to think that either you feel lousy because your immune system is revving up, or you had the bad luck to catch the flu before the shot had time to kick in and protect you.

Call your doctor for a prescription to one of the new antiflu medications that can stop it in its tracks. You are in an age group to which the flu can be dangerous.

Sexually Transmitted Diseases

Q: My brother is a twenty-six-year-old gay man who recently came out of the closet. I don't know much about his personal life, because he has his own apartment, but I get the feeling his relationships are pretty free-wheeling at the moment. Is he in as much danger of AIDS as he would have been ten years ago?

A: You have a right to be concerned, because, after a ten-year downturn, there is a resurgence of HIV cases among gay men. This has doctors at the Centers for Disease Control very concerned that many gay men may no longer view HIV/AIDS as a life-threatening disease. In fact, most men your brother's age were too young to watch friends die from this disease in the '80s and '90s.

A person can carry the virus for many years without having symptoms, and the CDC estimates that almost three hundred thousand people are HIV positive and don't know it.

The latest HIV and AIDS statistics also show that the fastest-growing numbers are among African-American and Hispanic gay men.

Try to talk to your brother about your concerns, and encourage him to make sure he is protecting himself. Just because someone tells him they don't have HIV doesn't mean he shouldn't be extremely careful. And if he's meeting men over the Internet, his antennae really need to be up—this can be very risky terrain.

Your brother also should know that there's a new twenty-minute HIV test, available at doctors' offices and public health clinics, so there's no need to be in doubt about the status of his health as well as that of a potential partner.

All that's needed for the test is a drop of blood from the patient's finger. However, if the initial test shows positive, more specific lab tests are required to confirm the results.

In the past, health agencies have struggled with attempts to control the spread of HIV because patients who took the old test had to wait a few days before getting results. Unfortunately, many people never returned to find out what their HIV status was.

Q: I saw a television program about a man with HIV fathering a baby after sperm washing. What is sperm washing?

A: Antibodies and other cells can cling to sperm and block its ability to be effective. Sperm washing is a chemical process used to separate sperm from the other cells in semen.

DID YOU KNOW?
WHY ISN'T THIS SCARY ANYMORE?

After a ten-year decline in new cases, HIV and AIDS are on the rise again in the United States, and an estimated 850,000 to 950,000 Americans are now infected with HIV. About 36 million people carry the virus worldwide. Some experts attribute the spike to "AIDS complacency"—people don't see it as a problem in the United States, they aren't being tested, and they are passing the virus along through unprotected sex and other practices. In the United States, HIV ranks fifth among the leading causes of death for all persons between the ages of thirty-five and forty-four, but second among Hispanic males of that age group and first among African-American males of that age.

We don't take each little sperm and scrub-a-dub-dub. We shake the semen and flush it with saline and other fluids to rid it of debris, including HIV. Sperm washing enables HIV-positive men to father children without passing the virus to the mother.

At one time, we thought HIV penetrated the sperm. It doesn't, but it does get into other cells that are floating in semen.

Q: I'm housesitting for a gay male friend, and another friend of mine is convinced I'm being reckless about AIDS. Even when I told her my friend is HIV negative, she didn't budge. Am I wrong about this?

A: No. You've got your facts straight, and your fearful friend doesn't. It has been proven again and again that you cannot catch HIV from objects or from the air. Nurses and doctors who touch AIDS patients every day and who are coughed on and sneezed on haven't caught HIV. Parents living for years in the same apartment with an HIV-infected child don't get HIV.

If your friend is in other ways a rational person, I can only conclude that she has a phobia about HIV, just as some people have phobias about spiders or heights.

Q: A good friend has just begun taking the drugs prescribed for HIV/AIDS, and he's worried about one of the side effects that can affect the fat in his body. This sounds really weird. What's he talking about?

A: The standard treatment for HIV/AIDS is a combination of drugs called Highly Active Antiretroviral Therapy (HAART). This has been a very effective treatment—but not a cure. It does have several side effects, and one of them is called lipodystrophy.

With this syndrome, large amounts of the body's fat can be redistributed in different places on the body, including the back—which creates a "buffalo hump"—lower stomach, breasts, face, buttocks, and arms. In other words, almost everywhere.

It is still not clear what exactly in the medications—or the combination of the drugs and virus—causes this syndrome. However, your friend needs to remember that not everyone experiences every side effect of a medication.

If he wants the latest research on this syndrome, he should look on the Internet.

Once lipodystrophy is fully understood, it could have a positive impact on other research related to body shape. When scientists figure out exactly how these drugs work, we will be taking a huge step in understanding fat metabolism.

Q: I got syphilis ten years ago from a sexual encounter, and I was treated with penicillin at the time. I have been married for four years and have two kids. Last month I donated blood and was found to have a titration value for syphilis. What does this mean? Is my wife in danger?

A: Your body is just indicating that you have antibodies against the syphilis germ, which is evidence that you had a syphilis infection in the past, just like it shows evidence of most past infections. This doesn't mean you have syphilis now. The living syphilis bacteria are not active in your body, and your wife is not at risk of getting it.

Q: I was diagnosed with genital herpes about ten years ago. About once a year, they break out at the base of my spine where the fold of my buttocks begins. I noticed that my baby's chicken pox sores look just like the sores I get. Do they have anything in common?

A: The chicken pox virus is called herpes zoster. The genital herpes virus is a different strain, called herpes simplex. Obviously these two are close members of the same family. But an outbreak of one is not related to an outbreak of the other.

The adult version of chicken pox is called shingles, which is also caused by the herpes zoster virus. It's most common in older people, and most people have only one outbreak. The virus infects nerves on your head or torso, and it appears as a rash that becomes small blisters. The rare and most dangerous form infects the eyes, nose, and face.

I do wonder if you have been properly diagnosed with herpes simplex, or if you may have instead had herpes zoster. Just a few years ago, we diagnosed herpes simplex on clinical evidence rather than actually testing to identify the specific virus.

The treatment for the two viruses is different, so it would be worth your while to have your doctor swab and culture your little sore to determine if it is shingles or genital herpes.

Q: Yesterday, I was diagnosed with genital herpes. I'm thirty-nine and have been married for twenty-one years. Is there another way to catch herpes besides sex? I have only had one other sexual encounter in my life; that was twenty-two years ago. My husband has had no sexual partners besides me. Having this big secret is painful for me. Can you help me understand how this could happen?

A: I've had many calls about this exact situation, so I don't find your story hard to believe. Don't start accusing each other and calling divorce lawyers.

Herpes is notorious for lying dormant for years. We have seen cases of seven or eight years of dormancy. Although it's a long shot, it is possible that you caught herpes twenty-two years ago and it's just now popping out.

Also, the herpes virus can move back and forth between the mouth and the genitals. Even without having visible cold sores, most of us carry the oral herpes virus, which can be transmitted to the genitals during oral sex. Clinically, we can't tell the difference, unless we swab the lesion and check the organism's DNA.

As many women do, you could have unknowingly had lesions before. In preparation for childbirth, we ask women about herpes, because the virus can cause life-threatening infections in infants. About 35 percent of these women who have herpes do not remember ever having a lesion.

Because a woman can have internal lesions, she may feel stinging and burning during urination and never identify that as herpes unless she gets a culture. Most women do not routinely examine their genitals with a mirror. It's a good idea, because both herpes and vulva cancer can be detected this way.

I want to give you the best medical facts I can, and I want to be realistic, too. I do always advise a spouse to consider the possibility that her husband has cheated, because we both know that that happens. Talk to your husband, and go with your instincts. It is possible that you guys have been faithful to each other all of your lives, and you still got herpes. Remember, your husband could have been infected with herpes long ago, not have lesions, and still spread it.

Q: My girlfriend has just been diagnosed with human papillomavirus (HPV), but I have never had any symptoms. So when she told me she was infected, I said, "Well, it wasn't me." Can I get a blood test to see if I have HPV?

A: I'm afraid that getting the definitive word is going to be very difficult. For one thing, this seems to be a virus that can stay put for a while, so your partner could have had the virus for many years without it manifesting until now. Men and women most often have no visible symptoms, but genital warts can be very subtle and inconspicuous, so doctors use a "vinegar test" on the genitals of both men and women and then look at the areas with a magnifying glass.

Another important fact to keep in mind is that the lifetime incidence of genital HPV infection is very, very high—more than five million people in the United States are infected each year. However, most people with a sexually transmitted HPV do not ever show symptoms.

So, before you do anything rash, take a deep breath and have a good, calm discussion with your girlfriend about your relationship.

As for being tested yourself, this may not clear up anything. A person can test negative and actually have the virus. We're only beginning to learn the life cycles and functions of HPV. The FDA has approved a test for the presence of HPV's DNA; talk to your doctor about its availability.

Sexually transmitted HPV is nothing to fool around with. It causes genital warts, cervical cancer, and other malignancies. You didn't say what your girlfriend's symptoms are, but the good news is that clinicians have an array of therapeutic weapons available to treat genital warts. And, although about forty of the more than one hundred types of HPV infect the genital tracts in men and women, the majority of HPV viruses carry virtually no risk of malignancy.

However, if genital warts do develop and are persistent, your girlfriend may be at a higher risk of cervical cancer or premalignant lesions, so she needs to get a gynecological exam.

Finally, you need to know that using condoms doesn't eliminate the risk of virus transmission, since we suspect that HPV also can be spread during foreplay and other sexual contact. It has been found under people's fingernails.

See more about HPV on page 79 in chapter 2.

Q: I've been fighting canker sores and cold sores for years. The minute I feel one coming on, I use a styptic pencil, and the sore goes away in one or two days. How can I tell the difference between canker sores and cold sores? If I bite my lip, I get sores, but I also think I have a virus that causes them.

A: Most canker sores are caused by a trauma to the inside of the mouth. Biting your lip would certainly do it. I get them all the time when I scrape my mouth with a hard bread crust or a taco chip. Canker sores are not infectious, and they take a long time to heal.

Herpes is the virus that causes cold sores. It's infectious, and usually breaks out in the mouth, around the gums and on the palate. But it can show up as a sore in the corner of the mouth. Canker sores are usually on soft tissue, such as the tongue, the lips, or the inside of the cheeks.

Staphylococcal and Streptococcus Infections

Q: My wife has had several serious bouts of streptococcus throat infections. They were so bad that she had to be hospitalized for several days and put on intravenous antibiotics. Her doctor doesn't seem to have any ideas about how to stop this from recurring. I haven't ever had this infection, and none of our kids have had anything like what she's experienced. What would you do?

A: Streptococcus can be very difficult to get under control, but every time your wife finishes with a round of antibiotics, the strep is gone from her body, so she has to be catching it from somebody or something. It's possible you or one of your children or a friend or relative could be carriers, without actually showing symptoms. Even a cat or a dog can be a carrier. Also, she could be getting it from her toothbrush.

You need to be a detective with this, and you still may not get to the source. But I'd start by having everyone in your family treated with antibiotics the next time she is infected. I would replace all the toothbrushes at that time, too.

Q: My friend's 11-year-old daughter was recently diagnosed with scarlet fever. I remember hearing about it when I was a child, but I realize I don't know much about it. Should I be taking special precautions with my daughter? Is scarlet fever contagious?

A: Scarlet fever is still very much with us, although its incidence has declined. It begins with a strep infection, which is caused by a bacterium, is contagious, and most commonly causes a throat infection.

Scarlet fever develops in 10 percent of strep throats, for both kids and

QUIZ

Streptococcus bacteria cause which of the following:
A) scarlet fever   B) cellulitis   C) toxic shock syndrome
D) impetigo   E) all of the above
(E: all of the above. Of course, it is probably best known as the cause of strep throat.)

adults, because, for some unknown reason, the strep germ secretes toxins and enzymes that cause a rash.

Strep is everywhere, but most kids develop immunity by age ten, so I don't think you need to take any special precautions.

Q: About four weeks ago, I had emergency surgery for an intestinal blockage. The doctors also removed my appendix. After the surgery, my wound became infected, so now I have an open incision that we're treating from the inside out to let it heal. Apparently I have three infections—an antibiotic-resistant staph infection, E. coli, and pseudomonas—but I'm not on antibiotics. Does this make sense?

A: There are two general kinds of infections—medical infections and surgical infections. In your case, the doctor is treating you for what we call a surgical infection, a term we use in medicine for infections that form a lot of pus.

A medical infection would be something like pneumonia or a bladder infection, and we routinely use antibiotics in those cases. But surgical infections can be a little different. Normally, a surgical infection begins with a wound, either from an injury or an incision from an operation. When a wound becomes infected, it doesn't heal, and a pocket of pus forms. The germs can come from your own skin or the hospital environment. It must drain continuously to the outside in order to heal. They're probably irrigating you, and, I assume, the bandages are changed regularly.

Once an infection exists, you can't stitch up this type of wound or let it heal over too soon, because if you did, you would seal in those germs, and, for

---

QUIZ

Which symptom could be a sign of a bacterial infection?
A) severe headache for more than twenty-four hours
B) fever over 100°F   C) very sore throat
D) phlegm that is yellow, green, rust, or brown-colored
E) all of the above
(E: all of the above. If the throat is just tickly or scratchy, and the headache and body pains are mild, you may have a viral infection.)

sure, they would wreak havoc with your body. Your doctor is kind of gutsy, yet he may be on to something. My guess is that, in general, we probably overutilize antibiotics in this situation, because draining off the pus is the most important part of the treatment.

It's difficult for an antibiotic to get to the center of a pocket of pus, because, with an antibiotic, you take a pill, the drug goes into your bloodstream, it circulates around and gets diluted heavily, and the bloodstream carries it to the wound. The antibiotic stops at the edge of the wound, because antibiotics don't really penetrate pus very well—once again, they're traveling in the bloodstream.

That said, the pseudomonas germ is very dangerous if it spreads beyond the wound. Although the germ's natural habitats are soil and water, it is frequently found in hospitals and is highly resistant to antibiotics. As with any medical situation where a patient has concerns about a course of treatment, you should call your doctor and talk to him about it. I think a good surgeon knows when a surgical wound is getting out of hand, and maybe he wants to save the antibiotics for more serious problems. If he had started with antibiotics in the beginning, and then you grew some germs in that wound, those antibiotics would be impotent against those germs.

See more about pseudomonas on page 426.

Q: Last week, I broke out in itchy, red bumps from head to toe. They were even on my eyelids. I had a sore throat and a fever, too. The urgent-care doctor said I had a very contagious chicken pox or a similar virus. The next day I went to my regular doctor who disagreed. He told me I had folliculitis, he prescribed antibiotics, and now I have mouth sores. I am healing, but I don't know what I had. Can you help?

A: I would never try to guess what caused your rash without seeing it myself, but I have to say that folliculitis, an infection of your hair follicles, doesn't sound quite right. It never occurs over the entire body, because the susceptible hair follicles are more common only in certain areas. The sore throat, sores inside your mouth, and a rash are more likely to be symptoms of a virus, and antibiotics aren't helpful for a virus. However, you could have had strep throat, which can be accompanied by a rash.

A good dermatologist can take one look at it and tell you in a second what you've got, so that's where I'd start.

Nowadays, doctors often don't even do blood tests to figure these things out, because most of these diseases are of such short duration. They will go away by themselves, and the insurance company doesn't want to pay for a test for something that has usually already healed.

Often, when we see a doctor we are at the peak of an illness, and we are about to start getting better anyway. But many folks are convinced that they must have antibiotics in order to get better, no matter what they have. However, as we say in the business: "A cold will get better in seven days; if you take antibiotics it will get better in a week."

Mononucleosis and Epstein-Barr

Q: Two weeks ago, my wife was diagnosed with mononucleosis. She went to her doctor because she was waking up tired, and staying tired all day, even after a good night's sleep. She also had a sore throat. Don't teenagers usually get this? How would she have caught it?

A: Your wife had two classic mononucleosis symptoms, and she is fortunate to have a doctor who tested her properly and could give her a reason for her fatigue. People are often mislabeled with chronic fatigue syndrome without being given even simple, basic tests for the myriad illnesses that cause fatigue, from thyroid disease to low blood pressure.

We used to call mono "the kissing disease," because it would run through college campuses where there's a lot of kissing going on. It is, in fact, highly infectious and seems to be spread by saliva. Almost all of us have been infected with the Epstein-Barr virus, which causes mono. We most likely don't even remember having it, because we caught it when we were little kids. If you get it as a teenager or adult, we call it "mono."

There is no medication to cure mononucleosis, but she will get better on her own with a lot of rest. The first few weeks are the acute phase, and most people sleep a lot. It is going to be anywhere from two to six months before she feels like her old self.

We're not quite sure why some people succumb to this virus that's around us all the time. Perhaps there's a little glitch in the immune system on that particular day, and the body gets knocked down by a viral invasion.

Many people have had mononucleosis without ever realizing it. They may have had a mild version, or mistaken their symptoms for the flu. Other people seem to be immune to it.

Q: My doctor says that the fatigue I'm experiencing is caused by the Epstein-Barr virus (EBV). Do you think I'm getting good advice?

A: I think your doctor is off base—unless you have mononucleosis and forgot to mention that. We used to think EBV was the cause of a controversial diagnosis called chronic fatigue and immune dysfunction syndrome (or simply chronic fatigue syndrome; see more on page 371, in chapter 8), but I don't know of any scientific evidence to support the existence of this illness. However, you won't have to look very far to find a lot of people who claim to have this illness, and there are M.D.s who treat it. While Epstein-Barr virus can cause mono (see previous question), there are specific tests to determine that, and fatigue associated with mono seldom lasts more than four months.

People with chronic fatigue often turn out to have viruses, bacteria, parasites, or other illnesses, like anemia or thyroid disease, that were missed by the initial diagnostic tests. An infectious disease specialist may be able to help you, because these doctors specialize in diagnosing stubborn infections. I want you to find someone who will stay with you to get to the bottom of this and treat you appropriately. Fatigue is the most common symptom for which people see their doctor. There are hundreds of causes, from depression to cancer, and you need to be methodical and persistent in order to find the cause of your tiredness.

Miscellaneous

Q: My church passes communal wine around to the congregation in a common cup. They do rotate the cup and wipe it with gauze, but with hundreds of people taking sips, that cup really makes the rounds. Can you arm me with any medical arguments to convince the church not to do that? I feel like our church is in the Dark Ages.

A: You might be surprised to know this question has been addressed periodically in religious and scientific journals since the late 1800s, obviously without any incontrovertible findings, since many churches still follow the practice.

The public health department would shut down a restaurant that had servers sharing cups among the patrons, and there is no doubt that germs can be transmitted this way, but who would know if the source of a flu or cold was the communion cup? We don't really have a statistical fix on how important a public health problem this is. I do know that some churches use disposable cups, and others use prepackaged wafers and wine. And at churches where there are both wafers and wine, some folks dunk the wafer in the wine rather than sip from the cup. However, there are germs on fingers, too, so you may not be avoiding anything by doing these things.

Q: Our favorite family weekend destination has a communal hot tub, which I use reluctantly. How germ-ridden are hot tubs likely to be?

A: A resort hot tub is likely to be better maintained than the hot tub in your backyard, so, most likely, it is free of disease. The same goes for public pools versus a home pool.

The laws vary from state to state, but most public hot tubs must have chlorination. In fact, if you can smell the chlorine, you know the tub has more than it needs. Some hot tubs are treated with ozone, which is effective when tub use is limited. However, chlorine should be added to tubs that see a lot of activity.

A bacteria called pseudomonas, which causes a really nasty skin infection called folliculitis, does sometimes like to cozy up in hot tubs, but to my knowledge it's only a problem in those tubs that aren't cleaned properly (see next question for more information).

People frequently ask me if they can catch a sexually transmitted disease in a hot tub. The answer is yes—if you have sex in a hot tub. However, I don't recommend that. When chlorine gets in the vagina, it can cause vaginitis.

Q: I've been itching for a month and a half from bites all over my body. My husband got them about two weeks after I did. It's not fleas, because we don't have any pets. We have a hot tub, and we've had that treated for pseudomonas.

QUIZ

What is a likely cause of a black tongue?
A) coffee   B) blood transfusion   C) antibiotics
D) too much licorice   E) strep infection
(C: antibiotics.)

Between the two of us, we've been to three dermatologists, and we still don't have an answer. My husband's dermatologist thinks it might be folliculitis, but my dermatologist says no. Can you shed any light on this nuisance?

A: I'm not sure you need a fourth opinion, but you might need an exterminator or a hot-tub expert.

First, I want to correct one point: You don't have to have pets to have a flea infestation. You could have introduced a piece of furniture to your house that had an infestation, or you could have been exposed to the fleas and brought them into your house.

An allergy to flea saliva, not the bite itself, causes the itchy rash. Two people can be bitten by fleas and if one is allergic and the other one is not, one will get itchy bites and the other one won't. Since you're both itchy, it's possible you're both allergic to flea spit.

One way to rule this out is to stick one big Band-Aid somewhere on your body. If you get the rash under it, then you know it's not fleas, because no flea is going to bite through that.

Folliculitis is an inflammation of the hair follicle, and there are two common types—one that is caused by staph bacteria, and a second, called "hot-tub folliculitis," that is caused by pseudomonas germs. It is visible as little bumps at the base of infected follicles, and it may be more intense on the skin covered by a swimsuit, because the contaminated water has more contact time with the skin. Sometimes the bumps are pus-filled, and sometimes they become dark red nodules. For severe cases, the treatment is usually antibiotics.

I know you had the tub treated, but pseudomonas can be tough bacteria, and it particularly loves wood hot tubs. If that's your problem, you need proper ongoing maintenance to keep it from returning. Start by running chlorine over every surface and every pipe of the hot tub, then make sure chlorine levels are maintained.

Q: During the SARS scare everyone seemed to focus on airplane travel as one way the illness spread. Do viruses and bacteria really spread that much more easily in a plane's closed environment than in an enclosed mall or a school?

A: The studies I have seen on this have reported conflicting results.

Although airplane cabin air is low quality in two regards—it is dry and it circulates in an enclosed space—I think the disease that does spread during air travel happens because a group is confined in tight quarters for a long period of time. If several hundred people on the ground were crammed into a building and stayed there for five or ten hours, they would probably spread around more disease than they ordinarily do.

By the way, you might wonder why airlines don't increase the amount of oxygen that circulates on planes to make flights more tolerable. After all, air is free, right? Well, not exactly. The air is cold, and heating it uses more fuel, which costs money.

I did read recently about a case of tuberculosis that was spread on a plane during a long flight. However, during the peak of the SARS (severe acute respiratory syndrome) outbreak, all the airplane scare stories I read—where one passenger was ill, and others started feeling ill during the course of a long flight—sounded more like cases of mass sociogenic illness (MSI) than the actual spread of any illness. (For more on MSI, see page 397.)

After all, viral illness doesn't spread from one person to another and cause symptoms in a matter of hours—it takes days. So a lot of people can only get sick at the same time if they were all exposed to the same source days before the flight.

Q: About a year ago I had gastric bypass surgery. About five months later, after I was hospitalized for mental confusion, lightheadedness, and loss of balance, one doctor told me I have Guillain-Barré syndrome, and another diagnosed my illness as a vitamin B12 deficiency. When I was hospitalized, the only test finding was extremely low vitamin B12.

I have some symptoms that are not symptoms of Guillain-Barré. I don't have elevated proteins, and, instead of deadened reflexes, mine are overactive. The doctors also think that either Guillain-Barré or the lack of B12 may have damaged the myelin of my nerves. I have numbness and paralysis in my feet.

QUIZ

True or False? You can remove bacteria from your mouth by brushing your tongue with your toothbrush.

(True: by removing the bacteria you also will freshen your breath.)

Can I expect to recover from this? I heard of one person who took two full years to recover.

A: Guillain-Barré syndrome is a type of autoimmune disease that, at its most severe, can paralyze a patient's breathing and cause death. It often follows an unrelated viral infection. We think that in making antibodies against the virus, the immune system goes into overdrive and attacks nerves.

This is a clear example of the danger of an overactive immune system, and anyone who buys supplements to boost the immune system should think again.

A vitamin B12 deficiency is a very serious thing. It can cause all the symptoms you described, and mental confusion is much more symptomatic of a B12 deficiency than of Guillain-Barré. People with vitamin B12 deficiencies have been mistakenly institutionalized for mental illness or hospitalized for Alzheimer's disease. With proper treatment, the mental dysfunction can be reversed.

This is caused by an inability of the stomach to absorb vitamin B12, so doctors usually give B12 shots. However, the newest research finds that large oral doses of B12 work, too. I think it's possible that the gastroplasty you had may have rendered your stomach incapable of absorbing B12.

I have every reason to be hopeful that you will see a recovery. Anything can happen in medicine, especially in a complicated case like yours, with so many unknowns. Myelin can be regenerated, as long as the insult to the nerves hasn't continued.

Neurology is a fascinating field where new discoveries are constant, and diagnosis and treatment are often a matter of finding the right doctor or university neurology professor who comes up with an explanation and a new perspective.

See a related question on page 307 in chapter 6.

Q: I'm having surgery a week from today to reverse a colostomy. I want to donate my own blood in case I need it during the operation, but my doctor says it's too late to do that. Am I at risk of getting tainted blood from a blood bank?

A: Blood banks test blood for hepatitis, HIV, and other serious diseases, and the possibility of tainted blood getting to you is very, very remote.

If you were to bank your own blood, you should give at least a couple of units, and yes, you are a bit late for that. You don't want to deplete yourself of red blood cells with surgery just a week away.

I was taught in medical school never to give a patient just one unit of blood. They either need more than that or they don't need it at all. This isn't a hard-and-fast rule, just a general principle to keep doctors from being sloppy surgeons, to spill as little blood as possible, and not to use the unit of blood just because it's there.

Most surgeons are very careful, of course. They don't go in trying to make you bleed. Sometimes bleeding during surgery just can't be helped, and a patient who has had prior surgery, as you did, may have fibrosis and scar tissue that make the operation a little more complicated.

Q: My nephew got a severe case of chicken pox when he was eleven. He had flulike symptoms and a high fever, and for a while he couldn't walk.

Eventually he regained his ability to walk, but, in the past four years, he has had three headache attacks that were so severe that he couldn't sit up completely. Both a CAT scan and MRI were negative. I feel like our family needs to know more about what's going on. What would be your next step?

A: A very severe chicken pox virus can cause encephalitis—a brain infection. That's why we recommend children be vaccinated against it. I suspect that your nephew has been struck with postencephalitic syndrome. This occurs in one in 1,000 cases of chicken pox, and while it can be fatal, it usually causes a variety of neurological problems that should go away with time.

You don't want to leave any stone unturned in getting a definitive diagnosis and treatment, so he needs to see a top-notch neurologist.

By the way, adults who didn't get chicken pox during childhood are susceptible to it. There is now a vaccine for chicken pox.

Q: I'm twenty-nine years old, and I was recently diagnosed with Crohn's disease in my intestines. Is Crohn's disease a bacterial infection or an autoimmune disease? And why does my stomach start to hurt and cramp even before food reaches my intestines? As soon as I begin to eat, I feel cramping.

A: The act of eating fires up what is called the gastrocolic reflex, setting the intestines in motion. This is a common experience that sends some people running to the bathroom as soon as they pick up a fork.

Also, we often begin eating meal No. 2 before the first one has made its way out of the intestines. After all, if you eat three meals a day, at any given time, there is food on board, because it takes at least a day for food to make its way from one end of the digestive system to the other.

In your case, as soon as you take in more food, your inflamed intestines begin to cramp. I could actually cut your intestines with a knife, and you would barely feel it, but stretching, which is what causes a cramp, causes horrible intestinal pain.

Crohn's is definitely an autoimmune disease. We don't know exactly what causes it, but it has been theorized that autoimmune diseases originate with bacterial infections. There is a strong genetic component and smokers are also at higher risk.

Many diseases begin when the immune system overreacts to germs. The antibodies that our immune system produces to attack germs sometimes attack healthy tissue, too.

You will able to find a lot of information and support about Crohn's disease on the Internet. I encourage you to do research online, because our knowledge is rapidly changing.

Q: Two years ago, I had a small lump removed from my neck, which was diagnosed as sarcoidosis. At the time, the surgeon told me that the disease might return and it might not. He also admitted he didn't know much about this disease. Should I be doing some follow-up? Is there anything new going on with this disease? I read about one woman who had an inoperable lesion, and it scared me.

A: Sarcoidosis is a condition in which areas of inflamed cells accumulate in a certain part of the body, most often the lungs. But, as you know, it can occur in many other places, including the lymph nodes, liver, and skin. Sometimes there are no symptoms.

It's a very unusual condition, because it seems to be an infectious disease and yet we can't find a source of infection. We don't know what causes it, but it has a genetic component. In the United States, the incidence of sarcoidosis is much, much higher among African-Americans, and their cases are usually more serious.

Sarcoidosis shows up on a chest X ray as excess tissue around the lungs. Under a microscope, it looks like tuberculosis or even lymphoma. Often it goes away by itself, but a small percentage of people end up with damaged lungs, and in some cases it is fatal.

So, yes, you should absolutely have a medical examination, and this time see a different doctor. Any surgeon who treats a disease he knows nothing about should send his patient to another doctor.

You need to see an internist and find out the status of your condition, because sarcoidosis can grow internally without your knowing it. Or, it could have disappeared, and you would want to know that, too.

Depending on which organs are affected, treatment for sarcoidosis ranges from doing nothing to taking steroids or immunosuppressant drugs.

Q: Is there a time of the year when I should be most worried about Lyme disease? And how do I know if I have the tick on my body that can make me sick?

A: Spring and summer are the peak of Lyme disease "season," and the incidents of this illness have jumped dramatically, so you are smart to be aware of it, especially if you spend much time outdoors in northern California, the northeast region of the United States, or Wisconsin or Minnesota. If you live anywhere else, your chances of encountering Lyme disease are much smaller.

Montana is the only state that has had no reported cases of Lyme disease, but they do have Rocky Mountain spotted fever, which is carried by ticks, too. And scientists are also looking at other possible diseases carried by these eight-legged creatures. So, when in doubt, check your body for ticks if you have been outdoors.

The deer tick is the carrier you want to watch for, and one way to recognize it—if you even see it—is by its smallness. It's about half the size of the average dog tick, or as small as a sesame seed. So you have to be diligent when you are checking your body after a day in the yard or out hiking or camping. If you do find a tick and remove it within the first twenty-four hours of exposure, you probably won't be contaminated—if the tick is even infected. In general, only one percent of deer ticks are Lyme-disease carriers.

The tick carries a spiral-shaped bacteria that leaves a very specific, bull's-eye-shaped rash at the site of the tick bite, followed by flulike symptoms, though the fatigue and achiness last longer than the flu. A small percentage of patients will develop neurological abnormalities, including Bell's palsy, which is a temporary paralysis of the facial muscles. Any single nerve—including the sciatic nerve—can be attacked initially, so any numbness—even a sore back—can be a symptom, too.

Most patients get arthritis as well, and, very rarely, heart problems will occur. At its worst, Lyme disease can be fatal. The standard treatment is antibiotics for anywhere from ten days to four weeks, depending on when the disease was caught. In some situations, the doctor may try antibiotics for many months. As you might guess, the sooner it's diagnosed, the better.

The one controversial aspect of Lyme disease is whether it can cause chronic, long-lasting symptoms, like fatigue and loss of concentration. Some doctors believe long-term mental and behavioral symptoms may be psychosomatic.

Scientists are exploring the possibility of a vaccine that would go after the tick, but that's not likely to happen soon. In the meantime, use a good insect repellent that includes DEET, and wear light-colored clothing (so you can more easily see the ticks) that fits tightly at the wrists and ankles. Pulling your socks over your pants may look silly, but it's a good way to block those access points. Closed-toe shoes and a hat are also recommended. Spraying repellent on your clothes is one more way to keep the critters off you.

Now you're ready to rake the backyard.

Q: Ever since the big breakout of the West Nile virus in Louisiana, my wife refuses to take a trip there. Should we avoid any place in the South that has mosquitoes?

A: I would not alter any travel plans because of the West Nile virus. If you think about the number of mosquito bites that occur in this country versus the number of serious cases of West Nile virus, I think you would be reassured. Most people who do get this virus have either no symptoms or mild, flulike symptoms. Between 300,000 and 400,000 cases of the virus occurred in 2002, but the serious ones numbered between 2,000 and 3,000, and there were about 250 deaths.

Mild West Nile symptoms include fever, headache, and body aches. In some cases, there is a rash on the trunk of the body and swollen lymph glands. Symptoms of a severe infection (West Nile encephalitis or meningitis) include headache, high fever, neck stiffness, stupor, disorientation, coma, tremors, convulsions, muscle weakness, and paralysis. People over fifty are at highest risk of a severe case of West Nile.

Symptoms can occur within three days of a bite, but it can take as long as fourteen days for the disease to make itself known. If you have severe symptoms, see a doctor immediately.

If you do visit an area where mosquitoes are abundant, take the standard precautions. Mosquito bites are not pleasant, and you should be able to avoid most of them with appropriate repellents and clothing (see specific tips in previous question). Enjoy the trip.

For more information about mosquitoes and other bug bites, see page 554 in chapter 12.

Q: I heard you say on one show that meat-processing methods in England in the eighties are a suspected source of mad cow disease, and that it is related to Creutzfeldt-Jakob disease (CJD). Well, my dad was a meat cutter here in America, and my mother recently died from CJD.

Her first symptom was that she had a terrible time sleeping, and, by the end, she was hallucinating and had dementia. One question: Why weren't the doctors more interested in figuring out where this originated? The only thing they questioned her about was whether she had taken a growth hormone.

A: You ask good questions about a very confusing and scary topic. And it's natural, when someone close to us dies, to want to know everything we can about what happened.

Fortunately, Creutzfeldt-Jakob disease is very rare in the United States. It is an attack against the brain by a mystifying organism called a prion, which is a unique life-form that is not a virus or a bacterium, but is suspected of spreading infection. Prions are misshapen proteins capable of changing other proteins into prions. They are a controversial topic among scientists.

CJD is considered to be the human variant of bovine spongiform encephalopathy (BSE), which has been given the common name of "mad cow disease." Research on this subject is particularly intense in Europe, and scientists are trying to determine the exact cause-and-effect relationship between the two illnesses.

So, your mom's doctor would just not have been equipped to track down the cause of her CJD. If there had been multiple cases at the same time, of course, the response would have been different.

The doctors asked about your mother's exposure to growth hormone because until we had synthetic growth hormone, we used to use human growth hormone from the pituitary glands of cadavers. Years ago, when I was a medical student, we removed the pituitary glands during autopsies and shipped them off to be ground up and injected experimentally into patients. We later found that we were transmitting Creutzfeldt-Jakob disease, because this prion lodges itself in nerve tissue.

Our first hints about CJD came from studies of cannibals who transmitted a CJD-like disease because of their dietary habits.

The disease can be transmitted by neurosurgical instruments, needles, and electrodes that have been contaminated by contact with a patient's brain tissue. Then there are sporadic cases for which we can't find an origin. But recent research indicates that blood transfusions do not transmit prions.

Although mad cow disease is a variant of Creutzfeldt-Jakob disease, meat is one of the last things I would look to as the cause of your mother's death. Fortunately, no American cattle have been infected with BSE. However, Canada had to deal with this problem in 2003 for the first time in ten years, and it's always possible it could cross the border. In Europe, brain tissue from infected sheep was found in cattle feed, and that's how the last outbreak started. We don't use that feed here.

Also, there is concern about a related infection called "chronic wasting disease" that is being found in wild elk and deer in several U.S. states. To date, research shows that it is unlikely this can spread to domestic cattle or bison.

Your mother's symptoms—sleep disorder and dementia—are classic for CJD, but it can be extremely difficult to diagnose. Mad cow disease can start differently, with symptoms like anxiety, depression, and disorientation. But remember, depression is extremely common and mad cow disease is extremely rare. Don't make yourself crazy about this.

Q: My seventeen-year-old son has had multiple warts on his feet and big toe, which were surgically removed. Now he's getting them on his hands, and he got one on his lip. Is this related to stress or hormones? And will they ever stop spreading?

A: A wart is a virus in the HPV (human papillomavirus) family, and eventually you develop immunity to the virus. That's why adults don't get as many warts. Kids have not developed their immunity yet, so they develop warts everywhere.

If you treat them very early, they come back often, because the body has not developed immunity to them. Getting rid of the virus, of course, is a tall order. I mean, just lasering it or scraping it or putting on a solution won't get rid of the virus, which is lying beneath the skin. So doctors have found that if you wait a little bit, the body builds up immunity. And then you treat them, and you have a much higher rate of cure.

In your son's case, it sounds like he has a bunch, and they're spreading. I think you should let the doctor keep after them with whatever treatment he prefers. No one treatment has a huge advantage except for mild chemotherapy, where the chemo is injected right under the wart. It seems to kill off the virus and the multiplying cells, which is what you want to do.

A lot of doctors use lasers and swear by them. Some use powerful solutions to chemically remove warts. Some doctors still freeze them off. No matter what you do, it seems, you get a similar rate of success. None of these solutions is foolproof. Warts are stubborn.

I'd go after the one on his lip, but I'd be careful. Make sure you deal with someone who knows what they're doing, because if you get scarring around the lip, you can get distortion, and I wouldn't want that to happen to him. Make sure his dermatologist is experienced.

See more about HPV on pages 79 and 419.

Q: For three days, I've had either the stomach flu or food poisoning. I'm nauseated, I have diarrhea, I'm weak, tired, and miserable. I don't have a fever, so I know I'm not dying, but this is not my idea of a bikini diet.

My husband and I ate the same exact meal at a restaurant, and he got sick, too, but not as sick as I did. Should I have gone to a doctor for antibiotics to stop the process when I first felt sick? Is there anything I can do for a quicker recovery?

A: Many people are shocked to hear this, but influenza does not cause stomach problems, and there is no such thing as the stomach flu. While viruses cause some stomach upsets, bacteria are often the cause.

The numbers for food-related illness in the United States are staggering. An estimated 76 million people have a food-borne sickness each year, with 325,000 hospitalizations and 5,000 deaths. And the cases are seldom as simple as just leaving the mayonnaise-laced egg salad in the sun for too long.

The Norwalk virus is a huge problem—that's what the cruise ship industry was dealing with just a couple of years ago, and it's the source of about 23 million stomach illnesses every year. The biggest bacteria troublemakers are campylobacter (from raw meats and poultry to milk and water), salmonella (eggs, meat, poultry, and more), and listeria (from unpasteurized milk and juices to cheeses and meats). And parasite-driven toxoplasmosis (from cats/cat litter to undercooked lamb, beef, and pork) is also a major concern.

Vomiting and some diarrhea usually indicate that a stomach problem is viral. Fever and bad diarrhea are stronger indicators of a bacterial infection, and for all other symptoms, take your pick on likely causes.

In general, the symptoms are short-lived, and people can treat themselves with over-the-counter drugs, though the vast majority of stomach bugs go away in a day or two without any medications. If needed, loperamide works so well on diarrhea that it's called "the cork."

Drink lots of fluids, too. A little salty broth is good, because dehydration, not the germ, is the real enemy of people with diarrhea. Dehydration from diarrhea kills thousands of children every year around the world.

Most doctors won't even test patients who come in with general gastritis, like diarrhea and vomiting, because finding the causative germ can be difficult, and by the time the lab results come back you've already recovered. Viruses are also difficult to identify. The body often does a better job of flushing food-borne illnesses on its own. Antibiotics are not recommended for most cases, because they can interfere with the process, and diarrhea is a main side effect of antibiotics.

However, antibiotics may be needed to treat severe symptoms. A patient whose symptoms last longer than a few days, or who has a fever or blood in the vomit or stool, should see a doctor immediately.

You should talk to your doctor, because it has now been three days out, and because he or she should be told about the restaurant. Of course, you don't know if other diners have been infected, but your doctor may have heard from other patients that week who ate in that same place. In that case, the public health department should know, and patients should be tested for bacteria.

Call the restaurant as well, because they may already know what caused the problem. If not, they should be told. A smart restaurateur knows that cooperation and honesty in these situations is the key to staying in business. Maybe the food supplier is to blame. The worst thing for the restaurant, and for the public, is to remain ignorant of the problem.

But, of course, you may have caught a virus from some unknown source, and the restaurant is not at fault. You can see how complicated this is.

Q: I've read that meningitis is being found at a high rate in college dorms, and some people are recommending vaccinations for college students. Is there a vaccination for meningitis?

A: Meningitis is not rampant. But when there is an outbreak, it usually

DID YOU KNOW?
CAN YOU SAY NO TO GUACAMOLE?

A trip to Mexico for a plate of tacos with a side of guacamole may not be as pleasant an adventure as you anticipated. A professor at the University of Texas Medical School, Houston, enlisted a bunch of colleagues to test assorted condiments from restaurants in Guadalajara, Mexico, and Houston, Texas, that serve Mexican food. The bacteria E. coli was found in 66 percent of the samples from Guadalajara restaurants and 40 percent of the Houston restaurants. But the levels of contamination were many hundreds of times higher in the Guadalajara restaurants *and* only the Guadalajara restaurants had the type of E. coli that causes diarrhea. In both cities, the guacamole was the most likely food to have dangerous levels of the E. coli. Tortillas, anyone?

occurs in places where people live close together, like college dorms and military barracks. Still, it is very uncommon.

Meningitis, which is the inflammation of the membranes covering the brain and spinal cord, is a broad label that is often misunderstood because it covers a slew of possibilities. Because viruses, bacteria, parasites and chemicals can all be causes of meningitis, we can vaccinate against some forms of it and not against others. Go ahead and get vaccinated.

Some types of meningitis are very dangerous, even fatal, and other types are not. Right now, I could find the germ that causes a very nasty form of it in many of people's noses and sinuses. It's there, but it doesn't bother you.

Then, for some unknown reason, once in a while, it will invade someone and kill them. That's what people remember—not how rarely that happens.

Q: I was a lousy student of science in college, but now I wish I had paid attention. Can you explain what a virus actually is and how is it that a new one can surface so quickly, like SARS did? And how is a virus different from bacteria, like anthrax?

A: The main difference between viruses and bacteria is, first, viruses have no sex life. Bacteria and viruses are both invisible, but bacteria are much, much larger, and they go along merrily dividing and exchanging DNA. Almost everyone has had to deal with bacteria at one time or another—they are at the root of everything, from staph and strep infections to gonorrhea, and you normally have ten times more bacterial cells in your body than your body's "regular" cells.

Viruses are intriguing, amazing organisms. What a virus will do, because it cannot reproduce by itself, is penetrate one of your cells, rewire the central DNA mechanism, and convert what might have been a perfectly healthy liver cell into a virus-factory cell. Once invaded, all that cell will do is manufacture copies of the original virus. In turn, those viruses then go and invade other cells and turn them into viral cells. This is how viruses multiply; they turn cells in your body into assembly lines to reproduce the virus.

We are now experimenting with introducing special viruses into the body to fix genetic cell abnormalities.

With most viruses, your immune system handles it perfectly well by attacking and killing them. But some viruses can mutate; in other words, their genetics are such that they produce viruses that your immune system does not recognize, or is just not as effective at fighting. So, even a simple flu virus that most of us can handle can mutate into something like the killer virus of 1918, which killed more than 20 million people around the world.

Infections in some organs can be viral or bacterial. A bacterial infection in the eye produces thick pus, whereas a virus produces a clear fluid. Pneumonia and ear infections also can come from either source.

Sinus infections, though, can start as viral and then turn into bacterial. Boils and abscesses are both. But colds and flus are viral. Some viral infections develop into secondary bacterial infections. Don't forget fungi, parasites, and those weird prions.

Now, about that pop quiz . . .

Q: I was turned down for insurance. The rejection letter says that I do not qualify because I have an "elevated cytomegalovirus." What is that?

A: I'm surprised they'd turn you down for that. Cytomegalovirus (CMV) is similar to the virus that causes mononucleosis. Around 80 percent of us have CMV without knowing it, because its symptoms are mild or nonexistent. In other words, most people who get this don't have symptoms or health problems.

The Edell Report

How Gross!

It's a nasty subject, but one we need to talk about: vomit.

Scientists looking at assorted outbreaks of illness have found that when viruses are the cause of a person's vomiting, that virus can spread far and wide every time that person throws up.

The drops of vomit can be "aerosolized" after they hit a hard surface, and a person can be infected with that virus simply by breathing in one of those drops of vomit. This seems to be particularly likely with Norwalk and Norwalk-like viruses.

Probably the most fascinating study of this phenomena involved an English restaurant where an unfortunate patron vomited at her table. Eventually dozens of other people became ill, and though the restaurant kitchen was suspected at first, it became clear it wasn't at fault.

Further research showed that the vomiting customer had brought the virus into the restaurant with her. And when table assignments were examined, it became clear that those tables located closest to the woman had the highest number of reported illnesses once the virus's symptoms started appearing about three days later.

So, if you think you are going to be sick, do everyone a favor and get to the bathroom in time.

However, newborns and people with compromised immunity caused by AIDS, chemotherapy, or other circumstances can be devastated by CMV. Also, one published study found that people with the highest levels of CMV antibodies were at greater risk for heart problems. Maybe that's what the insurance companies are worried about.

An insurance carrier who rejects you for a condition that 80 percent of us have tells you something about that company.

Yes, nowadays, carriers are being extremely conservative. They are denying coverage for reasons that I find unjustified. I think you're getting ripped off. I'd challenge them.

Q: I work with animals as my profession, and I've never given much thought to the germs I might be exposed to. Then, just yesterday, someone asked me if I ever worried about catching something. Should I worry? No one in our office seems to be constantly ill.

A: With the exception of rare and obvious diseases, like cat scratch fever and rabies, most of the time we wouldn't know if pets were transmitting infectious diseases to people. Doctors test very few viral infections, so the sources of many infectious illnesses are often unknown. There is no doubt that animals can pass their germs to humans. This is called "zoonosis"—the collection of all diseases that can be spread this way. From scabies in cats to rabies in dogs, it's worth being aware of—but no one should give away a pet because of this.

You make a good point, though, that by sheer volume of slurp opportunities, you and your coworkers are evidence that dog and cat licks are mostly harmless.

It's a good bet that the healthier the animal the less the chance of catching anything, so pet owners should be vigilant about vet checkups.

One disease, toxocara, which comes from a worm in dog feces, can be passed along to kids from backyard dirt that has been the dog's bathroom. The symptoms can be pretty unpleasant, although fortunately most cases don't cause serious problems. And pregnant women need to be aware of toxoplasmosis, a parasite that can be found in a cat's litter box.

Cats and dogs aren't the only pets capable of transmitting disease. Birds, turtles, and iguanas are among the creatures that are potential carriers of germs that can infect humans. Even prairie dogs can be a problem; remember the Monkeypox scare in 2003? So your best bet is to buy your pets from reputable vendors and make sure they are examined by your veterinarian.

Q: My ten-year-old granddaughter broke her right leg and her left ankle, so she has casts on both legs. Her mother wants to bathe her with this waterless, antibacterial gel. I heard you say that this gel is dangerous.

A: The use of all these antibacterials as a substitute for soap is a) unnecessary, because soap and water are up to the job, and b) likely to create resistant organisms. We have evidence that this is happening already. If germs start to resist antiseptics, we are in deep trouble.

So, the danger is not the immediate harm to an individual, but that we are

The Edell Report

Stop Washing Away the Bacteria

You may not know this, but most soap you buy contains antibacterial agents, such as triclosan, that can actually contribute to the spread of super germs.

What happens is that most people use a low level of the soaps, and this gives certain bacteria the ability to survive, build resistance to the triclosan or other agents, such as triclocarban, and flourish.

Researchers at Beth Israel Deaconness Medical Center in Boston analyzed data on national and regional hand-soap brands and found that about a fourth of all bar soaps contain antibacterial agents.

With liquid soaps, this figure zoomed to 75 percent for both national and regional brands, according to a report presented at a meeting of the Infectious Diseases Society of America.

This trend toward antibacterial soaps is a worrisome thing, because we don't really need such powerful germ fighters for washing our hands. It's the actual hand-washing that removes bacteria, and there's no evidence that antibacterial soaps can prevent infections in the household.

I'd suggest reading the labels on soaps and avoiding the antibacterial products, because germs can develop multidrug resistance from widespread use of these cleaners. A bar of plain soap is all you really need, and it's a lot cheaper than the fancy stuff.

As for those dirty bars of soap we've all come across in a public rest room at one time or another: Use them. They may have a few germs on them, but not nearly as many as you'll have on your hands if you don't wash them.

weakening our ability to combat disease-generating organisms in our environment.

Your granddaughter's situation is one in which using waterless cleaners makes good sense. Bathing a person who is wearing casts is a challenge. You have to avoid getting a cast wet, because water between the cast and the skin, or seeping into the cast, can cause chaffing and mold.

I would defer to her orthopedist's opinion, but I think using the gel is OK.

Q: My nine-year-old daughter has very smelly feet. What causes this?

A: Most people don't know that the soles of our feet have more sweat glands than any other part of our body. Smelly feet are the by-product of bacteria feeding happily on the food supply provided by the dark, damp world of a shod foot. The damp is moisture that comes from either freshly washed feet or sweaty feet. The bacteria are not fussy.

The germs that cause foot odor are very similar to the germs used to make Limburger cheese, which is why Limburger cheese smells like stinky feet, and stinky feet smell like Limburger cheese.

Odor also can be a sign of disease, but that's not very likely. The simple way to get to the bottom of this is to dab rubbing alcohol on her feet. The smell will disappear if germs are the source of it, because alcohol will kill the germs.

The solution, then, will be to keep her feet scrupulously dry. That means she should wear shoes that allow her feet to breathe.

Resource List

The Centers for Disease Control and Prevention has detailed information on everything from Rocky Mountain spotted fever to the West Nile virus. At the home page, just click on Health Topics A–Z: *www.cdc.gov*

For information on current AIDS clinical trials, go to the AIDS Research Alliance of America: *www.aidsresearch.org*

Find the latest news on HIV/AIDS in English and Spanish at the American Foundation for AIDS Research Web site: *www.amfar.org*

Before you head overseas, get the latest information on outbreaks and diseases at the Centers for Disease Control Travelers' Health Web pages: *www.cdc.gov/travel*

Find your local chapter of the National Multiple Sclerosis Society at *www.nationalmssociety.org*

Subscribe to the quarterly *Hepatitis Alert* from the Hepatitis Foundation International. The donation is $20 or whatever you can afford: *www.hepfi.org*

The Hepatitis B Foundation provides online information in English, Chinese, Korean, and Vietnamese: *www.hepb.org*

For information in English and Spanish on all hepatitis viruses, see the Centers for Disease Control Web site: *www.cdc.gov/ncidod/diseases/hepatitis/*

Extensive information on psoriasis and psoriatic arthritis can be found at the National Psoriasis Foundation: *www.psoriasis.org*

For comprehensive information about Crohn's disease and ulcerative colitis, go to the Crohn's and Colitis Foundation of America Web site: *www.ccfa.org*

For the latest information on all aspects of meningitis, go to the Meningitis Foundation of America: *www.musa.org*

For an update on lupus research as well as facts about this autoimmune disease, go to the Lupus Foundation of America: *www.lupus.org*

The National Institute of Allergies and Infectious Diseases covers a vast array of topics; just click on "information" and search by subject: *www.niaid.nih.gov*

For information on Lyme disease as well as links to a variety of Lyme disease material, go to the American Lyme Disease Foundation: *www.aldf.com*

The American Autoimmune Related Diseases Association has information on more than fifty illnesses: *www.aarda.org*

For related questions see chapters 2 and 11.

Chapter 10

Strange Lumps and Second Opinions

I can hear the fear in the voice. Someone has just been diagnosed with cancer, is in the process of being tested for possible cancer, or has a mother or brother or girlfriend—somebody very close to them—who has been told they have inoperable cancer and they are calling my show for advice. Always, there's disbelief. "She's so healthy," "He's so young," "How could this be?" Despite all we know and all the progress that has been made fighting this disease, "cancer" remains the most intimidating word in medicine.

I'm not going to try and sell you on the idea that cancer is a happy subject, or one to take lightly, but it's not always as bad as we assume it will be. Our outsized fear of it can be very unhealthy in itself, especially when it keeps us from taking advantage of everything available in the way of screening tests or, on the flip side, fills us with paranoia to the point that we rush to the doctor every time we cough or get a sore throat. I hate the scare tactics some doctors are employing to sell their expensive, full-body MRIs, leading you to believe they will find every little cancer cell in your body. Is the next step having a full-body scan every six months, just to be safe? That's ludicrous—but I have no doubt that cancer is scary enough for some folks that they would do that.

As far as we can tell, cancer has been with us since the dawn of time. It has afflicted all cultures in all periods of our history. All animals get cancer.

You may have seen a book on the best-seller lists telling you sharks don't get cancer and, therefore, you should eat shark cartilage to cure cancer. Don't believe it. Sharks do get cancer—and always have. It's just a book title.

Different groups of humans do seem to have different prevalences of cancer, though. For instance, in Asia, stomach and liver cancers are the most common. Colon, lung, and breast cancer are most likely to afflict Americans. And each cancer has its own set of statistics that define its virulence. Gallbladder and pancreatic cancers are probably the worst in terms of your likelihood of death, but that may be simply because they are more difficult to detect early, and by the time you detect them, they are more advanced.

Some cancers grow more slowly, even though they are true cancers and metastasize to remote parts of the body. Prostate cancer may be the most confounding of cancers. It grows so slowly that many doctors feel we shouldn't even screen for it, and not treat it when we find it. Skin cancers, other than malignant melanoma, stay in place and don't metastasize. Consequently they don't usually kill people, but they can deform you and must be treated.

The causes of cancer are myriad. But the two main factors are genetics and environment. Scrotum cancer in chimney sweeps was the first cancer for which a cause was discovered. Dr. Percivall Pott, a surgeon in London in the late 1700s, linked the cancer to soot and, from there, of course, we've learned about many environmental insults—from radiation to smoking—capable of causing cancer. But it's so much more complicated than that.

Basically, most cells in your body know what their job is and stay in their place. A liver cell is a liver cell, with many and multiple functions. When cancer happens, the genetic machinery of the cell is upset, and it begins to multiply wildly and randomly. Under a microscope, instead of seeing orderly and regular liver cells lined up like bricks in a wall, you see a swirling disarray of cells, and every cell looks different from the next—very different from how they looked before cancer developed.

This difference is what thwarts us in many of our treatments. Cancer cells can differ from one another in the same tumor, so when we try to treat them, each responds differently. In any given tumor, some cancer cells are easily killed with chemotherapy, but others are tougher. A tumor may shrink because so many cells have been wiped out, but the resistant surviving cells can live on to regrow the cancer.

While our fight against many cancers has been very successful—

leukemia is one example—with others, like lung and pancreatic cancer, the progress is slow. We are not going to wake up to a headline in the newspaper next week announcing that cancer has been cured. It's a slow and painstaking battle. One reason is that it's not one disease but more than two hundred different diseases. There are no quick fixes.

Some experts believe we will never eliminate cancer, and it's certainly doubtful that we will in this century. You should also understand that though cancer seems to be more common these days, we need to allow for the fact that we are living longer lives, and the older we get, the more likely we are to face some disease, including cancer.

The newest theories tell us that the price of suppressing cancer in our bodies is the overall deterioration of our bodies—what we call aging. We now know that there is a protein in our cells, called p53, that vigorously suppresses the cell growth that can lead to cancer. But that cell growth is how the body renews itself, and stopping that renewal process leads to the obvious—aging. The thinking is that aging is a side effect of the natural safeguards we have that protect us from cancer. In experiments, animals with too much p53 don't get cancer, but they do age prematurely. Kind of ironic, huh? But no one I know would trade their wrinkles, stiff joints, and gray hair for a case of cancer.

I personally feel that something similar is going on with hormones. When you are young, your body is bathed with hormones with no consequence. The hormones keep you young. As you age, your body becomes more sensitive to these hormones, and cells start turning into cancer, which is why hormones in an older person, while conferring some of the benefits of youth, increase cell growth, which ultimately leads to cancer. The high levels of testosterone that occur naturally in a young man cause no harm—but in older men it can cause prostate cancer.

This isn't meant to depress you, because we *are* making progress, slowly. The most recent global figures showed that at least one third of the ten million cancer cases now diagnosed worldwide each year are preventable, and another one third are curable. And there is a lot you can do to improve your odds. Most important, of course, is giving up those habits that can cause cancer—especially smoking and unprotected exposure to the sun—and maintaining a balanced diet for both children and adults.

Also, most people grossly overestimate their risk of cancer. For instance, a common cancer in women is breast cancer. The average lifetime risk for the U.S. female population at birth is 12 percent, or approximately one in eight. But, remember, that's *from birth*. The longer a woman lives without breast cancer the lower her ultimate risk is for the remainder of her life. A fifty-year-old woman has a 10 percent chance of having breast cancer, while a seventy-year-old woman has only a 7 percent chance.

In addition, many women are living scared, because they feel like so many of their friends are battling breast cancer or have died from it that it must be out of control. They usually don't know that the No. 1 cause of death for women, by a large margin, is heart disease.

Which brings me to just two of the many paradoxes of cancer: A higher exposure to sun decreases the risk of breast cancer but, of course, it increases your risk for skin cancer—melanoma. And alcohol is thought to increase the risk of breast cancer—but decrease the risk of heart disease. So, adopting any "extreme" measure to protect yourself—no sun, no alcohol—is not an approach I recommend, or which will keep you cancer-free. It's just not that simple. There's one exception, of course: No one has proven that anything about cigarettes is beneficial. They are killers, pure and simple.

Beyond the obvious relationship between tobacco and lung cancer, what is obvious is that, for many cancers, there is no one "strategy" for avoiding them. Overall, though, avoiding obesity and eating a diet lower in fat seems to be positive for lowering the risk of most cancers that we know of.

Early diagnosis is an important but complex issue. Colon cancer is one of the most high-profile—and there is no doubt that early diagnosis really helps. No one should skip a stool-blood-sample test or avoid a colonoscopy, because catching this cancer early greatly reduces mortality. Pap smears pay great dividends, and no one in this country should die of cervical cancer.

But we are very confused about both prostate cancer and now breast cancer. With prostate cancer, one of the big questions is quality of life versus need to treat. Some doctors are now advocating no treatment, because it is such a slow-growing cancer and treatments can be physically devastating. The good news is that in the United States, there is a survival rate of more than 80 percent for this disease.

As for breast cancer, despite many years of research, the once-accepted value of early detection has been thrown into question, with some studies showing that breast self-examination and mammography do not always reduce your chances of dying from breast cancer. One reason may be that when you get breast cancer, it's the cell type and its virulence that are more important than how early you detect the tumor. This is pretty scary stuff, especially since "early detection" has been etched into our consciousness over the past thirty years. But it's better that we know this than not know this.

For all cancers, the game is to stop it before it spreads or metastasizes. When cancer moves beyond its original site, your risk increases greatly, but it's still not hopeless, by any means. Unfortunately, we don't know exactly why some cancers metastasize early and some don't, which is another reason to be aware of warning signals and act on them promptly. There is nothing more painful than listening to a caller who has observed warning signs for months, but has yet to see a doctor.

Cancer confusion even extends to doctors and when they should tell you about your diagnosis. In Japan, for instance, only one in five cancer patients are given their diagnosis. In Spain, only one-third of the physicians tell their patients. In the United States, we prefer to address the topic right away, but we have found that sometimes the truth hastens a person's death. One survey in the United States says that 80 percent of the elderly want to be informed of a cancer diagnosis, but there are a significant number of us who don't want to know. Discuss this with your doctor ahead of time, especially if you would rather not know.

Perhaps the most upsetting of all cancer issues is that many people have not yet gotten the message that most cancers are curable—if treated early in the game. There is nothing more upsetting than to see someone with an easily curable cancer pursuing some wacky underground treatment—often at great expense. By the time they figure out they've been had, the cancer has often progressed to the point where even Western medicine won't help.

I don't blame anyone who seeks out alternatives when they are told they're incurable. That's human nature. But, think carefully when you or someone close to you is first diagnosed with cancer. This is the time to apply logic and basic statistics; you want the best chance of a cure and survival. Make sure anyone offering a treatment can give you real numbers. Don't believe anyone who says they cure all their patients; common sense tells you that isn't possible. Ask them for documentation and data; any reputable health-care provider should be able to do that. And, please, don't believe anyone who claims they are persecuted by the medical profession because doctors are afraid that this "cure" means they will lose business. That's a preposterous and offensive argument made by unethical folks seeking to take advantage of people at their weakest moments.

Remember that most of you will not get cancer. Yes, we have very high rates in North America: 1.5 percent of our population ages fifteen and older have been diagnosed with one of twenty-five different cancers within the past five years. The lowest rates in the world occur in Latin America and the Caribbean, where .4 percent is diagnosed with cancer. The reason, though, is simple: Higher incomes reflect longer life expectancies, and longer life expectancies mean more cancer.

Our society has become obsessed with what "causes" cancer, and I think that is unhealthy. Yes, it is stupid to smoke, and, yes, it is stupid to spend eight hours a day in the sun without protection. But we can't live in a vacuum, and it's absurd to live day to day trying to avoid everything that *might* hurt you.

As of 2002, the United States has 228 substances that are officially "known" or "reasonably anticipated" to cause cancer and, of course, they're worth avoiding. But I find it difficult to ignore one piece of information that supports the concept of the "naturalness" of cancer. Scandinavian researchers feel that natural radiation from the cosmos—and just rocks and minerals on Earth—is the most important cause of thyroid cancer in children. This natural radiation is what causes random mutations in our genes and is the prime force behind evolution and the mutations that drive evolution. Consequently, that radiation, though there is the cancer factor, is extremely positive and important to all mortals.

This seems to reinforce a constant message that we have trouble dealing with in health—that there are risks and benefits to everything. Nothing is purely a risk without a benefit, and no benefits are purely benefits without risks. People who are best able to balance that concept in their day-to-day lives are the healthiest, in my book. And remember, life itself is ultimately a terminal disease.

Colon Cancer: Don't Fear the Test

Q: I'm sixty years old and I have lost two uncles, one grandparent, and five good friends to colon cancer.

I asked my HMO doctor for a colonoscopy, and his response was to offer a barium enema instead. He said if that doesn't show anything suspicious, I'm probably OK. The research I've been doing says otherwise. Do you think a barium enema is good enough?

A: For diagnosing colorectal cancer, there is no comparison between a colonoscopy and a barium enema. A colonoscope looks right at the inside of the colon, but it's an expensive way to test asymptomatic adults.

Your health plan wants to do the easier, cheaper procedure. A barium enema can pick up colon cancer and polyps, which are precursors to the cancer, but only after the lesions have reached a certain size. A colonoscopy can find smaller polyps, and, with colon cancer, the sooner, the better. Polyps are growths, usually benign, in mucous membranes. If a patient has a polyp, it is cut out and sliced open to check for cancer. This is done at the same time as a colonoscopy. If a barium enema produces suspicious results, a colonoscopy will be done, and a biopsy is likely, too.

Cancer cells can also grow flat against the wall of the colon and will only be found with a colonoscopy.

With your family history, you may be at increased risk for colon cancer, and I agree that you are a candidate for a colonoscopy. It turns out that just one test after age fifty may be all that most people need. If the first test does not show any polyps, a person is unlikely to get colon cancer.

If I were you, I would get pushy and work the system. You can go in and say you've seen blood in your stool or you've had cramps.

Gastroenterologists have told me about people who save up their pennies to pay cash for their colonoscopies themselves. They say they are paying for peace of mind. Peace of mind can't be measured in a test tube or in dollars.

Doing the homework you've done gives you an advantage in pushing for the tests you need. HMOs have been successfully sued for skipping tests and treatments in the game of cost-effectiveness versus human lives, so they are sensitive to the issue. Good luck.

Q: I am a thirty-four-year-old woman, and I've just been diagnosed with colon cancer because I had a sigmoidoscopy. I feel pretty lucky, because my primary-care doctor attributed the blood in my stool to hemorrhoids, and no one in my family has had colon cancer. But there is a history of polyps, so I demanded to be tested. What I want to know is, what questions would you ask before the surgery?

A: You are a very lucky young woman. Knowing your age and symptoms, I, too, would have assumed that hemorrhoids were causing your bleeding, because that's the case 90 percent of the time. But you were right to mention the polyps, because most colon cancers begin as polyps. Some medical questionnaires only ask about a cancer history, but anyone who has a family history of polyps should inform their doctor.

Your situation is one that makes a doctor's job tough, because it isn't really cut-and-dried. Blood in the stool is always a reason to get checked, but colon cancer in your age group is rare.

Doing a sigmoidoscopy is easier, quicker, and cheaper than doing a colonoscopy, and much of the time the sigmoidoscopy is enough, because many colon cancers occur within that first couple of feet of the intestine that the sigmoidoscope probes. However, according to the *New England Journal of Medicine*, one study looking at the efficacy of occult blood testing, sigmoidoscopy, and colonoscopy found that the blood test and sigmoidoscopy both failed to detect advanced colon cancer in 24 percent of the subjects. And you are particularly lucky, because polyps can be lurking way down toward the other end of the colon, closer to the appendix, and only a colonoscope examines the entire colon.

DID YOU KNOW?
THE NO-CANCER ZONE

Do you know where on your body there has never been a cancer reported? The lens of the eye and the inner structure of the cornea of the eye have been cancer-free throughout the history of medicine. What sets them apart from the rest of the body? Well, for starters, there's no blood supply in these areas, which might make you think that cancer comes in the blood. That's a viable theory and it's partially true. When a cancer-causing toxin gets into your body, it's delivered to your cells by the blood supply.

But what also sets the lens and cornea apart are their very slow growth. In fact, they barely grow at all, and therefore may be less susceptible to cancer. These are the kinds of hints, of course, that we hope some day to capitalize on to develop effective therapies and preventive strategies for all cancers.

So, a sigmoidoscopy saves money, but medicine must confront the truth that some people pay with their lives for the cost cutting.

As for what questions to ask about surgery, it really depends on your case. Only after a doctor has opened you up and looked at the colon will he or she know the important stuff, like how likely it is that the cancer has spread, and how many inches or feet of the colon will need to be removed. The basic questions would involve recovery time, diet, daily activities, and what to expect postoperatively.

After the surgery, your doctor also may recommend that you start taking aspirin daily. Ask him or her about two recent studies involving aspirin and baby aspirin. In both studies, polyp recurrence was reduced somewhat for those on an aspirin regimen. We are hopeful that aspirin will prevent their occurrence altogether, though that's not proven yet.

Q: A couple of days ago I had a routine sigmoidoscopy. I had problems with both the procedure and the doctor.

The forms I signed said I'd feel mild discomfort. Well, the doctor didn't give me any kind of medication, and the sigmoidoscopy was positively the most painful experience I've ever had. At the beginning of the test, the doctor ignored me when I asked him to back off a little bit, because it hurt. I actually reached my hand around and started to push him away. His assistant told me not to do that. However, once the scope was all the way inside, and I was able to relax, I was absolutely comfortable. Is this a typical experience? What would you have done?

A: First, you never want to push the doctor away. You don't want him to lose his aim.

However, you're not alone in being troubled by this procedure, although your case goes beyond the standard squeamish reaction that people have. You should have been adequately premedicated to make you as comfortable as possible. It's bad medicine to let a patient be in pain.

The sigmoidoscopy tube goes in just a short way—about two feet—taking advantage of the fact that most colon cancers are going to be found within 60 centimeters of the anus.

The colon does not have the same pain receptors as our external parts, but stretching it does hurt. When the tube goes in, air is used to inflate the colon so all the surfaces and little hidden pockets can be seen, which is in your best interests. However, the air can stretch the colon quite quickly, and that hurts. Once it's actually blown up, it relaxes, and that's why you got more comfortable.

Some people do have heightened sensitivity to cramping and stretching of the colon—they may feel more pain than others do for the same degree of stretching. Yet doctors tend to lump everyone together: "Wow, the last guy I had in here didn't make a peep, so what's wrong with this one?"

From what you've told me, you weren't premedicated just right, and such behavior can hurt the cause. You're certainly not going to want to go back for another sigmoidoscopy, and the millions of people who listened to you on the radio are scared now. Well, a sigmoidoscopy can be a lifesaver, and a doctor has an ethical obligation to listen to his patients and to make the procedure as comfortable as possible.

Even with the gentlest care, this procedure is not something you can sell tickets to, but if it's done right, most people don't have trouble with it.

Q: I am thirty-one years old. Am I too young for a colonoscopy? During routine physical exams in their early fifties, both my father and his sister were diagnosed with colon cancer and were successfully treated.

A: Unless you have symptoms, most gastroenterologists would consider you too young for a colonoscopy, but you should, of course, get your own doctor's advice. Of course, as an earlier question proves, people in their thirties can get colon cancer, and your overall risk is elevated because of your father's and aunt's cases.

Blood in the stool is a symptom of colon cancer, and I recommend that you do an annual test for that. Some folks make a big deal out of the stool-smear tests that you do at home—the test looks for microscopic amounts of blood that you can't see. If you find this test distasteful, you can substitute a test you can buy at the drugstore where all you have to do is toss a testing strip in the toilet and check its color.

You can also be tested for the gene for colon cancer, although that won't give you a definite answer, because it does not automatically follow that you will get cancer if you have the gene. You will know, though, that your risk is higher.

If it will give you peace of mind, you may want to go ahead and have a colonoscopy anyway. It will do no harm, although there is a very slight risk of perforating the colon. Plus, it is expensive, and because you are so young, your insurance company will fight paying for it.

Prostate Cancer: We Need to Know More

Q: I have just been diagnosed with prostate cancer, and I'm torn about my next step, either surgery or radiation. Neither one sounds all that great, but I know I need to do something. I'm fifty-eight and in good health. My doctor is recommending surgery, but I'd like your opinion. I know you've talked about this in the past, but I never paid attention, because I didn't think it would happen to me. What should I be thinking about?

A: You are right, I've talked about this a lot, because I feel like this is one disease that isn't getting the research attention it deserves. And it's pretty staggering when you go to a Web site like the one for the National Prostate Cancer Coalition and they have information on decision-making software and a cancer calculator. That's intimidating, but it tells you just how complicated this cancer can be to treat and understand. In general, the big questions are what the quality of life will be after treatment ends and whether to treat at all because it's such a slow-growing cancer. At your age, though, I think most doctors would treat you.

Two of the most frequently used treatments are a radical prostatectomy, which is where the doctor takes it all out and you're likely to wind up impotent and incontinent, or brachytherapy, radiation treatment involving the implantation of radioactive seeds, which, so far, seems just as effective but not as invasive. However, one study showed that when comparisons were made between prostatectomy patients and brachytherapy patients, the latter reported more limitations and lower quality of life, because of side effects like inflammation of the colon and rectal areas.

Prostatectomy patients did have higher incidences of urinary incontinence and erectile dysfunction compared to those who had radiation therapy, of whom, say, 6 to 7 percent reported urinary incontinence and 55 percent reported erectile dysfunction. Of those who had a prostatectomy, 80 to 90 percent reported erectile dysfunction. Bowel problems were reported in 30 to 35 percent of the radiation patients versus 6 to 7 percent of the prostatectomy patients. At the end of the study, the researchers stated that they could not recommend one treatment over another.

Since your doctor is recommending a radical prostatectomy, you want to find a surgeon who has done a lot of these operations. A study from the University of California, Los Angeles, examined the relationship between complications and the experience of the surgeon. If your surgeon has done more than forty such operations a year, your risk of complications is about half that of other patients.

Also, ask your doctor about treatments that combine surgery and radiation, as well as nerve-sparing surgery where doctors try to preserve the erectile nerves. We also are optimistic about newer therapies, like high-intensity ultrasound, radiofrequency tumor destruction, and cryosurgery (freezing the prostate), but it's too soon to know about long-term results.

Q: I am fifty-four years old and I have a PSA (prostate specific antigen) test every six months. It leveled out around eleven for about a year and a half, then it jumped up over the last five months. I've had two biopsies—they took about seven samples each time—and they both were negative. An ultrasound didn't show anything either. The urologist said certain people have a high PSA. Is there something else that would affect my PSA? And what would be your next step?

DID YOU KNOW?
YOU CAN DO IT: PROSTATE SELF-EXAM

It's easy for a man to feel his own prostate gland. It's a walnut-sized organ at the base of the bladder. It can be felt with the tip of a finger inserted into the rectum. Its texture and firmness should be similar to that of the flesh between your thumb and the rest of the hand when you make a tight fist. If you feel anything that is as firm as the knuckle, then that needs to be brought to a physician's attention.

How you reach the prostate, of course, is up to you. Some men may do the exam in the shower, where soap can be used as a lubricant. This can be a little tricky, because you need to get the palm surface of your finger in contact with the prostate, although the fingernail surface can be used for a cursory examination. You may feel more comfortable if you wear a thin latex glove. Or you may say, "Let the doctor do it."

A: The PSA test is making doctors and patients crazy. For those who've yet to face prostate problems, PSA is a protein produced by the prostate gland, and elevated levels of it can be an indicator of prostate cancer, but several other things can affect the reading, too.

We once thought it varied with something as simple as sex and exercise. If you take a PSA after a man has ejaculated or run a marathon, you may get a slightly higher number. Another warning: A recent study in the *Journal of the American Medical Association* found that one-third of men with elevated PSAs had a normal reading if the test was repeated four to six weeks later. So, in general, it's a good idea to repeat the test before agreeing to any further treatment, because there's a one-in-three chance you will be spared a biopsy.

What can cause a man's PSA to be higher is an inflamed prostate. Inflammation and an elevated PSA could be caused by trauma to the prostate. The trauma caused by cycling may be enough to alter the PSA (see more about this in chapter 1). We also know that just having an exam can cause a PSA to rise.

In your case, the primary thing we know is that if you do have prostate cancer, it's very small, because seven needles going through your prostate are missing it.

Second, even if cancer is found in the next round of tests, not all doctors would agree on what to do about it. I think it's difficult for us to accept the "do nothing" approach. Yet we're conducting studies to see whether doing nothing is better than some standard treatments or if there are surgical procedures that may not create the mayhem that many guys experience with both radiation therapy and radical prostatectomies.

So, for now, you obviously don't have an aggressive, rapidly growing tumor, and I'm not sure there's anything you should or could change about your lifestyle. While it's disturbing when the PSA suddenly goes up, the evidence is unclear about what to do next.

The bottom line is that a 2003 Harvard study found that the PSA test misses most cancers. For instance, men under 60 with biopsy-proven prostate cancer had normal PSA levels 82 percent of the time. For older men, the test missed tumors 62 percent of the time.

One solution being considered is to lower the level at which a PSA is considered abnormal. While that might pick up more cancers, it will surely lead to more unnecessary biopsies. Like I said, this is a mess.

Q: My husband had radical surgery for prostate cancer. I've been trying to do what I can to help, including lots of research, and I'm wondering if home-cooking rich in tomatoes, selenium, and vitamin E could help. What do you think?

A: These seem to play a role in preventing prostate cancer, but the big question is: If a substance can prevent cancer, is the substance also beneficial when you already have cancer? We don't know the answer.

I don't see any harm in enhancing his diet with these foods, but because we have found that certain vitamins may make cancer grow faster, you certainly don't want to overdo it. Cancer is a voracious cell—it likes to eat. You don't want to provide it with a nutritious meal.

Studies were done to discover the effects of vitamin C, vitamin A, and beta-carotene on prostate cancer. Well, vitamin E popped up as more effective than any of them. The others turned out to be worthless.

The news about the ability of lycopene in tomatoes to do battle with prostate cancer has been very exciting (see next question). And selenium is an important micronutrient, except that the health-food people want to sell you way too much of it. I'd be very careful about pushing it.

Breast cancer and prostate cancer have similarities. A recent study on breast cancer found that lowering fat in the diet did not help, but consuming more fish and chicken, and not eating red meat, did lower the death rate.

So, if your husband is a heavy beef eater, I'd cut back on that and increase fresh fruits and vegetables.

Your husband is fortunate to have such a supportive wife. For a better understanding of all the issues related to dealing with cancer, you might want to read *The Human Side of Cancer*, by Jimmie C. Holland, MD, and Sheldon Lewis.

QUIZ

Twenty years ago, the survival rate for prostate cancer was 67 percent. Based on the most recent statistics, the survival rate is:

A) 77 percent   B) 83 percent   C) 89 percent

D) 96 percent

(D: 96 percent for all stages; the five-year survival rate is almost 100 percent for men diagnosed in the local and regional stages.)

Q: Most health journals advocate antioxidants to prevent cancer. Now I've been hearing that antioxidants might actually help the cancer grow faster. My husband has prostate cancer, so he's been taking lycopene. Are antioxidants a good or bad choice?

A: Nature supplies us with the correct balance of antioxidants in foods. The body has thousands of antioxidant systems at work, so I've got to question what possible effect one more antioxidant, in the form of an expensive pill, will have. Antioxidants neutralize free radicals—the toxic forms of oxygen that come from the body's normal metabolism.

Evidence shows that antioxidants and lycopene in a diet rich in tomatoes, carrots, and a wide variety of other fruits and vegetables have cancer-preventing potential. But we don't know what the impact might be for patients who already have cancer.

And, yes, you heard right. I'm glad the word is getting around that some antioxidant vitamin supplements may have the absolutely undesirable effect of helping cancer grow. For instance, beta-carotene may turn into a free radical in some people's bodies and increase rates of lung and colon cancer in certain situations.

Of course, we'd all love to have a pill that wipes out disease. I don't blame anybody for giving their all to fight cancer. That means gaining knowledge about what the studies say we should and shouldn't do for men with prostate cancer.

Fortunately, because prostate cancer is usually very slow-growing, we have a measure of control over its growth. Statistics back me up in feeling very positive about your husband's prognosis.

Breast Cancer: Men and Women Need to Be Watchful

Q: My wife is forty-two years old and has just been diagnosed with breast cancer, specifically ductal cancer in situ. Thank goodness I had heard about a sterotactic biopsy on your show. That's how it was found; the needle biopsy had missed it.

We have seen two different doctors, and one recommends a mastectomy, but the other, a radiologist, sketched out a different plan for a lumpectomy and radiation. You've helped us once, can you help again? What should we be considering?

A: Well, I'm always thrilled when my advice produces such immediate results, and I think I can help again.

Although DCIS is a noninvasive cancer that has not spread outside of milk ducts in the breast, the *Journal of Clinical Oncology* reported in a study that women younger than forty-five whose DCIS was treated with lumpectomies and radiation had a much higher recurrence of cancer than did older women. Younger women have denser ducts, so the supposition is that the cancer has more opportunity to spread.

I have personal knowledge of a physician with DCIS who chose a mastectomy over the breast-conserving surgery. She had a type of breast reconstruction called TRAM and feels very secure with her decision.

A transverse rectus abdominus muscle (or TRAM) flap is costly, state-of-the-art reconstructive surgery. Most insurance companies don't offer it. The surgeon reconstructs the breast using muscle, fat tissue, and the blood supply from the woman's own abdomen.

I advise you to do research and get several opinions on a treatment plan. I'm happy to tell you that regardless of what you do, the success rate is going to be high. DCIS is a tiny cancer usually caught in the early stages, and it has a very good recovery rate.

The sterotactic biopsy is a good example of how medicine has been impacted by computer technology and eliminated the need for an incision at this step in the diagnostic process. A special biopsy needle that is linked to a computer is inserted right into the suspicious area with a high degree of accuracy.

Q: I had breast cancer, and my oldest daughters, who are thirty-two and thirty-seven, have been diagnosed with it, too. I have two more daughters, and I'm worried about them. My daughters who have cancer are both marathon runners, they eat lots of soy and have always been very careful about what they eat. Is there anything my other two daughters should be doing to avoid this scary legacy?

A: I am sorry you have to watch your children go through this, but everything we are learning seems to confirm that most cancer can be influenced by both environment and genes. Many cancers seem to be strongly influenced by environment—smoking and diet, for example. But in the hormonally related cancers, like breast and prostate cancer, genetics seem to be a much more powerful factor than lifestyle.

All of your daughters need the best genetic counseling they can find (see the Resource List on page 485 for more information). A genetic expert can look at the entire family history and give you specific odds. Also, testing for breast cancer genes is warranted. And if you want a good book on this subject, look at *Assess Your True Risk of Breast Cancer* by Dr. Patricia Kelly, a medical geneticist.

Too much soy may not be a good thing, though this topic still needs more research. The isoflavones in soy are a weak form of estrogen that mimics naturally occurring estrogen. They have complicated effects and can, in some instances, fight breast cancer and, at other times, stimulate the growth of cancer cells. On the flip side, women in Asian countries—where soy is a dominant element of diets—have a much lower risk of breast cancer than American women. But soy may have nothing to do with Asian women's lower rate. You can see how this is confusing.

The Edell Report
Don't Blame Yourself!

There is one aspect of our response to cancer that makes me crazy: We want to assume that it's our fault, that somehow we could have prevented it. Yes, for some cancers personal habits play a role; smoking is probably the best example. But for the vast majority of cancers, we have done nothing to cause them.

In one study of four hundred breast cancer survivors who have been disease-free for an average of nine years, 42 percent cited stress as one of the main causes of their breast cancer. You might think that's good, but let's read on. Only 27 percent of women felt genetics was involved, 26 percent attributed it to environmental factors, 24 percent blamed hormones, and 16 percent said it was diet.

Sixty percent of the women felt a positive attitude helped them to keep the breast cancer from returning, followed by 50 percent of those who believed that diet kept them cancer-free. Other factors that these

Soy supplements are especially suspect, because they contain an inflated amount of isoflavones, so avoid those.

It might be best for your daughters to avoid grilled meat and limit their alcohol consumption as well. Though the hypothesis about grilled meats increasing the risk of cancer is still being debated, combining that potential risk with your family's genes is not a chance I would take. The same goes for alcohol. A recent study by researchers at the University of California at San Francisco found that women who had at least two drinks a day were diagnosed with breast cancer at twice the rate of women who drank less. And with three drinks a day, the numbers soared.

The other standard risk factors to be considered by your daughters include keeping their weight down, having children earlier rather than later, breast-feeding those children, and exercising regularly.

---

women believed prevented the cancer from returning were a healthy lifestyle, 40 percent; exercise, 40 percent; prayer, 26 percent; stress reduction, 11 percent; alternative medicine, 11 percent; luck, 4 percent; and tamoxifen, at the bottom of the list, was 4 percent!

In fact, there is no real evidence that your personality, stress, or emotions have anything to do with cancer. But you will hear otherwise from some doctors.

According to a report in Psycho-Oncology, *the lead clinician on this study said that these beliefs did give these women a sense of control over the disease. The researcher said that these attitudes can be helpful in getting women to switch to healthier diets, etc., but also pointed out that these beliefs can backfire by giving women a feeling of personal failure if the disease returns, despite all they did to stop it.*

Well, we've got to stop this thinking! Breast cancer is not your fault, and you didn't cause it by having unhealthy thoughts and feelings. And anyone who thinks stress plays a bigger role than genes and other known lifestyle factors needs to chill out.

Most important, though, is constant vigilance. And be prepared for some doctors to suggest prophylactic mastectomies, if they haven't already.

Q: Both my mother and sister died from breast cancer a few years ago. I have been getting mammograms for the last thirty years. Should I get a sonogram or one of those new breast scans, too? I have a PPO health plan that I consider comprehensive, but none of my doctors has mentioned a sonogram. Should I insist on it?

A: Research is showing that a sonogram, when combined with a mammogram, improves the accuracy of breast cancer diagnosis. It is most effective in premenopausal women, whose breasts are more dense and fibrous, which is a bit of a hindrance to the penetration of X rays in a mammogram.

I want to be clear that mammograms alone are the best overall tool we have, and sonograms should never substitute for them. A sonogram is especially beneficial in telling whether a growth is a hollow cyst or a solid tumor. Solid tumors are more likely to be cancerous than cysts.

Of course, an additional test costs more money, and it's not routine, so even a PPO (Preferred Provider Organization) may balk at approving it. But, considering your family history, I think it would be foolish of them to not pay for such a test. What I don't know is if there is a recommended age for having both tests.

Finally, recent studies indicate breast MRIs may catch tumors that are missed by mammograms and sonograms, but they have a higher number of false positive readings, where there is no cancer but you need additional tests including a biopsy before you know for sure. So MRIs should not be used for primary screening. See what your doctor thinks about having one done.

Be careful when you hear advertisements for newer "scans" and thermograms. While these may formally take their place in the diagnostic armamentarium one day, so far there is no proof they are better than what we have.

Q: I saw a doctor yesterday to have a small lump checked out. It's about the size of a pea. The doctor says it's very unlikely that I have anything to worry about, especially since I'm only thirty, and she did not recommend a mammogram. She wants me to come back in six weeks. In the meantime, she wants me to give up caffeine to see if the lump will go away. I'm highly skeptical that coffee has anything to do with it. Do you know of any relationship between caffeine and the formation of breast lumps?

A: In my opinion, there is no relationship between caffeine and breast lumps. Yet many physicians may think otherwise.

Breast lumps are very common, and so is coffee drinking. That fact, along with a small study many years ago by an Ohio surgeon who did think there was a link, has created a lot of confusion about caffeine and breast lumps.

Based on a biochemical justification of how methyl xanthines—caffeine's chemical classification—could result in breast lumps, larger studies were undertaken. To my knowledge, no connection was substantiated, but the retraction hasn't sunk in.

The lump you have may or may not go away on its own, but I don't buy into the idea that your life hinges on quitting coffee. I have known doctors to make these kinds of suggestions to a patient just to get her involved in her own care.

I do want to compliment your doctor for trusting her clinical judgment and going against the tide by not recommending a mammogram. In the current environment, most doctors order a mammogram and a biopsy for any lump to protect themselves legally. Presumably, your doctor is making her call based on her examination of the lump and on your medical history and youthful age rather than on a formula.

I don't blame you for not wanting to give up your coffee, so you might want to go back to the doctor, mention you've done some research on the Internet, and ask her how strongly she feels your problem is due to caffeine. There is controversy here, and maybe you can have your cappuccino and drink it, too.

Q: I am planning to get breast implants, because I'm barely an A-cup. Do breast implants make mammograms hard to read? Could I be taking a risk of letting a tumor go undetected?

A: I know you'll like this answer. Not only is there no risk, but the barely-an-A-cup woman will actually get a better mammogram with implants. The process for a mammogram is to squeeze breast tissue between two mechanical plates. Well, the implant pushes the breast tissue way forward, which makes it easier to get enough tissue from a small-breasted woman between the plates.

It is true that X rays can't penetrate the saline, but mammographers know this and take extra care to position the breast properly to get the picture they need. Just make sure they know that you have an implant. Breast implants of the future won't block X rays, resolving this altogether.

By the way, women with breast implants seem to have a lower incidence of cancer. This doesn't imply that breast implants *prevent* breast cancer, but they certainly don't *cause* it, which remains one of the war cries of the anti–breast implant crowd.

See more on breast implants on page 333 in chapter 7.

Q: I am forty-two years old. A little over six months ago, I had a light, rust-colored discharge from one breast. The discharge is still happening, but it is now yellowish. I had a mammogram and a smear, and both came back normal. I have seen three doctors and received three different recommendations, from a repeat mammogram to duct removal to, finally, a ductogram.

My question to the last doctor was "What would you do if this were you?" And she said, "I would not have my duct removed. I am not seriously concerned by the color and consistency of this discharge." She wants me to see a surgeon for a ductogram.

A: I agree with that recommendation. It's one way to find out what's going on. The ductogram is done by injecting a little bit of dye into the ducts in your breast and then taking an X ray. It's similar to swallowing barium to get a view of the intestines. If you have any growths, they will show up. Then you will know what you're dealing with.

One other option—the newest way to go after this—is ductal lavage, where the doctor puts a tiny tube into the nipple and flushes out cells, which he then examines under a microscope.

Breast discharge is not uncommon. The colors range from clear to milky to rusty. We're happiest with clear or milky. Rusty concerns me, because it's a sign of blood, which can mean papillomas, which are benign tumors. But it can also mean cancer.

Since the discharge was rusty at some point, you are right to pursue the tests necessary for a diagnosis. When you get a clear mammogram but have a symptom like this, you don't want to just say, "OK, I pass, I'm healthy." A tumor can be very, very small. It can hide, and it can be missed.

Q: I am a thirty-two-year-old man with a lump in my left breast. I went to the doctor to have it checked out, and he sent me for a mammogram; I was the only guy there. Then I went to a specialist and he recommended having it cut out. Needless to say, I'm not crazy about doing this. Would they normally remove something like this in a guy?

A: Sitting in a mammogram center is not any guy's definition of fun—even if you're providing emotional support to your wife. But, of course, mammograms are nothing to be embarrassed about.

Breast cancer happens in men, and breast cancer in men is worse than in women because of our disbelief that this is happening to us. So we put off seeing the doctor.

Well, men do get breast cancer! If the mammogram shows, say, a cystic structure or some extra fatty tissue or something typical, they would probably not recommend removing it. The fact that they do means that your clock is ticking, and you shouldn't fool around. The odds are it will be OK and will not be breast cancer. But it happens enough in men that I have no doubt exactly what you should do. Get it out now.

Q: I am a man who was diagnosed with breast cancer about a year ago. My first symptom was that my left nipple was inverted—it was pulling in. That began to increase, and then it became very painful. One night, it hurt so badly that it woke me up. That's when I went to my doctor, who sent me on to a surgeon.

The surgeon didn't think I had breast cancer, but he tested me anyway and found out that I did, and the tumor was removed. Why was there so much doubt about the possibility of cancer?

A: The "pulling in" that you describe can be a symptom of breast cancer in either a man or a woman. This pulling also can affect the skin. It's called *peau d'orange*—"orange peel"—and it should be taken seriously, as should a lump in either gender.

Nonetheless, I would expect that some doctors would not give your symptoms a complete assessment, because you are a man. Fortunately, your doctor had a top-notch response that may have saved your life.

Breast pain is more likely to be something other than breast cancer, but, as your case illustrates, that's not always true.

Q: The results of my recent mammogram were inconclusive, so I have an appointment in three weeks for another one. I'm freaked out and don't know what to think.

The advice nurse said that the mark on the X ray could be a cyst or fatty tissue. What's the difference between a cyst and a tumor?

A: A cyst is a hollow growth in body tissue. They are sometimes filled with air, fluid, or pus. A cyst is rarely cancerous, but a cyst can cause a tumor. A tumor has both benign and malignant forms, and it's a growth, a bump, or a lump. A pimple is a tumor.

The vast majority of mammograms are normal, and doing a second one is routine if something unidentifiable shows up in the first sweep. Fatty tissue and fibrocystic tissue can make a reading unclear.

If your doctor saw something highly suspicious, he or she would have had you back immediately for a needle biopsy. A sonogram should easily distinguish a cyst from a solid tumor.

Q: I'm about to begin chemotherapy for breast cancer, and my doctor is going to have me come every two weeks, because of new research that found that more frequent sessions will increase my chances for survival. I looked up the study on the Internet and it sounds significant. Do you agree?

A: First, anyone who heard about this study needs to know that each cancer has its own chemotherapy timing, so what works for breast cancer may not work for lung cancer.

As for breast cancer treatment, it's hard to argue with this study, which involved two thousand women at a major research facility in New York. If your doctor thinks it is right for you, I wouldn't argue with that decision.

The general thinking about this treatment timing is that the tumor cells have less time to return before the next infusion of drugs. In the past, the three-week waiting period between sessions was designed to let the body—and the white blood cells—recover from the treatment. This new plan also is much more expensive, because it includes another drug—Neupogen—which stimulates white-blood-cell growth.

The study found that cancer recurrence after four years was 18 percent in women who had the every-two-weeks treatment versus 25 percent for women who had the conventional treatment. And the rate of death in the first three years dropped from 10 percent to 8 percent.

I hope it works for you.

Gynecological Cancers: Be Informed

Q: A forty-year-old woman I work with was recently diagnosed with ovarian cancer, and the prognosis is not great. She seemed perfectly fine

right up until she got the news. Now all the other women in the office are scared, especially since we don't know much about this disease. What are the key signs?

A: I can understand the sense of panic in the office, because one of the reasons ovarian cancer can be such a bad cancer is that there aren't any discernible symptoms early on. And there is no early test for it, but a gynecological exam can find it.

Every year some 23,000 women develop it, and because it is not easy to recognize, most women do not receive a diagnosis until the cancer has advanced. Approximately 14,000 women in the United States die from it each year.

In one study, researchers at Memorial Sloan-Kettering Cancer Center in New York asked 186 women with ovarian cancer and 251 healthy women how often they experienced bloating, abdominal pain, nausea, lack of energy, and lower back pain.

Of course, both healthy women and women with ovarian cancer can have these symptoms, but they were more common in women with ovarian cancer. Researchers noted that women with ovarian cancer experienced these symptoms almost constantly, while healthy women experienced them intermittently.

As for the back pain, this fits into something that I feel very strongly about: If you have back pain, don't go to a chiropractor first. And don't go to an acupuncturist, either. Go to a physician and get an internal exam, because an internal exam is about the only way a doctor will be able to tell if you have ovarian cancer—by feeling your ovaries. There is also a blood test that some doctors advocate, but, in my book, it's not consistent enough to be a definitive step.

Q: My mother died from Paget's disease. Is this the same as cancer of the vulva? Is there anything I can do to protect myself?

A: Paget's is one of the more confusing names in medicine, because it can relate to diseases of the bone, breast, or vulva—all of them different.

In the breast, it is a rare form of breast cancer that starts around the nipple. It looks like a scaly, eczema-like, raw irritation, and, unfortunately, it is often ignored.

In the vulva, Paget's is almost always found in postmenopausal women, and it is also rare. It usually appears as a red or pink velvety area dotted with white spots of tissue. It can be oozing or scaly—it doesn't always appear exactly the same way. It is usually treated with surgery, and its cause is unknown. It can be aggressive.

The Edell Report
When the Husband Flees

I think most of us would like to believe that serious illness brings out the best in couples, but the fact is, love and commitment in America don't always survive a diagnosis of cancer.

A study of married patients with malignant brain cancer contained staggering findings. Married women with malignant brain tumors are eight times more likely to undergo a divorce than married men with malignant brain tumors.

In other disease categories, it's the same. Women with multiple sclerosis are seven times more likely to be separated or divorced than male patients. And the rates of women diagnosed with systemic cancer who experience a divorce is twelve times higher. But statistics for brain tumor patients may be the saddest. From diagnosis to death, the patients in this study lived an average of thirteen months, and many of their marriages ended within that time frame.

There are exceptions, however. We once thought that husbands commonly deserted wives who had breast cancer, but, in fact, it's the opposite. Even eight years after diagnosis, the illness seemed to strengthen marriages. It seems that women can be empowered by a diagnosis of breast cancer—there are great support systems for women with breast cancer, more so than for most other cancers.

However, according to a report in the Journal of the National Cancer Institute, *many men are not equipped to be caregivers to spouses with higher-maintenance illnesses, such as brain cancer, where dementia may eventually become a factor. Husbands of terminally ill patients also are at a higher risk of depression. Why? Because they have much less social support for caregiving when the diagnosis is catastrophic.*

As a society, we don't instill men with the capacity to provide the kind of care that they should provide. We need to fix that—for everyone's sake.

Cancer of the vulva accounts for three to seven percent of all malignancies in women, and it can be deadly. Yet many women never know what hit them, because it is often overlooked.

I think women should check their genitalia monthly, just as they do with their breasts. Don't be afraid, it won't bite you. Armed with a mirror, and in a well-lighted space, look at the skin around the vagina, particularly the labia. Common symptoms can be as minimal as a rash, or include a lump or a mass. If you notice any abnormalities, don't put off seeing your doctor.

The rate of vulvar cancer is increasing, and we are very frightened about this. It may have something to do with the human papillomavirus (HPV); we're not quite sure (see more about HPV on page 79 in chapter 2 and pages 419 and 435 in chapter 9.).

Postmenopausal women are at greatest risk, but I encourage all women to keep on the lookout.

Lung Cancer: A Big Killer

Q: My brother has lung cancer. The doctors said they can't operate, because he waited too long and the cancer is in the lymph nodes. He already went through all the radiation and chemotherapy. Why are the lymph nodes so important? I feel like they are giving up.

A: We operate to remove cancerous tumors before the cancer cells have spread beyond the organ itself. In other words, if a woman has uterine cancer, we can take out her uterus. But if the cancer has spread into her intestines, then the surgery won't get it all.

Many cancers spread to the lymph nodes first. The lymph nodes have to do with the circulatory system, which is a pathway that cancer cells can take as they spread. Once cancer is traveling through the lymph nodes, removing the lung may not improve chances of survival.

At that point, bombarding the entire body with anticancer treatments, like chemotherapy or radiation, is all that can be done.

Unfortunately, we have a low success rate in curing lung cancer at this stage, because we often don't catch it before it has spread to the lymph nodes.

Q: I have a sixteen-year-old niece who is in permanent remission from leukemia—she had it eight years ago—and I am scared because I caught

DID YOU KNOW?
THE SMOKING GUNS

How many reasons do you need not to smoke? Well, try these:

First, more Americans die each year from lung cancer than from breast, prostate, and colorectal cancers combined. An estimated 154,900 Americans died in 2002 from lung cancer, accounting for 28 percent of all cancer deaths.

Second, if the lung cancer doesn't get you, then watch out for stomach cancer. A large U.S. study, reported in the *International Journal of Cancer* in 2002, found that both men and women have a much higher risk of dying from this cancer if they smoke or use any other tobacco product.

If serious cancer doesn't impress you, how about impotence and wrinkles? Nicotine constricts blood vessels all over your body, including the pelvic area. And if you're already at the wrinkled stage and you're considering a facelift, forget about it. Plastic surgeons won't do facelifts on smokers.

Smokers overall have more surgical complications, including post-operative infections, and facelifts require a very robust blood supply to the facial skin. Smoking impairs that circulation, which can compromise the vitality of the tissues after the lift. Translation: There's the potential for patches of gangrene on the face.

---

her smoking. Since she had leukemia, does smoking put her in greater danger? You can imagine how angry I was when I saw her, because I remember her in the hospital, totally medicated. I said, "How can you do this to your body?" I am an ex-smoker, and I'm wondering what else I can say that might resonate.

A: I hate to fan any fear needlessly, but your instincts are right on the money. Even though we consider surviving more than five years to be "in the clear," her illness can return. That's why she should still go for regular check-ups. Leukemia survivors also have higher rates of certain other cancers later in life. By no means is it common, but they are in a higher risk group than the general population.

With all we know about smoking, we don't know exactly what about it causes cancer. I'm not aware of any association between smoking and leukemia, but, of course, she shouldn't smoke.

Giving kids tools to resist peer pressure has been shown to be the most successful way to keep them from starting and for helping them quit. The least successful approach is to talk to them about their health—even when they've had a life-threatening illness. They all believe they can quit at any time, and that, of course, is the delusion that gets everyone who has ever smoked in trouble.

Use your experience to approach her about smoking, and listen to what she says. Ask her why she's smoking and what got her started. Although most kids won't respond to health horror stories, you might mention that she's exposing herself to an increased risk of breast cancer, too. A Canadian study found that girls who begin smoking as teenagers were 70 percent more likely to get breast cancer than nonsmokers.

If that doesn't catch her attention, appealing to her vanity might work. Most girls don't like to hear that smoking can encourage premature wrinkles and gives them horrible breath. Most guys, on the other hand, could care less about such matters. She is probably addicted at this point, so getting her help to quit is reasonable.

Good luck.

QUIZ

Which state has the highest rates of lung cancer, for both men and women?
A) Kentucky   B) New York   C) Texas   D) West Virginia
E) North Carolina
(A: Kentucky; approximately 121 men and 57 women per every 100,000 residents, according to the latest statistics from North American Association of Central Cancer Registries.)

Q: There's such a big to-do about smoking and cancer, but people smoke marijuana and call that medicinal. I was told that the heat from the smoke causes cancer among tobacco smokers. But then wouldn't smoking marijuana cause cancer, too?

A: You'd think we'd know by now exactly how smoking causes cancer, but we don't. Some of the theories focus on tars, polonium, and, as you mentioned, the burning process.

The tars in cigarette smoke do contain known carcinogenic chemicals, but those chemicals don't really accumulate where lung cancer occurs.

Polonium, which is radioactive, builds up in tobacco leaves as a result of fertilizers. In a chronic smoker, polonium accumulates in the bronchial tree, which is also a location for cancer. If the fertilizer causes cancer, maybe organically grown tobacco would make a safe cigarette.

Burning any vegetable matter produces known carcinogens, too. But marijuana, which is certainly vegetable matter, doesn't seem to cause lung cancer when it is burned, based on what we know so far. Pretty curious, huh?

Carcinogenic substances also are produced when we barbecue. And those substances are more abundant in marijuana and hashish smoke than in tobacco smoke.

However, a cigarette smoker often smokes twenty to thirty cigarettes a day; a marijuana smoker smokes one or two at the most. The quantity might be the difference between cancer and no cancer.

One of the main reasons we can't pinpoint what part of smoking causes cancer is that cigarette companies have a big secret. An incredible loophole in the law allows them not to disclose about five hundred of the ingredients in cigarettes. Maybe the burning of one of those ingredients causes lung cancer. But we can't test it, because we don't know what it is.

Coping with Radiation and Chemotherapy

Q: The radiation and chemotherapy that my friend had to treat her breast cancer seem to have been successful; all her tests are negative. Now, the problem is that she won't eat at all. This has gone on for several days. What are the ramifications?

A: Getting patients to eat is an ongoing challenge in oncology. First, there's the loss of appetite, because radiation and chemotherapy often make people feel sick—and when you are nauseous you aren't hungry. Then there's the fact that cancer itself actually secretes substances that suppress the appetite.

This is one of the reasons many people are in favor of medical marijuana, because marijuana increases appetite as well as suppresses nausea.

The body is well prepared to handle a lack of food for the short term. But as more time goes by for your friend, her body will first raid its own fat stores for energy, and then her muscles will begin to waste away as her body burns up protein. Obviously, this is very dangerous.

Make her doctor aware that your friend isn't eating, so the doctor can monitor her nutrition. She may be angry that you did this, but she'll get over it once she is healthy again.

Q: My wife is fifty-six years old. The aggressive chemotherapy and radiation that she had ten years ago to knock out her breast cancer also knocked out her allergies. But this spring, the allergies are back. We are thinking about moving away from Northern California. Do you know which areas of the country have the least pollens?

A: The reason your wife was allergy-free after chemotherapy may be because chemotherapy stops the immune system—among other things—and an overactive immune system is what makes one susceptible to allergies.

Before you do anything as drastic as moving, you need to find out what she is allergic to—which isn't very hard—and where it grows, which is trickier.

An allergist can tell what she's allergic to, and, based on that, you can begin looking for places to live. This is a good excuse for a spring vacation. After doing your research, visit a few of the safe zones and see how she does.

Also, your wife should keep her eyes open during the season for what's blooming and when, and her reactions to it. For example, acacia blooms very early in Northern California. If she starts sneezing as soon as those yellow flowers bloom, she'll have one allergen figured out.

Arizona used to be reputed as *the* destination for the allergy prone, because the desert doesn't naturally support a lot of plant life. However, residents have planted all kinds of things that aren't native to the area, so even there you've got to watch out.

We can be allergic to indoor allergens, too. It would be a shame to move across the country—unless you're itching to leave California anyway—only to find that it's house dust or pillows that make your wife sneeze. We now suspect that synthetic pillows may have more allergens than do feather pillows.

You have some detective work to do.

Q: Several weeks ago, my seventy-three-year-old mother was diagnosed with a malignant tumor on her sciatic nerve. The doctors started the surgery to remove it, but decided the tumor had engulfed too much of the nerve, so they left it in. Now they want to try radiation. I'm perplexed about why a knife is too risky and could damage the nerve, but radiation is not.

A: A malignant tumor can bind to the nerve and create scar tissue, making removal very difficult. You want to remove every speck of cancer, but with a scalpel there's the risk of cutting or nicking the nerve.

A surgeon faces the same problem in cutting away a tumor from a man's prostate. The challenge there is to preserve the nerves to retain potency and still get all the cancer.

The tremendous benefit of radiation is that while tumors are very sensitive to it because they are such rapidly growing cells, nerve tissue is very resistant to it. You can blast a lot of radiation at the brain and at nerve tissue without harm, but it can kill the tumor.

Sometimes doctors charge in like cowboys, without properly scanning the territory. There is a time for that type of aggression and a time to use another approach. In your mother's case, it seems to me they are doing the right thing.

Q: My sister-in-law had radiation with iodine therapy. The doctor told us to stay six feet away from her for two to five weeks. I am having all the relatives to my house for Thanksgiving dinner, and they are worried. Will my sister-in-law be a radioactive danger?

A: Her doctor is operating by the book. The guidelines say that no amount of radiation exposure is acceptable, but the practice is that people ignore this rule all the time, and no increased rates of cancer come from it.

Your sister-in-law took a much bigger and direct hit of radiation than anyone standing or sitting near her could experience, and she will not show an increased rate of cancer. Compared to her exposure, everyone near her gets only the tiniest amount. But we have guidelines about radiation, just like we do about outdated drugs, and the doctors must communicate them.

So, in my opinion, there is nothing to worry about in this situation. Give thanks for having the family together and pass the cranberry sauce.

Moles and Skin Cancer: Be Aware

Q: Some years back, I had a basal-cell skin cancer removed from my neck. I now have a mole on the inside of my arm that changed from tan to black to red. It has gradually returned to a normal tan mole color, but its shape is different. Do you think this is another basal-cell cancer?

A: No, but you should be clear on the difference between basal-cell cancer and malignant melanoma, which can occur in moles.

Basal-cell and squamous-cell skin cancers are not very dangerous, because they are relatively slow-growing, they can be removed, and they rarely metastasize. However, each year untreated squamous-cell skin cancer causes a few deaths by burrowing deep into the skull.

A change in the color or shape of a mole can also be a symptom of another type of skin cancer—malignant melanoma, which is a major killer. The process your mole has gone through makes me think you might have whacked it, and that caused it to bleed inside, which is what turned it black. But any change in a mole should be examined without delay.

Get yourself to a dermatologist—not a general practitioner—ASAP. Every month the dermatology journals have photos of malignant melanomas that look like ordinary moles; identification is not easy. I have been humbled so many times myself that I don't even try anymore. I just go to the doctor.

Many dermatologists don't take chances with any suspicious moles; they just remove them, along with the skin around them. That can be in your best interest, because you can't judge a mole that has changed by looks alone. It needs to be removed and examined by a pathologist. If you just whack the growth off, its roots can flourish underground, just like those of a tree stump. Malignancies of the skin can have roots, too, that can be cancerous, so, again, this is nothing to fool around with.

QUIZ

Where are you most likely to find the most risky moles?
A) arms   B) legs   C) back   D) neck   E) hands
(B: legs; and if you have more than twenty moles on the trunk of your body, make an appointment with a dermatologist to have them checked out.)

DEAN'S LIST: LOOK AT YOUR SKIN

Skin cancer is nothing to fool with. If you notice any of the following, get yourself to a dermatologist:
- a sore that won't heal
- a smooth bump indented in the middle
- a reddish patch that doesn't itch
- a shiny growth or scarlike spot

Q: Is it acceptable medical practice for a physician's assistant to perform cancer surgery? I recently had mole surgery to excise skin cancer on my face, and I was kept on the table until the pathology report came back. Finally, the doctor told me that only a few cancer cells were left on two margins, and then he left the room. The physician's assistant proceeded to finish the procedure and to suture the wound. At the time, I was so shocked I was speechless. Now I'm angry. Was this appropriate?

A: You and I have both experienced what is called Mohs surgery, a very specialized treatment that, in one operation, removes malignancies to a depth that is microscopically free of cancer. And, in my case, I was sent to a dermatologist who specializes in this.

With this type of cancer, the doctor has to be very careful about interpreting the margins of the growth and how much tissue should be removed. As the cells are excised, he or she is constantly assessing them for malignancy and going back for another little slice until all the cancer is gone.

So, I would say you have a legitimate beef, especially because your doctor wasn't even in the room and also because he just sprang it on you. If a doctor believes his assistant is qualified to do a procedure—and, in some states, physician's assistants are not legally allowed to perform surgery—the doctor should first say to the patient, "My assistant is perfectly able to do this, and, at a point in this operation, he'll be doing this simple step." Still, I don't feel it's the "simple step" phase when cancer is still being removed from the margins—stitching up the wound, maybe, but not the last of the actual Mohs surgery.

Tell your doctor about your concerns. At the very least, he should be preparing his patients if he's not going to do the surgery himself.

The Last Stages

Q: My father has bone cancer and is no longer on chemotherapy because it's no longer effective. The morphine and Percocet that he's taking for pain are leaving him without an appetite, because they make everything taste like diesel fuel. Is there something to take away this side effect of the pain medicine?

A: Marinol, the FDA-approved pill form of marijuana, might increase his appetite. Talk to his doctor about it. And there are alternative prescription medications to help his appetite if the idea of a marijuana pill scares him.

Once your father's appetite is stimulated, the awful taste might let up. A dry mouth can also cause a loss of appetite and strange taste sensations. This is a difficult time as it is, but you hate to watch someone get even weaker because they don't want to eat.

Q: My ninety-two-year-old mother-in-law has cancer in her gallbladder and liver, which was discovered when we took her to the doctor because of pains she was having. She had surgery, and she is now pain-free. We've been told to keep her comfortable at home and to keep her weight up. She has always eaten a lot of vegetables and fruit, but that's not keeping pounds on her. I actually think junk food would help, but the doctor says it has no nutritional value. She likes beer, too.

Now, we've been called to the hospital for two full days of tests. Is it going to help her? How much longer will she live? We have been very close for fifty years.

A: I cannot tell you exactly how much longer she has, but if the cancer originated in her gallbladder, you need to know that gallbladder cancer kills very quickly.

Physicians are poorly trained to deal with death. Death is the enemy. Cancer is the enemy. Our instincts are to fight a battle to the bitter end, and that isn't always in our patient's best interest.

One battle that may be worth fighting is to open her bile duct if the cancer is blocking it, as gallbladder cancer can sometimes do. A blocked duct will hasten demise. Opening the duct can make her more comfortable and give her more time. Since she was in pain and isn't any longer, maybe this was done in the surgery.

Ask the doctor about the condition of the bile ducts and about the necessity of the tests, because I know that you're concerned about the quality of her life for the time that she has left. Unless some helpful action can be taken based on the test results, I, too, question making her miserable by putting her through any more.

She's lived to age ninety-two, so I'm certainly not going to worry about what she eats. You should ask her for guidance. As far as I'm concerned, she can eat all the burgers and fast food she wants. And let her have some beer!

Appetite can be a serious problem. See the previous question.

You are on the right path. The idea is to make her as comfortable as possible during the remaining time she has with you. This time of passage can actually be a very positive experience. But keep a watchful eye against doctors jumping in and causing pain and disruption.

Miscellaneous: Scans, Lumps, and Second Opinions

Q: I have a friend who mentioned that he found a lump on his right testicle. It wasn't on the scrotum itself; it was on the testicle. He didn't get any more specific about the location because you know how it is: Guys don't talk about this much. I suggested that he go to a doctor immediately. I also told him that I have another friend who had testicular cancer, and he had one of his testicles removed, and later on he got an implant. My friend is twenty-nine, and I'm sixty, so I think he does listen to me about such things. Is there anything else I can do?

A: You did the right thing. Of course, he needs to see a physician. As you noted, men are terrible at this stuff. This conversation should have never happened. But you would feel terrible if you advised him to relax about it, and he wound up dying of testicular cancer.

This is the No. 1 cancer killer of men in this young age group. But sometimes men do get confused about what they are touching when they examine their testicles. There is a structure in the back of men's testicles called the epididymis, which normally feels like a lump, and most men who have not examined themselves carefully don't even know it's there. They discover their epididymis, and they go running to the doctor fearing cancer.

That could be what your friend has found, but he needs to see a doctor immediately to be sure. No man should die of testicular cancer. But they do die of it because, in general, guys don't like to go to doctors.

More important, men don't examine themselves. But they should, and if they can't do it themselves, they should get a partner or wife to do it. I think this can be a fun thing, for both sexes. A hospital near where I live used to advertise classes for breast self-exam where you could bring along your mate to learn how to do it together. Four hands are better than two, right? That's my homily for this chapter.

Q: During his shower a few days ago, my friend felt a growth under his arm. It's bigger than a golf ball, and, he says, it's tender. He's been losing some weight, too, but not very much. By coincidence he has a doctor's appointment ten days from now, and he plans to wait. I think he should go immediately. Do you agree?

A: Yes. With weight loss, even a little, and a mass under his arm, he should push to see a doctor. The doctor will want to take a biopsy, which is going to take some time, so he should get started.

What you're really asking is, could ten days make an overall difference? If he happens to have cancer—perhaps lymphoma—it only takes one little cell to escape from the main mass of malignancy, travel through the lymph system, and implant someplace, and that could later cost him his life. Statistically, the longer he waits, the more chance the cancer has to spread, so he should do something as soon as is reasonable.

Most of the time, a lump in the armpit turns out to be a swollen lymph node, but they are usually not as big as you are describing. If the growth is red and sore, it's not likely to be cancer. But it could be an infection, which should be treated right away, too.

QUIZ

In the 2002 government update of known or likely carcinogens, what was labeled "known" for the first time?
A) wood dust   B) steroidal estrogens
C) broad spectrum ultraviolet radiation   D) all of the above
(D: all of the above; the carcinogens list is updated every two years.)

Q: My husband's father is dying of esophageal cancer. He had lots of chronic indigestion in his life, and my thirty-seven-year-old husband has the same pattern. Should he have his esophagus checked preventively?

A: There certainly is precedent for chronic irritation leading to cancer.

Indigestion by itself is not a precise term—it's hard to know exactly what is meant by it. Most of the time, it's a heartburnlike syndrome, as acid gets up into the esophagus.

The vast majority of the billions of people with heartburn out there—like 99.9 percent—do NOT get esophageal or stomach cancers.

Esophageal cancer is slowly becoming less common. It's a generational thing that may be linked to foods or diet, and does not seem to have a strong genetic component. However, it would be prudent for your husband to mention it to the doctor, and the doctor can decide how to respond.

Usually, by the time we catch esophageal cancer, after it causes symptoms, it has often invaded adjacent structures, so you can see how it could be a pretty bad cancer. But a doctor can do screenings to look for it.

And if your husband has indigestion, he should have some diagnostic testing anyway, simply because of his symptoms. He needs to know the cause of it.

He may have reflux esophagitis, which should be treated. Treating that with acid-reducing drugs may spare him any slight increase in esophageal cancer risk that might result from the reflux, but we're not absolutely certain about that.

He will certainly feel better, and that's worth something.

Q: My two-year-old had a CT scan a couple of months ago. Then just last night I heard a story on the news about a relationship between CT scans and childhood cancer. I'm concerned. Also, is a CT scan the same as a CAT scan?

QUIZ

Your body has nine ounces of bone marrow. How many cells does that marrow make every second?

A) two hundred   B) two thousand   C) twenty thousand
D) two million
(D: two million cells.)

A: Yes, they are the same procedure. Maybe they quit saying "CAT scan" because people made too many jokes about cats and dogs.

A CT scan uses radiation to generate three-dimensional pictures as well as two-dimensional slices of the body. It's as if we put the body in a bread slicer. It is a fabulous technique that gives us information we just can't get any other way. It also involves more exposure to radiation than a simple chest X ray.

Children may be more susceptible to radiation than adults, because their cells are growing rapidly, and we think cancer develops more easily in these kinds of cells. Still, the risk of a two-year-old getting cancer is very, very small. Even if a CT scan doubled that risk, the odds are still minuscule.

The decision to give a child a CT scan is yet another example of the importance of weighing benefits and risks. Because of the risk, it should never be done lightly, but it has powerful abilities to diagnose a sick child. It can save a child's life.

Also, the radiation level can be cut back during a child's CT scan. Many facilities don't do this, and they should. A child should be getting the minimum effective dose.

Nothing is risk-free. We are all exposed to radiation from the cosmos, and even that is not 100 percent safe. We think that cosmic X rays may trigger gene mutations, some of them horrible, as well as some cancers.

Q: My thirty-nine-year-old daughter, a mother of two, has been diagnosed with lymphoma. It was found first in her neck, and her doctor referred her to the Stanford University Medical Center, where they found more in her abdomen. Is it possible that my daughter's diagnosis is a mistake? Should she get a third opinion?

A: Lymphoma is a cancer of the lymph cells, which are a type of white blood cell. Because it can sometimes be a tricky disease to diagnose, and the

---

QUIZ

Cancer can be caused by a virus. True or false?

(True: certain types of the human papillomavirus [HPV] can cause cervical cancer.)

rate of error is higher than with other cancers, I usually do advise people who have been diagnosed with lymphoma to get another opinion. However, the fact that something has been found in her abdomen lowers the chance of error.

Your daughter has been to one of the best medical institutions on the West Coast, so your best bet is to ask her doctors about the possibility of a mistake. The rate of error in pathology is pretty low—one study found an error rate of about 1.4 percent in evaluating biopsies—but, of course, if that occurred nationally, it could be thirty thousand misdiagnoses a year.

It's human nature not to want to believe bad news. But the best thing you can do now is to help your daughter with her day-to-day challenges of taking care of two kids while she wrestles with emotional and physical challenges of her life at the moment. Overall, lymphoma is a highly curable cancer.

Resource List

For general information about all types of cancer, as well as access to a comprehensive search engine that will find all clinical trials for a specific cancer within twenty or fifty miles of your zip code, go to the The National Cancer Institute Web site: *www.cancer.gov*

At the People Living with Cancer patient-information Web site of the American Society of Clinical Oncology, you'll find oncologist-approved information on more than fifty types of cancer: *www.peoplelivingwithcancer.org*

Assess your risk for about a dozen of the most common cancers at the Web site for the Harvard Center for Cancer Prevention: *www.yourcancer-risk.harvard.edu/*

The Women's Cancer Network provides the latest news reports on all cancers that affect women, and the Web site allows you to search by zip code for gynecological oncologists: *www.wcn.org*

For information on lung cancer in both English and Spanish, go to *www.lungcancer.org*

Cancer Care provides free professional help to people with all types of cancer through counseling, education, information, and referral, and direct financial assistance: *www.cancercare.org*

New York's Memorial Sloan-Kettering Cancer Center has specialized in cancer research and care for more than a hundred years: *www.mskcc.org*

Find the Cancer Survivors Network, medical updates, and more at the American Cancer Society Web site: *www.cancer.org*

The Leukemia & Lymphoma Society Web site offers support, research, and much more: *www.leukemia-lymphoma.org*

For a directory of genetic counselors around the United States, see the Web site for the National Society of Genetic Counselors: *www.nsgc.org/*

For information about free and low-cost mammograms and Pap smears, call 1-888-842-6355 or go to The National Breast and Cervical Cancer Early Detection Program at the Centers for Disease Control Web site: *www.cdc.gov/cancer/nbccedp/index.htm*

The National Breast Cancer Foundation has information in both English and Spanish on everything from breast cancer myths to research: *www.nationalbreastcancer.org*

Find a breast cancer support group anywhere in the United States at the National Alliance of Breast Cancer Organizations: *www.nabco.org*

For the latest information on prostate cancer, subscribe to *Aware*, a free twice-a-week electronic newsletter from the National Prostate Cancer Coalition. This organization's Web site also has lots of information on a variety of treatments: *www.4npcc.org*

The National Ovarian Cancer Coalition Web site is packed with information, including state-specific listings for additional informational in your region: *www.ovarian.org*

For information about clinical trials and the latest treatments, go to the Colon Cancer Alliance Web site: *www.ccalliance.org/*

For related questions see chapters 1, 2, 3, 4, 6, 7, 9, and 11.

Chapter 11

The Hard Facts on Booze, Grass, Paxil, and the Patch

My day cannot begin until I hear the friendly clunk of a mug hitting the coaster on my bedside table. Yep, it's coffee time, and I'm an addict. Thanks to my wife's early-morning efforts, I can keep my head on the pillow until I know the coffee has cooled to just the right temperature, ready for my first sip.

I love the warm feeling of the cup and all the physical ritual that surrounds this experience. After a few mugs' worth, when I've been at my desk for a few hours, it's time for my broadcast—and my last cup of the day. That one is mostly drunk with need and desperation; I wonder if I could even do my radio show without that cuppa joe.

Caffeine is the most widely used mood-altering drug in the world. It is, in its pure form, a white powder, and if it came on the market today, no doubt it would be considered illegal. But, in reality, as addictions go, it is pretty harmless.

That's not the case with most addictions, and one of the difficult issues facing American society today is how to deal with the abuse of both legal and illegal substances. We have drawn moral lines in the sand, and we are paying dearly for them.

We are spending an outrageous amount of money on our prisons, filling many of the cells with people who need treatment for alcohol and drug addiction. We watch college kids die because of binge drinking and driving under the influence. We regularly witness the downfall of Hollywood celebrities, sports figures, and politicians who have yet to come to terms with the fact that their habits could ruin them. And in too many corners of our society, addictive behavior is still viewed as personal failure, not serious disease.

So treatment programs are consistently underfunded or nonexistent, and only the wealthiest families have access to residential facilities where their sons and daughters and husbands and wives can face their demons. It would seem that everyone else is on a waiting list, in jail, or living on the streets.

I've worked in drug and alcohol rehabilitation centers, so I've seen just about every type of addiction, and I refuse to make medical assessments based on what's legal and what isn't. I think this has confused the issue and is preventing us from making any progress on such an important subject. The bottom line is: You're in trouble with any mood-altering chemical if it interferes with how you want to lead your life. If it is getting in the way of your social, professional, and familial relationships, then you have a problem—whether the substance is legal or not.

There's no doubt in any expert's mind that the most dangerous drug in our society—the one that causes most mayhem and death—is alcohol. The number of homicides, wife beatings, child assaults, and other violent acts committed under the influence of alcohol—and its impact on our emergency medical care and police and social services—is so huge that it is a wonder that it is legal.

Of course, most people use alcohol responsibly and, indeed, you would have to be living on another planet not to know that alcohol—in moderation—is good for your health.

But if it came on the market today, it, too, would probably be illegal or sold to you by pharmaceutical companies. And therein lies the catch: It's not the drug itself, but how people use it that causes all the problems that we associate with drug abuse.

Marijuana may be the best example of the contradictions that exist in our current laws. Research has confirmed that, like alcohol, it has medical benefits. It can help everything from chemotherapy side effects to migraine headaches, and it has not been linked to violent activity. In fact, everything we know indicates it is a pretty benign drug when used in moderation.

However, our society judges that it should be illegal, so people suffering from nausea after chemotherapy don't have access to it because being thrown in jail is not good for your health, either.

Even nicotine as a drug has medicinal qualities, and that's why it was originally used by the Native American population. People who smoke may have lower rates of Parkinson's disease and certain forms of colitis. Nicotine may actually even be good for your heart. However, there are way too many downsides to justify its casual use. Does that mean I think it should be illegal? Absolutely not.

Why humans pursue altered states of being is another matter. There is a well-known UCLA professor, Dr. Ronald Siegel, who has documented most animal species (from the mongoose to the water buffalo) experiencing the effects of "drugs" like opium poppies and loco weed. He considers this to be a "fourth drive," that the pursuit of altered consciousness is as human as our hunger, thirst, and sex drives.

Mental health and addiction are so closely intertwined that it's sometimes difficult to draw the line between them. When teenagers become alcoholics at a young age, they are often self-medicating depression. If your child needs therapy or an antidepressant, isn't that better than watching him get drunk every weekend and begin a lifestyle pattern that will be harder and harder to change?

Children and adults use drugs excessively, because they make them feel better. The issue that has to be addressed is: Why does ordinary, day-to-day life not feel as good as life when you are high?

I don't think that "just say no" was ever a good idea, and I'm not a fan of D.A.R.E., either. Drawing hard and fast boundaries only works on maps, and sometimes that's not even true. We need to talk sensibly to our children, we need to acknowledge the pleasures and the dangers of alcohol and marijuana. We also need to be familiar with the young-adult environment and understand the role of peer pressure when it comes to alcohol and drugs. We need to know whom they are spending time with, and we need to know where they are after school.

In many European countries, for instance, they teach children how to consume alcohol as part of the family ritual at mealtime—not as a tool to make fools of themselves in a bar or to bolster self-esteem. Drinking alcohol is seen as a family pleasure; that's not how we handle it here.

It's also interesting to note that most mood-altering chemicals, when left in their original states, don't seem to cause the problems that we have with them. Coca leaves have been chewed by natives in South America for thousands of years. But when extracted as a white powder, it can be a killer.

We've also entered the era of designer drugs, with chemists creating compounds that nature never created on its own. Ecstasy—no matter what the name might promise—is not a good thing. Yet I suspect that the typical twenty-two-year-old who takes this drug—or any of the other "club drugs"—doesn't begin to think about the unknowns.

There is no doubt that it is easier for some people to fall into the black hole of addiction than others. A family with a multi-generation history of alcoholism shouldn't ignore that fact. And yet we still don't know why some members of one family might be more likely to be addicts than others. Until we do, it's a matter of understanding the use/abuse curves and recognizing when you or a friend or family member is in trouble or on the cusp of danger.

While it is possible for some people to quit alcohol, nicotine, and other addictive drugs on their own, why do that to yourself—or expect someone you love to do that—when there are doctors, medications and support groups that can make the process more bearable? And keep in mind that success does not always come on the first try. In fact, the statistic for smokers is stunning: On average, people have six relapses before stopping for good.

The other aspect of drug abuse that never fails to confound and amaze me is the line that's drawn between prescription drugs and alcohol, cigarettes, and the illegal stuff.

Why is it that even the more dangerous and useless drugs—for instance, amphetamines—can be used by sleep-deprived fighter pilots, chubby bridge players, and chronic fatigue patients with the backing of the medical profession, yet outside those narrow models you'll go to jail for many years if caught with the drug?

And why is it that some people won't use the term "drug addict" when the drugs being abused are prescription medicine? An addict is an addict, whether the problem is gambling, or crack, or wine.

In terms of benefits and risks, some drugs stand out as particularly dangerous, and that's how I view cigarettes. Even though most smokers don't die of lung cancer, it still seems to be a drug where the odds are stacked against you. And don't forget other quality-of-life issues, from how you smell every day to the number of wrinkles on your face to loss of erectile function.

There are mysteries, too. You can give a smoker nicotine in the form of gum, patches, inhalers, and sprays, but that doesn't always seem to get smokers to want to quit. There's something to the hand habit. I understand that.

I grasp my coffee mug, feel its warmth, and wonder whether it would still feel as good if there were just hot water in that mug.

I'm lucky, because I know my addiction isn't killing me. The same might be said of gamblers, though research indicates that maybe one half of all compulsive gamblers have a substance-abuse problem, too. Unfortunately, most addictions are doing serious, irreversible damage to our bodies. And, along the way, we lose family and friends. Is there any bigger price to be paid?

Alcohol and Alcoholism

Q: My husband is an alcoholic, though he would never agree with that statement. He gets drunk at least three times each week, and he's been having bad abdominal cramps lately. I don't think he's been straight with his doctor about how much he drinks, and the doctor recently put him on Paxil—and that scares me. What can I do?

A: I have heard similar stories from spouses and children throughout my career. There is no simple answer for most of these difficult situations.

First of all, let's address the easy part of your question: Anyone with unexplained abdominal cramps should see a doctor. And this can be a very serious symptom for an alcoholic. The hemorrhaging of varicose veins around the esophagus is one possibility, a bleeding ulcer is another. Cramps coupled with other symptoms, like throwing up coffee ground—like material, are even more ominous.

Dragging a guy to a doctor can take an act of God to begin with, and dragging an alcoholic in denial is harder still. Then there is the problem you mentioned: Patients like your husband tend to underreport their drinking problems to their doctors, which can lead to the doctors writing prescriptions for drugs that are inappropriate for the person, because they don't mix well with alcohol.

There is only so much you can do. You love him, and you want to help him, but if he's his own worst enemy, it's difficult to stop him. If he has a close friend, you might consider asking that person to talk to your husband about getting help.

During medical training at teaching hospitals, which care for indigent populations, most doctors learn more than they want to know about the devastation of alcohol. It truly is our most dangerous drug. I've been at many surgeries performed on alcoholics and seen the bleeding hole in the stomach; seen the varicose veins in the esophagus that can cause an instantaneous and fatal hemorrhage; seen the swollen, bulging, sclerotic livers and abdominal cavities full of fluid.

Your husband needs to get help by calling his local chapter of Alcoholics Anonymous. If he objects, and you can afford it, ask him to consider in-patient treatment at a private facility. If he rejects both of those suggestions, I think you should call his doctor and tell him what you told me. It's possible the doctor will not want your input, but you need to try. If your husband finds out you called, he is sure to be angry, but it's better to have an angry husband than a dead one. And your husband's life could be on the line.

Take care of yourself, too. Al-Anon is a worldwide support group for families and friends of alcoholics. You'll find the Web site in the Resource List on page 527.

Q: I think I might be an alcoholic. After a night of partying, I shake a lot the next morning, and my voice is shaky, too. I've tried to stop drinking, but I feel awful when I don't drink. Yet I get to work every day and I don't drink during the day. Could I be sick with something else?

A: I was taught that if a patient asks you if he is an alcoholic, you can presume that he is. You describe the classic morning-after symptoms, so I have no doubt that you are an alcoholic. And you're not alone. Alcohol goes unrecognized as the most common drug-abuse problem in our society.

Start with Alcoholics Anonymous; they're the best. Meetings are free, they are everywhere—see the Resource List on page 527 for the Web site—and they have the most experience. No, AA isn't perfect—some folks object to the reli-

---

DID YOU KNOW?
WHAT'S AN EXCESSIVE DRINKER?

The National Center for Health Statistics defines excessive alcohol drinkers as those who consumed five drinks or more in a day at least twelve times in the past twelve months. Using that measure, almost 10 percent of the adults in the United States drink too much, and men far outnumber women in all age groups.

gious references—but it's the best place to begin. They know all about denial. They know how to help you, and they know where to send you if you need more help than AA can provide.

There is a simple self-evaluator for alcoholism, called "the CAGE test": C is for Cut Down, A is for Anger, G is for Guilt, and E is for Eye-opener. Each letter is associated with a question, and a "yes" to any of them indicates a drinking problem:

—Have you tried to Cut Down on your drinking?

—Do questions about your drinking make you Angry?

—Do you feel Guilty about your actions when you drink?

—Have you ever taken a drink as an "Eye-opener," that is, to calm you down or get you going in the morning?

You called because alcohol is affecting your body, and most likely, if I questioned you, we'd find that it's also affecting your work—even though you make it to the office every day. And your social life is being affected, even though you may not know that either.

In general, doctors do a terrible job of diagnosing alcoholism. Researchers have sent alcoholics to see doctors, and most of them do not get diagnosed.

You are one giant step ahead of many alcoholics, because you are willing to consider the possibility that you have a problem. The first step is to end the denial, and you sound like you're ready to do that.

Q: What's your opinion of Alcoholics Anonymous? I am very concerned about my wife's drinking habits, but I'm not sure what to do next. We are not a religious family, and I know that AA does get into that. Would she have any options, if she agrees she has a problem?

A: I think Alcoholics Anonymous is a wonderful program if it's a fit with the person who needs it (see previous question). Many people object to the religious and spiritual aspects of it, and I'm glad to see similar nonreligious groups arise, like Women for Sobriety, and the Secular Organization for Sobriety.

If you think your wife is an alcoholic, and she doesn't think so, you're in the same boat as a lot of other folks. Most alcoholics have a primary problem called denial. Getting them past that is critical. If your wife isn't in denial about this and is willing to get treatment, encourage her to look at her various options—you can learn a lot online these days.

If denial is a big factor, you may want to set aside the religious issues for the moment, since getting treatment for her is the highest priority. You could talk to AA representatives about coming to your house for a meeting with her. This isn't going to be easy, so hang in there. She has to believe that she is being controlled by alcohol before any group can begin to help her.

Q: My fourteen-year-old son was in the car with me, listening to you. He likes your suggestion that alcohol be introduced as a family thing. My husband and I have always shied away from giving alcohol to the kids, because their two grandfathers, two uncles, and two aunts are alcoholics. Is there something like an alcohol gene that could increase our kids' chances of becoming alcoholics if we expose them to it while they're still growing?

A: There is no single alcoholic gene, but we do believe that family history is a risk factor. We have more questions than answers, though, about the interplay of genetics and environment in fostering alcoholism.

Some studies have found that even before they've had their first drink, the children of alcoholics metabolize alcohol differently than do children from non-alcoholic families. Children of alcoholics are not as sensitive to alcohol. They can handle more without getting sick or drunk. It's possible that they drink more to get the buzz, and that hooks them.

One piece that doesn't fit the gene puzzle is that humans have consumed alcohol for too brief a time for an alcohol gene to evolve. And why do some people who do have a biological tendency toward alcoholism become responsible drinkers?

I think that what is inherited is a personality predisposition. Certain personalities, including risk takers, moody people, and anxious people, appear to be predisposed to mood-altering substances. And teenagers who are wrestling

QUIZ

Children under twenty-one consume what percentage of all alcohol consumed in the United States?

A) 7 percent   B) 16 percent   C) 25 percent   D) 31 percent

(C: 25 percent, according to The National Center on Addiction and Substance Abuse at Columbia University.)

DID YOU KNOW?
ALCOHOL AND PREGNANCY

For anyone with doubts about the effects of excessive drinking on a fetus, here's sobering proof. A study by researchers at the University of Washington spanned more than twenty years and looked at children born into more than four hundred families that were first surveyed back in the 1970s. At that time many mothers-to-be drank a lot more than they do today. The study found that the children of women who had even one episode of excessive drinking (five or more drinks) during the pregnancy were three times as likely to have alcohol problems at the age of twenty-one. Does anyone really want that for a son or daughter?

with depression may mask that illness with alcohol or drugs. The sooner parents figure that out and get their son or daughter treatment, the better.

A small but growing group of physicians is saying that we should adopt the European approach to alcohol. That instead of banning liquor before the age of twenty-one, we might let a teenager have a sip of wine at a family dinner. Teach him that a drink is a pleasant part of a meal, not something we drown our sorrows in at a bar.

We've got to break this terrible chain. Because right now, our young people go off to college and hey, you're not a man unless you can drink a six-pack and vomit all over yourself. Binge drinking among high school and college students kills kids every year. Something's wrong here, folks.

Q: I was diagnosed with gout about twelve years ago. I take allopurinol and colchicine, but they don't knock it out. Now it's really bad in my big-toe joint, and sometimes it actually leaves my toe and goes into my right hand, into the knuckles. It's getting progressively worse. Do you think that changing my drinking habits and my diet might help? How much alcohol is too much?

A: Gout is usually successfully controlled by the drugs you mentioned, so changes in diet have taken a back seat as treatment for most cases.

But, since you've had it for twelve years and it's getting worse, you ought to cut out all drinking immediately and also change your diet.

Gout is the result of an overproduction of uric acid, which is linked to alcohol and foods rich in purines—organ meats like liver, and also anchovies, herring, and mackerel. Carrying extra pounds can aggravate gout, too.

And gout can travel all over the body. Kidney stones are one result, and, in the ears, the uric acid shows up as white clumps of crystal. All in all, this is not stuff you really want to fool with, is it?

Colchicine comes from the autumn crocus, and it was an herbal medicine in the time of Hippocrates. Now it's a manufactured pharmaceutical.

By the way, Hippocrates once said, ". . . it is more important to know what kind of person has a disease than to know what kind of disease a person has." I would say that applies to your case, wouldn't you? Talk to your doctor honestly about your drinking and eating habits and get this gout under control.

Q: I'm a lifelong alcoholic, and I have a couple of questions about alcoholism. I've quit drinking twice in my lifetime, both times thinking I could do it. I was wrong.

Question No. 1: Is there any hope for an alcoholic to drink moderately? Question No. 2: What's the cause of a drinking problem? I have this strange, daily cycle where I feel fine in the morning and all during the day, but by six at night, I feel terrible; I'm morose, I have low energy, and so on. Life is just not fine. For me, alcohol is what I use to fix the problem.

A: Although your situation may seem bleak to you and to your loved ones, you have a lot of insight, and that's a very positive thing. I want to work backwards from that, because your last thought is extremely important.

A vast number of people who are alcoholics are actually self-medicating depression. You used the word "morose" to describe your evening time, when you are drinking, and this is one alcoholism pattern. Some alcoholics don't touch liquor during the day, because they're on the job and, usually, that means you are involved, with people, with projects. But at night, or just on weekends for some alcoholics, real life hits you in the face, and it's just too much to consider while sober.

You may be a person who could really benefit from antidepressant medications, in terms of helping you with alcohol, and you should talk to your doctor about this.

It wasn't that long ago that alcoholism was considered to be a moral failure. We've since, of course, reclassified it as a disease, and, as I mentioned in a previous question, certain personality traits may be linked to higher risk of alcoholism. You may never know, as an individual, whether it's genetic or environmental.

As to your question about drinking moderately, the classical thinking about alcoholism is there is no such thing as an ex-alcoholic moderate drinker; you have to quit completely. The twelve-step program of Alcoholics Anonymous reflects this attitude. However, I constantly see medical literature challenging that, and I think there are some successful moderate drinkers out there who are ex-alcoholics. But they are in the minority, and this is very risky business. Obviously, you tried to drink again—I'm assuming you had hoped to be a moderate drinker and didn't plan to abuse alcohol the second time around—so I seriously doubt that moderation will work for you in the future.

You must ask yourself why it is that you want to drink moderately, and you have to admit to yourself that you can't quite give up your drug. You are giving yourself the excuse that you can control it. So, you need a substitute, something to fill in that blank. You need to deal with the depression. You need to find an activity that will be good for your body and your mind. But start first with the depression. It takes a while for the medicine to kick in, but you may be amazed by the results.

Q: I gulped some NyQuil for a bad cold. Shortly afterward, I got into an accident while driving, and, at the scene, the paramedic told the police officer that I had alcohol on my breath. He gave me a Breathalyzer test, and I came really close to flunking it. Could the NyQuil have that much impact? I had not been drinking.

A: You are lucky. People are supposed to take NyQuil—the "nighttime" medicine—just before they go to bed, because it has a decongestant, a pain reliever, and other stuff that will help them SLEEP. What were you thinking?

NyQuil, and lots of other cold and cough medicines, definitely contain alcohol, and alcohol is definitely a cough suppressant. Alcoholics commonly die from spitting up while passed out. They inhale stomach acid rather than coughing it up, because alcohol has shut down their cough reflex.

Aside from suppressing the cough, alcohol is also a great organic solvent for the other active ingredients, additives, and dyes in the cough medicine. Plus, it induces a pleasant, foggy feeling.

You say you "gulped" the NyQuil, which leads me to believe you drank more than the recommended dosage. If you also had an empty stomach when you gulped, it's possible that the alcohol rushed into your bloodstream, temporarily spiking to the edges of the legal limit for driving.

Next time you have a cold, if you must take something and you want to drive, get a "non-drowsy" medication.

Q: Is it possible to become an alcoholic later in life? I'm in my forties, and, over the last four or five years, I find myself drinking more and more. I've become a completely different person and I have blackouts.

A: It is possible to become an alcoholic at any age, and it certainly sounds like you are there. As I said in an earlier answer, anyone who recognizes they have a problem has a great head start on beating this addiction.

Looking at your situation, I would recommend two things. One, find out where the AA meetings are held in your community and start going right away. If you need help with that, look in the white pages of your phone book or go to the AA Web site (see our Resource List on page 527).

Two, see your primary care doctor right away to make sure there's no other cause for the blackouts, and, while you are there, get a recommendation for a psychologist or psychiatrist. You want to identify what's happened in the last several years that made you want to drink so much.

Nicotine, Cigarettes, and Chewing Tobacco

Q: I've been an ex-smoker for about twelve weeks. I had a pulmonary exam that showed I have a 69 percent lung capacity. Will it ever improve?

A: Congratulations. At twelve weeks, you've made it through the tough part.

First of all, no one has 100 percent lung capacity. When we exhale, some air is still left behind in our lungs. When we inhale, we don't inhale fully. We breathe in until we have enough air, and then we breathe out. When we exercise, we need more oxygen, so we breathe in more deeply.

The permanent changes that smoking causes to the lungs are complicated.

Your lungs will never return to what they were, but they may improve. By quitting, you are sparing them further damage.

Smoke in the lungs destroys the walls between tiny spongy air spaces, creating larger bubbles. They hold the same volume of air as many small bubbles do, but because there are fewer of them and they're larger, they don't have as much surface area for the exchange of oxygen. This is why people with emphysema and lung disease have to breathe rapidly and have an increased respiratory rate.

I wouldn't focus too much on the lung-capacity number. If you do need an incentive to stay away from cigarettes, remember that you don't want to cause any further damage. Being tied to an oxygen tank, gasping for air with every breath, is not how you want to spend your last years on earth.

Q: I quit smoking cold-turkey five days ago, and I'm at my wits' end. I have had terrible mood swings, I'm hypersensitive and easily aggravated. Last night, my boyfriend dumped me because it got so bad. Is there anything I can do to decrease my irritability?

A: Any guy who can't endure five days of bad moods for such a good cause isn't worth having around, right? So, stick with it, and yes, I think you can address the grouchiness. It will pass, but if it's just too much, call your doctor immediately and see about getting a nicotine patch, gum, inhaler, or even an antidepressant, like Wellbutrin. All of these seem to improve the success rate for kicking the habit.

What's interesting is that some quitters climb the walls—becoming as close to psychotic as sane people can be—and others don't have any mood swings.

You are doing the right thing. Good luck.

QUIZ

Once a smoker quits, how long does it take to lower his or her heart attack risk to that of a nonsmoker?

A) two years   B) four years   C) five years   D) never
happens

(*A: two to three years.*)

DID YOU KNOW?
THE NUMBERS ON SMOKING

The number of U.S. smokers age eighteen or older declined 2.7 percent between 1997 and 2002, but more than one fifth of the adult population (22 percent) still smokes. Most teens who smoke will have their first cigarette by the time they are fifteen. And one study found that teenage girls who are focused on being thin are four times as likely to smoke as girls for whom thinness is not an important issue.

Q: I'm hoping to get pregnant soon, and I'm a smoker. What's the worst thing that could happen to my baby if I can't quit?

A: We know that smoking during pregnancy increases premature delivery and low birth weight, and those alone should be reason to quit. The risk for some birth defects, including clubfoot, also increases.

Fortunately, many women have gotten smart on this issue; the numbers of pregnant smokers had dropped dramatically by the end of the nineties. However, that wasn't true for pregnant teens.

One other thing to keep in mind: If you have a baby, don't you want to watch it reach adulthood? As long as you smoke, you are cutting your odds for a long life.

Q: I am a smoker who is also an active runner and walker. I have cut back from thirty cigarettes a day to ten a day. I just can't quit completely. Several months ago, you talked about a study that found the damage to your health was the same whether you smoked five cigarettes or two packs a day. Should I just smoke a pack and a half a day and not bother to cut down?

A: Sorry—you don't get to use that one study as an excuse. I have a difficult time believing that five cigarettes a day is just as bad for you as two packs. And that study only looked at one health aspect of the smoking issue— heart attacks. We know that smokers also have lousy dietary and exercise habits, and there are other health issues.

Researchers looked at "chippers," people who have cut their smoking to three or four cigarettes a day. Doctors found that even they have an increased rate of heart attacks. But this is just one study.

You may not believe this, but I think it is probably more difficult to cut down to ten cigarettes a day than it is to quit altogether. Psychologically you are facing constant temptation, and physiologically your body is going through the ups and downs of nicotine withdrawal. You are subjecting yourself to unrelenting addictive tension, so to speak.

Talk to your doctor about the last step. You are so close that it's crazy not to go all the way.

Q: I smoked for thirty years, and the patch helped me quit. I am now totally smoke-free. I completed the patch cycle two weeks ago. So when am I going to start feeling normal? I feel really spacey, like I'm on the outside looking in. I have good days and bad days, but will this ever stop altogether?

A: Yes, the spacey feeling will stop—eventually. It's to be expected after thirty years, and you need to be patient.

Smoking is a very complicated addiction that is not ruled by nicotine alone, otherwise everyone who uses nicotine gum, patches, and inhalers would give up cigarettes. Smoking is also a hand habit, a social habit, and an emotional habit.

Smokers smoke for a variety of reasons: to beat depression, to stifle anxiety, or to mask insecurity. When you quit, you go back to the person you tried to turn away from. So, some emotional consequences are normal. Don't let this discourage you, but it usually takes about six months to get back to your normal self.

When you're having a bad day, remind yourself that the good days will come around. You have been able to quit and that's a real triumph. Stick with it one day at a time. Online meeting rooms for people recovering from addictions have also become popular; the QuitNet Web site focuses just on smoking. For more information, see our Resource List on page 527.

Q: My surgeon told me to stop smoking six weeks before my breast reduction surgery. Doesn't nicotine clear out of the body in a week?

A: It's not the nicotine. The surgeon is concerned about your constricted blood vessels. He or she wants your vascular tone to return, and that takes longer than simply clearing nicotine from your system.

Smoking constricts blood vessels and decreases your oxygen supply. You need all the oxygen you can get when you have an operation like this, so the tissues are healthy and can heal properly. You don't want gangrene in your breasts.

Facelifts, in particular, are treacherous for smokers, and many plastic surgeons won't operate on a smoker.

Finally, never lie—believe me, I've seen it happen—and tell a plastic surgeon that you quit smoking when you haven't. That truly is playing with fire.

Q: I have ulcerative colitis, and I know that studies have found that nicotine has a positive effect for people with ulcerative colitis. I quit smoking ten years ago. Of course, I know that smoking nicotine isn't the solution, but what is?

A: While smoking may reduce the risk of ulcerative colitis, and even Parkinson's and Alzheimer's diseases, there are no major studies about using it for treatment. Of course, you could talk to your doctor about nicotine gum or a patch, and see what happens.

Another, cheaper source of nicotine is Swedish oral snuff (see more about this on page 505). But most doctors would rather give you a patch, because the nicotine absorption can be more carefully controlled.

There is some confusion about the dangers of nicotine in noncigarette form. Some research suggests that smokers who switch to an alternate nicotine source get healthier hearts, suggesting that something else in cigarettes—like carbon monoxide—is the cause of heart problems.

Q: Are there any harmful effects of chewing Nicorette gum long-term? Nicorette helped me quit smoking years ago, but I've had to fight against

---

QUIZ

If you have a two-pack-a-day cigarette habit and you quit at age thirty, how many years have you added to your predicted life span?

A) almost two years   B) five years   C) almost eight years

D) ten years

(C: 7.83 years.)

overeating all this time. I'm thinking of chewing Nicorette again to cure this food craving.

A: You got off nicotine once, so I'd hate to see you bring it back into your life and your system. Since you have a positive association with gum, maybe you can fool yourself by chewing plain old gum.

There are lots of unanswered questions about nicotine. For one thing, why are cigarettes addictive but the gum, which gives you the same blood level of nicotine, seldom hooks anyone?

And we are wary of nicotine's ability to constrict blood vessels, which carry oxygen throughout the body. Another bit of scary news about nicotine is that recent research indicates the body may turn it into a cancer chemical.

I encourage you to remain free of any dependence on nicotine.

Q: My seventy-five-year-old mother, who quit smoking thirty-five years ago, has been diagnosed with COPD. Is this lung cancer? Also, since she quit so long ago, why didn't her lungs heal?

A: COPD is not cancer. It stands for "chronic obstructive pulmonary disease," and it is the diagnosis used to describe lung damage, which is most often caused by smoking. Both emphysema and chronic bronchitis are COPDs.

COPD occurs when the partitions between the air sacs of the lung break down, and the amount of the lung available to absorb oxygen decreases. The vast majority of COPD cases (between 80 and 90 percent) can be attributed to smoking.

One of the worst things about smoking is that it does irreversible damage. Quitting saves the smoker from continuing destruction, allows some healing, and decreases the smoker's risk of disease, but the lungs never return to their presmoking condition.

COPD symptoms include chronic coughing, chest tightness, shortness of breath, difficulty breathing, and increased mucus. As the disease progresses, in most cases, breathing becomes more difficult and the coughing increases, eventually restricting even basic daily activities.

Because your mother's lungs are so impaired, she should definitely keep current with her flu and pneumonia shots and do everything she can to avoid catching a lung infection. She should also talk to her doctor about what exercise might be appropriate because even a small amount could be beneficial.

Q: I'm sixty-six years old, and I'm a smoker. The fingernails of several

fingers on both of my hands have been curving downward for the past three months. Do you know what causes this?

A: If we did not cut and file our nails, they would grow in curves toward our palms. However, a type of curve called "clubbing" is not natural, and it can be a sign of lung or heart disease. Since this is a newly developed symptom, I want you to pay attention. Perhaps this is the incentive you need to quit smoking.

The way to distinguish clubbing from the nails' natural curve is to look at your fingernails from the side and examine the place where the nail bed meets the cuticle. In healthy people, that place is a little valley, a dip, and the nail curves slightly up from there.

When clubbing occurs, that angle between the nail and the cuticle flattens out, and the valley disappears. We're not certain, but we think that reduced oxygen to the fingertips is what causes the unusual shape.

You should see your doctor and ask her or him directly, "Is this clubbing?" If so, you need further examination of your lungs and heart.

There is also Buerger's disease (*thromboangiitis obliterans*), which only smokers get. It causes gangrene in the fingers, toes, hands, and feet. Nicotine constricts blood vessels, which is why smokers often have cold fingertips. In extreme cases, you can lose your hands and your arms.

I've seen fingerless people find ways to grip cigarettes, because they can't give up the habit. Of course, *thromboangiitis obliterans* is a very rare result of smoking, but it is definitely due to the lack of oxygen caused by constricted blood vessels.

Q: Is the habit of chewing tobacco more difficult to kick than smoking tobacco? My husband has been chewing tobacco for more than ten years now, and he just can't stop. Is Zyban or Wellbutrin effective in helping chewers quit?

A: Yes, there is evidence that chewing is harder to quit than smoking. Of course, fewer studies have been done on chewing tobacco, but possible causes of the deeper addiction are oral habits and taste, as well as the higher, more steady dose of nicotine that chewing zaps to the blood.

I don't think the effectiveness of Zyban and Wellbutrin in helping chewers quit has been studied. Nevertheless, I encourage him to give them a try, because they might work.

One potential method I know for kicking the smoking tobacco habit is

Swedish oral tobacco—called snus. It's not available in the United States, but you can order it online.

The tobacco comes in a little package to put under your lip. It delivers the tobacco flavor and nicotine without causing oral cancer, according to researchers. It may be the way to go for someone who absolutely craves the flavor of tobacco.

Q: I had a chest X ray recently, and three doctors called me to talk about it. I'm thirty years old, and I've been smoking heavily for seventeen years. I was recently on an inhaler, because I wheeze so much. One doctor said that my lungs look like I'm a year away from having emphysema and needing an oxygen tank. She talked to me for twenty minutes, and everything she said was really scary. Do HMO doctors call you just to scare you like that, or could she have been telling me the truth?

A: You're lucky that you have an HMO doctor who is able to spend that much time with you. And if three doctors called me to discuss my health, I'd darn well pay attention. These days no doctors have time to play games.

If the stories that scared you were about emphysema, terminal lung disease, and the unending feeling of suffocation, then you were getting the truth.

Some people have a type of metabolism—and women are more prone to this than men are—that, when combined with heavy smoking, will prematurely tear up the lungs. Once the little walls break down between the air sacs in your lungs, they don't heal.

If the wheezing and the inhaler haven't convinced you about your deteriorating lungs, what will? I find that I can get men's attention by telling them that smoking is linked to impotence, and I can get some women's attention by telling them that smoking makes them wrinkle. And that's no scare tactic, either.

Smokers look about ten years older than their actual age, and Japanese researchers recently figured out that nicotine alters the breakdown of collagen and elastin in the skin. In studies, research subjects have been deadly accurate in picking the smokers from the nonsmokers in a group of photographs.

Cold turkey is the single most successful way to quit smoking. Millions have done it, and so can you. Don't listen to negative messages about struggle and failure. Take a shot at it. If you fail the first time, try again.

Marijuana: The Medicine and the Illegal Drug

Q: I have hepatitis C, and I'm getting ready to start the interferon/ribavirin therapy. As an occasional marijuana user, I was hoping to continue smoking it to help me get through the loss of appetite, and restlessness at night. Is there any danger in the way that it is metabolized?

A: Marijuana, like most medications, is metabolized in the liver. With active liver disease, a little dose of marijuana may go a long way. In addition, street marijuana has such variability that predicting its effect is difficult.

I know of no contraindication, and I'm in favor of medical marijuana, but I'm uncomfortable recommending an illegal substance to a person with a serious illness.

You must ask your doctors about this and, believe me, you won't be the first person to do so.

People with worse illnesses than yours have used marijuana to fight nausea with no negative consequences, and any anti-nausea drug that the doctor gives you will be metabolized by the liver. I feel more secure with your liver trying to handle marijuana, because Marinol, the FDA-approved pill form of marijuana, has shown no toxicity to the liver.

I would estimate marijuana to be as safe as anything else. Interferon and ribavirin are a pretty hefty combination that can be curative in a significant percentage of cases. It's basically all we have for hepatitis C. Interferon can make you pretty sick, but ribavirin is fairly easy on you. They are both antiviral drugs.

Q: I just found out I am pregnant, but my husband and I have been smoking a lot of marijuana and I'm worried about it causing birth defects. I've stopped smoking it now. Will my baby be OK?

A: Marijuana does not seem to cause birth defects, so I think you can relax about that.

Clinically, it's difficult, because when you study women who use marijuana, there is almost always other stuff going on, such as alcohol consumption or the use of other drugs.

The literature is mixed. One study done in Jamaica found that babies of mothers who smoked marijuana during pregnancy were bigger, healthier, happier babies. I believe the reason there was sociodemographic—women in Jamaica who can afford pot have more money and deliver healthier babies.

As a parent, I know that a child's bad grades in school are frequently the sign of other problems, from depression to drug use to family issues. Well, these facts add fuel to that fire. One study found that youths who reported an average grade of D or below were more than three times as likely to have used inhalants during the past year as youths with an average grade of A. Those same kids were more than four times as likely to have used marijuana in the past year. So, if your child is seriously struggling with school, don't automatically assume drugs are involved, but do get to the bottom of the problem.

The one thing they've seen clinically in mothers who smoke pot heavily throughout pregnancy—which you're not going to do—is that their babies have sleep disturbances after they're born and may develop learning problems.

Q: Over the holidays, my son came home and found out that his dad, who is fifty-five, smokes marijuana to sleep better. My son had a fit, and the two of them got into a heated argument over it. The funny part is, the kid had bought your book, *Eat, Drink, and Be Merry*, as his dad's Christmas present. What is your opinion on using marijuana to get to sleep?

A: It's a strange world we live in. It would be perfectly legal—and probably acceptable to your son—for your husband to waste his money on melatonin or other supplements that don't help people sleep.

The fact is, he's spending money on an herb that evidence finds to be very effective for sleep, has a higher safety profile than sleeping pills, and doesn't seem to cause a hangover. Yet it is illegal.

Many upstanding and responsible Americans, who have jobs and raise kids, use marijuana. The key word here is *"use,"* not "abuse." Cancer patients use it to fight nausea and increase appetite, multiple sclerosis patients use it to fight spasms, glaucoma patients use it to decrease pressure, and insomniacs use it for sleep.

If the old man were a pothead, smoking all day long, I'd say that's a bad thing. But as far as we can tell, light users don't seem to have medical problems. Yet I can't advise the use of an illegal drug, and one survey found that in homes where parents are perceived as having lax views about drugs, children are more likely to use drugs themselves.

I can't help but wonder what your son's reaction would have been if he had discovered that his dad was a regular user of prescription sleeping pills.

Of course, neither pot nor pills are ideal. It would be much better in the long run for your husband to learn how to sleep without medication.

Q: I injured my eye at the age of fifteen. Just recently the pressure in it increased to around thirty. The ophthalmologist gave me medication and the pressure now varies between eighteen and twenty-three, but I don't have vision in that eye anymore. I asked the doctor about using marijuana to decrease the pressure, and he is pretty much against it. He says I would have to stay stoned all the time for that to work. Do you agree?

A: The approach we take to the problem of a damaged eye depends on whether we are trying to save the eye or to save vision.

If you lost your sight due to glaucoma caused by excessive pressure on your optic nerve, once the pressure decreases, some sight may return if the nerve damage is not permanent. That's unlikely, though.

If you lost your sight because of the original injury, nothing is going to change that.

Normal pressure ranges from eleven to twenty-one, and there are several simple surgeries that might control the pressure. Talk to your doctor about that.

Although marijuana can lower eye pressure, I agree with your doctor—you would probably need so much that you would be stoned all the time. And there are other medications that do the same thing, without that side effect.

It is often recommended that an eye with no vision be removed if it becomes painful, because, for some reason, eyes in that condition have high rates of melanomas and cancers. The cosmetic results are better with a prosthesis than with a blind, diseased eye, too.

Q: Do you think marijuana is a useful herb for treating alcoholism and heroin addiction? I'm now thirty-five, and I've been addicted to both for more than ten years.

A: I think that marijuana could probably be used to calm down alcoholics who are going through withdrawal, the way Valium is now used. However, you are talking about alcohol and heroin, so your situation is much trickier.

While swapping a deadly addiction for a safer one may seem like progress, the big goal is to be addiction-free and find out who you really are, to get to know the person who ten years ago had reasons for going down the dark path of addiction. With a lot of courage and help, you can face your demons.

One of the controversies in the addictions field has been the use of illegal and/or dangerous drugs to treat the primary addiction. Before LSD was criminalized, it was showing promise in research on treating alcoholism—however, I don't recommend you go out and try it. Ibogaine, which is a similar type of psychedelic, is being tried in research nowadays to treat addictions.

Methadone has been successfully used for heroin addicts, and newer treatments include buprenorphine and rapid detox.

Whatever you do, don't try to tackle these addictions by yourself. Start with a visit to your doctor, because more can be done from the doctor's office than ever before. He or she will help you to start moving in a healthier direction.

See more heroin-related questions on page 516.

Q: I'm comfortable asking you this question, because I can remain anonymous. In preparation for an upcoming hand surgery, I got an instruction sheet from my doctor that says I shouldn't smoke for three weeks before or after surgery. Does that apply to marijuana, too?

A: I can't act as your doctor and give you specific advice, but I can tell you that the reason patients should stop smoking cigarettes weeks before surgery is because smoking constricts the blood vessels and interferes with healing.

Nicotine is a vasoconstrictor; it narrows your arteries. This is one reason why smokers commonly have cold hands. And while I don't want to aid an illegal drug habit, I don't know that marijuana has the same effect as cigarettes. I haven't seen many studies on the effects of marijuana on surgery.

Hands are far from your heart, and during surgery you want as much oxygen as possible to run through your arteries, so my gut tells me you should follow the instruction sheet on all counts.

Caffeine is also a vasoconstrictor, and I have wondered why people aren't told to back off of coffee before surgery. One reason may be that, after surgery, patients would wind up with major caffeine-withdrawal headaches, and caffeine's effect on arteries only lasts a few hours.

I urge you, just as I urge people who take herbs, to ask your doctor. The anesthesiologist is the best person to ask. I've seen anesthesiologists try to put someone to sleep and run into difficulties because the patient has been using herbs or other kinds of substances.

I would hope a patient would feel safe letting her doctor in on her personal habits, because it's a bad idea to be secretive about your health needs. Yet I understand that many of you have legitimate fears about what information employers and insurance companies might be able to get from your medical records.

Try asking the question anonymously, in a phone call. You might get your answer that way.

Q: I have a family member who swears by marijuana for relieving debilitating headaches. She claims that taking a puff of good marijuana when she feels a headache coming on does the trick nine times out of ten. She'd much rather do that than take codeine, or the pill-form marijuana, Marinol, which doesn't do anything for her. Is this possible, or is she just justifying her pot use?

A: I have a pharmaceutical text from the 1930s that puts migraine headaches at the top of a list of diseases that marijuana can treat, so marijuana as a potential treatment for headaches is nothing new.

For a couple of reasons, smoking marijuana works better than swallowing Marinol. The delivery system is key. When your relative smokes marijuana, it goes right to her bloodstream and her brain, calming her arteries. The absorption of Marinol takes about half an hour.

Also, while marijuana as a natural product has a slew of active ingredients, Marinol is a synthetic version of just one of those ingredients, and it could be missing some of the effective components of a joint.

If your relative's headaches are migraines, they are often preceded by nausea. As she has found, marijuana may help that, while swallowing a Marinol pill may not. But you should encourage her to see a neurologist, because there are new migraine medicines in the market that have proven very effective. And, of course, marijuana makes you high—an undesirable side effect for most people.

The big problem with the medical marijuana issue is the smoking of a cigarette. I don't know of any medicine that you smoke. If researchers ten to twenty years ago had been given a green light by the government to develop

DID YOU KNOW?
CAFFEINE COUNTS

What do you think contains more caffeine—espresso or instant coffee? Coca-Cola or Mountain Dew? The answers might surprise you. Here is the caffeine content of several common foods, beverages, and medicines:

No-Doz Maximum Strength; Vivarin (one tablet): 200 mg

Brewed or percolated black coffee (8 ounces): 80–200 mg

Celestial Seasonings Iced Lemon Ginseng Tea (16-ounce bottle): 100 mg

Instant coffee (8 ounces): 85–100 mg

Starbucks shot of espresso (1 ounce): 90 mg

Ben & Jerry's No Fat Coffee Fudge Frozen Yogurt (1 cup): 85 mg

Red Bull energy drink (one can): 80 mg

Jolt (12 ounces): 72 mg

Iced tea (12 ounces): 70 mg

Excedrin (one tablet): 60 mg

Maximum Strength Midol (one tablet): 60 mg

Mountain Dew (one can): 55 mg

Coca-Cola (one can): 34 mg

Hershey's Special Dark Chocolate bar (1.5 ounces): 31 mg

alternate delivery systems for marijuana, I'm sure there'd be many inhalers, pills, patches, and "conduits" on the market right now that contain the active ingredients of pot. As it is, pharmaceutical companies have these products in the final phases of development, and I think the medical marijuana issue is going to go away when these new treatment options hit the market.

Unfortunately, the government's close-mindedness on this topic once made marijuana research extremely difficult.

Methadone, Cocaine, Amphetamines, and Heroin

Q: I'm in my early forties, and I recently did some cocaine at a party. Now, I'm worried that the cocaine will show up in my upcoming health-insurance blood test. How long does cocaine show up in the blood?

A: I'll postpone the lecture for a moment and jump to the answer. Research conducted on heavy users shows that cocaine is undetectable in the urine within three to seven days—and sometimes sooner. Now, this is in urine, which is what your insurance company is more likely to test. In hair it's detectable for months. You are dealing with an illegal substance, of course, so we lack information. Doctors aren't taking people into the back of a lab to load them up on cocaine and see what happens.

As for your party habits, you need to take a hard look at the risks involved. Just one snort can stop your heart. It is a very dangerous drug, and anyone who uses it is gambling with their life.

Q: I'm forty years old, and I'm wondering if all the speed and cocaine, and especially the freebase cocaine, I did back in my late twenties will shorten my life span. Can a heart scan tell me anything?

A: I don't think we know the answer. The problem is, if you do study the people who abused speed and cocaine in their youth, they've often used lots of other things. So, when you find medical problems, how do you know if it's the cocaine or something else, like genetics or even bad eating habits?

Then you face the question you really want answered: Am I going to live as long as everyone else? Well, we'd have to take a bunch of people who did what you did, and put them in cages, and then take a bunch of people who didn't, and put them in cages, and control everything in their environments and follow them along for eighty years to really know the answer.

Cocaine and amphetamines constrict blood vessels and speed up the heart, making the electrical systems of the heart hypersensitive, so you understand how they can kill you. And you really put your heart through hell with the free-basing, but you've survived those tests, and my guess is that you'll probably be OK. However, no one should take that as my endorsement for using these drugs.

As for the heart scan, it won't tell you anything. The scans you're talking about look for calcium in the coronary arteries; that's hardening of the arteries and has nothing to do with drug usage.

I think all you can do is put your wild youth behind you, consider yourself lucky, and move on and enjoy your life. I know of no evidence that you would be at a higher risk. If you start again, that is different. People chronically using substances like that are putting their life at risk.

I would recommend a hepatitis C test. If you've ever snorted cocaine in a group with a rolled-up hundred-dollar bill or a tube, you are touching the noses of people who likely have fresh blood in their noses. Cocaine causes bleeding in the nose. You are then coming into contact with another person's blood, and that can transmit hepatitis C.

Anyone who has ever been around cocaine should get a hepatitis C test, and if you don't want to go to the doctor, you can do it with a home test.

Q: I just did a backpack trip in Peru, where we had coca leaves in Machu Picchu—everyone was chewing them—and it helped a lot; everyone was talking about how strong we felt. Now that I'm home, I have one worry: How long does it stay in your system?

A: Yes, you would test positive, but not for long—maybe two to three days. However, if you have to take a drug test, try to put a week between usage and the test, just to be sure.

As you discovered, the coca leaf works as a minor stimulant that can help with altitude sickness, curb your thirst and appetite, and allow you to work harder. Your body also requires less oxygen—which is why it's great for a climb on the Inca Trail.

Chewing it is not at all like snorting a big fat line of concentrated powder cocaine and overdoing it, the way people in the Western world do. Native populations have used the leaf appropriately for thousands of years without harm.

At the turn of the century, coca leaf was an ingredient in tonics used by little old ladies, safely. And the original Coca-Cola formula had cocaine in it, as did all cola drinks at the time. But by 1929, coca was no longer part of the recipe.

Q: I was addicted to methamphetamine for about eight years, but I stopped using it more than ten years ago. I've also recently quit drinking. But now I'm scared. I saw a study that revealed just how bad speed really is, and I think it explains why I have a hard time remembering things. I'm thirty-eight, and I have a hard time selecting the right words, and now I am dealing with depression. That's why I loved speed, because it made me feel better. But now I am on Prozac, and it helps somewhat. Will anything else help me?

The Edell Report
LSD, Chapter Two

I became a doctor in the sixties, so I saw my share of folks on bad acid trips and other drug experiences who found their way to the emergency room. Everyone was talking about—or experimenting with—hallucinogens. Timothy Leary lost his teaching position at Harvard because of his adventures, and Ken Kesey would become a sixties legend, thanks to a bus full of "Merry Pranksters." Even Life *magazine was there: "LSD: The Mind Drug That Got Out of Control."*

By 1966, LSD was banned in California, and, in 1970, the FDA had declared it a "schedule 1" drug, which is where you'll find hallucinogenics and opiates—most of which are illegal for any use beyond approved medical research.

Flash-forward to a new century, and I can't believe I've lived to see the day when doctors are once again studying the medical potential for LSD and other hallucinogenics. It tells me that all of us who grew up during the sixties are now in charge, and we're changing the world with our attitudes. We have finally gotten past the fact that an abused drug is not automatically a bad drug.

Researchers from Harvard to Purdue are now looking at how hallucinogenics may be useful in treating everything from psychiatric illnesses to pain. Will LSD ease the fear of dying patients? Can symptoms of obsessive-

---

A: You're in a tough spot, because it's hard to say whether anything you're observing today is related to what you did. I'm not downplaying the danger, especially with drugs like that. But speed—and that's a generic term, as you know—encompasses a variety of pharmacological agents in similar categories. Diet pills are amphetamines, of all different sorts and kinds, that we legally peddle hand over fist to people who want to lose weight, and they seem to do OK.

It's never too late to start dealing with who you are, and that's what you need to keep doing—deal with your problems. Speed is really attractive to

compulsive disorder be impacted by psilocybin (derived from Mexican mushrooms)? Can the peyote cactus help alcoholics stay sober?

Aren't you interested in knowing this? I know I am. Yet we continue to allow our politicians to practice moral pharmacology. The Drug Enforcement Administration classifies hallucinogens as drugs with no known medical value, purely drugs of abuse.

That's baloney. Can anyone name a drug that is purely a drug of abuse? I can't think of one. Heroin, cocaine, marijuana—they all have tremendous medical uses, but because they've been abused they've been demonized.

Many of the people who are in scientific power today came of age during the sixties, and they, unlike their parents, are not as afraid of these substances. I have lived long enough to see a changing of the scientific guard to more open minds!

Of course, we also know a lot more about the brain than we did thirty years ago, and hallucinogenics may work by changing the brain chemical called serotonin, which is just what Prozac does. Brain systems can become more sensitive, kind of like turning up the volume on your radio; suddenly you can hear very weak stations.

This research is still in the earliest stages, but I plan to stay tuned in. Remember, I am advocating not illegal drug use but legitimate research to help sick people.

---

people who have depression. So is alcohol. So, you quit drinking and you quit speed, and now you are on Prozac. That's a good start, and now I would encourage you to look at what is going on in your life today that works for you and what doesn't—and go from there, with the help of a therapist, if possible.

I've never seen a good study that would say your memory problems have to do more with the speed than just being alive on earth today. We all think we're losing our minds and that Alzheimer's is just around the corner. Well, for the vast majority of us, it isn't true.

Q: I'm just getting off of heroin, and my doctor wrote a prescription for buprenorphine. Because I live in rural Colorado, I couldn't get methadone here, but my doctor says this is much better than methadone. Is this true?

A: Until the fall of 2002, heroin addicts had to go to a treatment clinic for help. General practitioners had their hands tied, because a regular doctor couldn't prescribe methadone—which was considered the treatment that worked best.

But buprenorphine was out there—it had been approved by the FDA as a pain reliever, not as a treatment for heroin addiction. So some doctors were using it "off label," because they knew that studies had shown that it worked.

The FDA eventually approved both buprenorphine and buprenorphine/naloxone. The combination drug, known by the brand name Suboxone, is for addicts who are already in some type of treatment. What you are using, which has the brand name Subutex, is for people who are just starting treatment. Go for it.

Q: I am withdrawing from heroin, and I get something my doctor calls "restless leg syndrome." He hasn't been very helpful about treating it. Is there anything I can do?

A: Restless leg syndrome is a condition that causes tingling and twitching in the legs at rest. Typically, it starts when you try to settle down in bed at night, and the sensation—like ants crawling under the skin—makes lying still impossible. The person has to move; he's got dancing feet. It's not painful, but it's extremely annoying.

The medical community is divided over restless leg syndrome. Some think of it as a "mini-seizure disorder" that needs medication, while others say that hot packs and stretching exercises will take care of it.

I haven't heard of a specific connection between opiate withdrawal and restless leg syndrome, but, as you well know, withdrawal causes a lot of neurological agitation. Because you've been there, you know more than I do about the spasms and tremors.

It's also possible that you've had restless leg syndrome all along, and now that you've stopped using heroin, you're feeling it for the first time. Alcohol, marijuana, and other mood-altering chemicals mask pain and other conditions that are revealed once the habits end. I guarantee you that opiates would mask restless leg syndrome.

Knowledgeable treatment for opiate withdrawal is a neglected specialty. I am convinced opiate addicts could probably be helped more successfully than cigarette smokers and alcoholics, but society shuns them.

You can get more information online from the Restless Legs Syndrome Foundation (*www.rls.org*).

Q: Several kids at my daughter's high school were just expelled because they had Ecstasy in their possession. And then I saw it mentioned on the TV show *West Wing*. Can you please tell me why this drug is so popular right now? And how dangerous is it?

A: Any drug abuse is a bad thing, and this is a dangerous drug in high doses and with repeated use, but I can understand why kids would want to try it.

Ecstasy's medical name is MDMA, and it's a synthetic stimulant drug. One of its nicknames is "love drug," because it is known for filling the users with a sense of profound closeness and intimacy. Which explains, of course, why it's so popular.

What worries me about the current fervor over Ecstasy is that in our zeal to stamp out drug abuse we are also stamping out legitimate research.

MDMA is a fascinating molecule. Any drug that can induce the emotional feelings ascribed to MDMA is worth knowing about. Researchers used it in divorce counseling, before it was made illegal. Videotapes made of couples on the verge of divorce—before and after the use of MDMA—were astounding. Their psychological insights and understanding of each other when under the influence of this drug make it worthy of further research.

It's not a sexual drug, as many have characterized it, but a drug that seems to enable the user to drop the normal boundaries and barriers we have for expressing intimate feelings. This may sound rather mushy, but it's exactly how psychiatrists who have had experience with this drug describe its effect on people.

To find that a single molecule can approach the feelings that most of us would call love is so interesting that it would be a shame for this drug to be banished forever simply because we want teenagers to stop using it. Laws never stop people from committing dangerous acts, and I'm not convinced that a heavy program of education about the dangerous aspects of MDMA isn't a better way to go.

Nevertheless, there are organizations that are beginning to get grant money to try and understand how this drug alters the human brain.

Prescription Drugs: Vicodin, Viagra, Nasal Sprays, and More

Q: I have been addicted to Afrin nasal spray for about four years. I use it once every two hours. I asked my doctor about it, and he told me to just stop using it, but he didn't tell me how. I've tried, but I can't breathe. It affects my concentration, and I can't work. I'm considering taking a week off work just to get over it. Do you have any helpful ideas?

A: You're right, you can't quit nose spray cold turkey. You stuff up immediately, and you can't breathe. For starters, you should find another doctor, more committed to helping you, because this one is not giving you appropriate care.

Afrin is one of many brand names for oxymetazoline, and it is notorious for this problem. When the label says to use it only once every twelve hours, there's a reason for that.

One way to wean yourself off this is to use saline nose drops, which are easier to quit. Slowly begin to decrease the amount of your nasal spray by substituting the saline spray. Another option would be cortisone drops, which will reduce the inflammation that will occur when you cut back on the oxymetazoline. You'll have to see a doctor for a prescription for the cortisone drops.

As you begin using the saline spray, try expanding the time between all doses of spray. Go from every two hours to every two and a half hours for a few days, then up it to every three hours. Gradually build up until you are spraying every twelve hours, and keep on until you reach once a day and then not at all.

When you've stopped using the original spray altogether, taper off the

---

QUIZ

The "club drug" MDMA—so-called because it's popular at all-night dance parties—also goes by what other name?
A) Ecstasy, XTC, and X   B) Adam   C) Clarity
D) Lover's Speed   E) all of the above
(E: all of the above; MDMA is a synthetic drug that surfaced in the early 1990s, and its use has skyrocketed. It can increase heart rate and blood pressure and can also lead to dehydration, hypertension, and heart and kidney failure.)

saline and the cortisone, so you don't get hooked on those, and you'll be fine.

One other thought: See if simple over-the-counter oral decongestants relieve the stuffiness enough to allow you to kick the habit.

Properly used, nasal sprays are the best way to directly target that most annoying of cold symptoms, the stuffy nose. Cold pills flood us with more drugs than we need when we're just going after a stuffy nose.

So I recommend nasal sprays, but stick to the directions. "Every twelve hours" never means "every time I need it."

Q: I love Vicodin. I think it's one of the best drugs on the planet. The problem is, I think I'm addicted. I took Prozac for a time, but Vicodin is a much better attitude adjuster. Is there any research on making a drug that has all of Vicodin's power and none of its addictive ingredients?

A: If you think you are addicted, you probably are. And I'm afraid the drug is keeping you from getting at the root issues in your life—or your health—that have put you in this situation. A life without mood-altering chemicals will be a lot better for you, and I advise you to find help to get off the Vicodin.

Over time, larger and larger doses are needed for Vicodin to be effective. And, very often, you get hooked on taking it, not because it's making you feel better, but because going without makes you feel worse. When you stop taking it, you may be surprised to find that you don't need it anymore, or you may realize just how profoundly it has been affecting you.

Opiates, the classification of drugs that Vicodin falls under, are phenomenal medications that have eased man's psychic, physical, and spiritual ills for thousands of years. There is no doubt it's the king. If only we could get rid of that pesky addiction problem.

You are hardly alone in wanting a better drug, one that has everything we want and nothing that we don't. Every year or two, a new flock of drugs comes on the market, promising to have the power of opiates, but not the addictive potential. So far the promises have fallen flat.

Ironically, a lot of terminally ill cancer patients, including children, suffer unnecessary pain because the government hounds doctors with the largely overblown fear that those on opiate pain medications will become addicted. So, many very sick people are undermedicated when it comes to pain. This is ludicrous. If you're dying, so what if you become addicted?

As you have probably figured out, the body tolerates opiates very well. People who are taking prescribed morphine and other heavy opiates don't appear stoned, can function, and can drive—things a drunken person could not do. Of course, for some folks, this makes it easier to justify the addiction.

Q: I have chronic back pain and had surgery three months ago. At my checkup today, my doctor switched me from Dilaudid to methadone. Isn't methadone for heroin addicts in recovery? I'm not a heroin addict. I have been doing fine on Dilaudid, for three months, and suddenly I can't take it without throwing up. Isn't methadone a dangerous alternative? My doctor told me not to worry.

A: Heroin, Dilaudid, and methadone are all opiates. Vomiting is a common side effect of opiates, but it occurs less frequently with methadone, which is probably why your doctor made the switch.

Yes, methadone is given to recovering heroin addicts, but it is also a very powerful pain medication along the lines of Demerol and morphine. Some doctors think it's the strongest painkiller we have. The problem is that methadone and all the other opiates are addictive. You may be staying on methadone forever.

In treating chronic pain, you want to find the least powerful drug that will do the job. Your doctor must have started you on the lighter-weight painkillers, ibuprofen for example, which is fairly mild but can be helpful in targeting a specific source of pain. If that didn't work, you would have moved up to the next most powerful analgesic.

A complicated situation like yours would really benefit from a review by a pain-management specialist. These doctors are very underutilized, and their expertise should be used for pain, like you use an orthopedist for back care or a neurologist for migraines.

Doctors who are not pain specialists will often prescribe chronic use of opiates with the best intentions of relieving their patients' pain. However, they are putting their patients at risk for addiction. Yet, statistically, pain patients usually don't get hooked on their meds. It takes a certain personality for that to happen.

Q: My friend tells me that the biggest drug on the streets these days is Viagra. How does Viagra affect a healthy male? Is it dangerous?

A: It didn't take long for Viagra to become a recreational drug—which means guys are not using it for erectile dysfunction but for fun. However, one of its potential side effects is an erection that will not go away without the services of a doctor with a needle. How fun is that?

I'm not sure what folks who are playing with this drug think they are going to get out of it. After all, an erection is an erection. Viagra doesn't turn you on; you have to turn yourself on. Maybe it boosts confidence, but it does not alter libido.

Apparently, there is Viagra use among men who are also taking amphetamines, cocaine, and MDMA (a.k.a. Ecstasy). That's dumb and dangerous. Some of these drugs really fire up the libido, but they also make you impotent. They give you the will but not the way.

Speed drugs constrict blood vessels, while Viagra dilates blood vessels. We don't really know what this combination can do, but Viagra has caused some blood-pressure problems that have been fatal.

Q: My husband has been diagnosed with chronic fatigue syndrome by several doctors—he's had the Epstein-Barr virus—and he's on a ton of medications. He takes Lipitor for elevated triglycerides that are hereditary and not related to the chronic fatigue problem. He takes Norvasc for slightly elevated blood pressure. He takes Xanax for anxiety and Ritalin for energy. He takes Tylenol with codeine and aspirin with codeine three times a day. At night he takes Restoril to get to sleep. Does this make sense? And what are the long-term effects of the drugs?

A: Your husband is being grossly mismanaged. I have never heard a worse list of contradictory medications. Of course, I am not his doctor, and there could be something I don't know, but here's a breakdown of what's going on with the drugs he's taking.

Ritalin should perk him up. Xanax should make him tired. This is like being on an amphetamine and Valium. What doctor would prescribe something like that?

Throw in an opiate like codeine, and a tranquilizer like Restoril, and you have an alphabet soup of pharmaceutical garbage.

But let's begin with the diagnosis: I don't believe that chronic fatigue syndrome has yet been determined to be a single real disease. At one time, a link was suspected between the Epstein-Barr virus and chronic fatigue syndrome. After extensive testing, infectious disease experts have concluded that the suspicion is unfounded. While it's true that 95 percent of chronic fatigue patients tested positive for Epstein-Barr virus, consider the fact that 95 percent of the general population has had Epstein-Barr virus, most with no symptoms.

Very often these sick people have other undiagnosed diseases, such as a thyroid or heart problem, low blood pressure, or parasites. By the way, if your doctor decides to test you for parasites, remember that most doctors don't test aggressively enough for these microorganisms. Consider seeing an infectious disease specialist. With so much uncertainty, it is crazy to pummel your husband with so many medications.

He needs one doctor who has the guts to take over his case and start from scratch. Don't do this on your own. Withdrawal from even codeine can be tricky, to say nothing of this cocktail they've got your husband on.

His blood pressure is probably the most important symptom to treat, and yet it can be treated with lifestyle changes like weight loss, exercise, and a sodium-restricted diet. The doctor may still want to keep him on blood pressure medication and one for the cholesterol problem. He's likely to drop everything else: the Xanax, codeine, Ritalin, and Restoril.

See more about chronic fatigue syndrome on page 371 in chapter 8.

Q: I have two questions about Valium. Can Valium, in and of itself, cause ill effects, if taken over a long period of time? Will someone who has taken Valium for many years ever be able to stop?

A: Of all the sedatives, Valium is probably the most highly studied, and it seems to be eminently safe. Its most common side effects are drowsiness and fatigue.

Molecules in the brain called gamma-aminobutyric acid, or GABA, regulate anxiety. Valium interacts with those molecules to help a person whose level of anxiety is out of whack.

Valium is also used to help people get off other medications. We give it to alcoholics to offer some relief from the nightmare of detoxification.

Of course one can stop taking Valium, but it is a physically and psychologically habit-forming drug. Over time it takes more and more Valium to have the effect that was previously attainable at a lesser dose. Addictive is a strong word, and manufacturers hate to hear it, but the truth is that Valium can be hard to quit. So, I would call that addictive.

Many people who do quit are surprised to find that life without Valium is just the same as life with it. It is so gently effective that people spend years of their life on it when they don't need it anymore.

For most people, quitting cold turkey is too difficult. To stay on an even keel, I recommend that anyone trying to quit should notify his or her doctor and then cut down on the dosage bit by bit, week by week.

Q: My husband had back surgery four months ago. He is still getting fentanyl for pain through a transdermal patch. Now, he gets ill if he doesn't wear the patch. How can he break his dependence on the fentanyl?

A: He should go to his doctor for help, because he can't stay on the fentanyl forever. After all, he went through the surgery to be pain-free and drug-free.

Q: I use OxyContin recreationally, and I plan to stop taking it when I see that it's becoming a problem. In the meantime, what can I do about the constipation that this causes?

A: Well, let's start with your basic premise—that it isn't a problem yet. You're wrong. Using a narcotic painkiller that you don't need, just to have some fun, is a problem. And if you happen to be using it while you're drinking, you could kill yourself. So, whom are you kidding here?

Abuse of OxyContin has become such a problem that many states are looking at legislation to create databases for pharmacy transactions that would be available to police when they are investigating a doctor or user.

You need to stop worrying about the constipation and start looking at why you need to take this drug for fun.

Miscellaneous

Q: Can a person become addicted to Tylenol PM? I have been taking it almost every night for about a month and a half. Once or twice I went out for dinner and a cocktail in the evening, and I fell asleep without it. But on a regular night at home, I take it. I feel anxious that I won't fall asleep without it.

A: Tylenol itself is not addicting. The drugs that make up the PM part of it are mild antihistamines that are unlikely to cause physical addiction, but you can start to believe that you can't sleep without them.

Long-term, daily use of Tylenol, especially when combined with other pain medications, is associated with kidney disease, and you should not be taking it as a sleeping pill. You can get the part of it that makes you sleep in pure form—something like Benadryl—and avoid taking Tylenol. Benadryl is totally safe and will continue to work if you use it once in a while. If you take it all the time, it loses its effectiveness.

What I would most like is to see you learn to put yourself to sleep with sleep hygiene techniques. Research has found them to be more effective in the long run than medication. If you feel you need help achieving this, check out the Web site for the American Academy of Sleep Medicine, which has a directory of sleep centers in the United States (*www.aasmnet.org*). You can find more information about sleep hygiene on page 533.

Q: **I walked out on the chance for a good broadcasting job today because I refused to take a drug test. I know I would test negative for drugs, but I am ethically opposed to this invasion of my privacy. The terms were that I would hand over a urine sample to an unnamed lab, and sign a form releasing my test results to the employer and all its affiliates. The company would notify me if I passed or failed, without giving me any details.**

I can understand that people who are responsible for public safety might need to be tested. But broadcasting?

A: My personal feeling is that the policy you described is unethical, and recent research shows it is also ineffective.

I feel so strongly about this that if the company I worked for required a drug test, I'd do the same thing.

My other main objection is that like the D.A.R.E. program and this country's so-called War on Drugs, these mandatory drug tests don't work—serious drug users know how to cheat—and the tests can be plain wrong or biased. They also have the potential to be seriously misused.

Some companies do a drug test with hair, and everyone should know there is a racial bias with that test. One study in a forensic medical journal found that cocaine accumulates in dark hair and is detectable longer there than in light hair. So black people and people with pigmented hair are at a great disadvantage compared to blond people.

Mandatory drug testing should not be unleashed on the American public until it has reached a level of extremely high reliability. Tests that give a false positive just because the test-taker ate a poppy-seed bagel or took a cold pill should not cost people their jobs and impact their lives. In addition, we have not proven that testing in the workplace reduces drug abuse. And a recent federally funded study of 76,000 high-school students found that schools with drug testing did not have lower rates of drug use.

DEAN'S LIST: THE BENEFITS OF CAFFEINE

Everyone who has listened to my show knows I love coffee. From a purely medical perspective, here are just a few reasons why. However, do keep in mind that coffee, like any stimulant, does not affect everyone the same way.

Coffee:
- increases the size of brain cells
- can cut risk of suicide
- great headache reliever
- may reduce risk of gallbladder disease and colon cancer
- often increases metabolism and may help with weight loss
- improves stamina for long-distance events

Of course, the key is moderation. Too much coffee can be dangerous.

Yes, drug abuse sucks; it's a terrible drain of America's talent. But common sense says that before we implement programs, they should be evaluated objectively to see if they can solve the problems they are designed to tackle.

Q: My teenage son and his friends are taking over-the-counter caffeine pills to stay awake and complete their homework assignments. Is there any harm in this?

A: Caffeine is like anything else: Too much of it can kill you. If you pumped fifty cups of coffee all at one time into your body, you'd probably die. If your son and his friends are overdosing on the pills just to get a buzz, I would be concerned.

However, if they really are behind on their homework, you've got to teach your son to break this bad habit, get his homework done ahead of time, and get some sleep.

Now, as a parent, I know that kids don't want to listen to us. But do what you can to discourage his reliance on a stimulant in order to meet his responsibilities. Once these kids go on to college, they'll be tempted to try some more serious drugs to keep them awake.

If he still needs a little boost, see if you can get him to drink coffee instead of taking pills. At least then you will know the amount he's drinking, and coffee has less caffeine than the pills do.

Q: I found my teenage son in a state of hallucination from inhaling gasoline fumes. How dangerous is this? He is on medication, too. Will that have an even stronger effect on him?

A: Huffing is very dangerous, and you have to do what it takes to put a stop to it. Inhaling gasoline fumes—I'm not talking about the occasional whiff that floats our way at the gas station—is treacherous.

Gasoline is extremely toxic to our major body systems, including the liver and the lungs. Our liver detoxifies drugs in our bodies, so, yes, if your son is taking medication, huffing could be putting an added strain on a liver that's already working hard.

One piece of luck is that it's often easy to get kids to stop huffing, because it really makes them feel sick. But you might also want to haul him to his doctor, who can explain in detail what his life will be like if his liver fails.

Huffing is a good example of how criminalizing substances and waging drug wars doesn't work. Kids who huff are hurting themselves with stuff they can buy at the local hardware store.

Q: My girlfriend attributes her soon-to-be-ex-husband's philandering to a sex addiction. Is there really such a thing?

A: If you define your life by talk shows, it looks that way, but professionals are classifying excessive sexual behavior as a form of obsessive-compulsive disorder rather than an addiction.

By strict definition, addiction relates to behaviors and substances that are external to our biology. We don't have biological needs for alcohol, drugs, or cigarettes, for example. We can live without them.

But we can't live without food, and the species can't survive without sex. Eating and having sex are life-sustaining biological drives, so urges for food and sex are not addictions. Can they be dangerously compulsive? Absolutely.

Human sexuality is vast in its expression, making "normal" impossible to define. But sex crosses the line from biological urge to compulsive behavior when it puts your safety, your social life, your family life, or your job in jeopardy. Then it's something to take a look at.

Resource List

For information on clinical trials, fetal alcohol syndrome, common questions, and answers (in both English and Spanish), and the latest alcoholism research, visit the Web site of the National Institute for Alcohol Abuse and Alcoholism: *www.niaaa.nih.gov*

Alcoholics Anonymous now has real-time online AA meetings in six languages (English, German, French, Spanish, Finnish, and Swedish) as well as online meetings for men only, women only, and gay and lesbian members. The Intergroup of Alcoholics Anonymous Web site includes AA organizations in twenty-one countries: *www.aa-intergroup.org.* For all other Alcoholics Anonymous information go to *www.aa.org*

Looking for a free online community of people who have just stopped smoking or are about to do so? Check out QuitNet, a private company that operates in association with the Boston University School of Public Health: *www.quitnet.com*

For information on Chronic Obstructive Pulmonary Disease, see the Web site for the American Lung Association: *www.lungusa.org*

The National Council on Alcoholism and Drug Dependence's services include the National Intervention Network, with operations in eighteen states. At the NCADD Web site you'll also find a list of affiliates that provide treatment programs: *www.ncadd.org*

The National Institute on Drug Abuse has information on current clinical trials as well as links to NIDA-related Web sites dealing with marijuana, steroid abuse and "club drugs": *www.drugabuse.gov/NIDAHome.html*

If you need help coping with a family member or close friend who's an alcoholic, check out Al-Anon and Alateen. For information on meetings in your community, go to *www.al-anon.org*

Women for Sobriety is a self-help organization focused solely on women with addictions: ***www.womenforsobriety.org***

For information on the network of nonreligious self-help services for substance abusers, check out the Council for Secular Humanism's Web site for the Secular Organizations for Sobriety (SOS): ***www.secularhumanism.org/sos***

SoberCity is a free online community for people dealing with alcoholism and other addictions. It is not affiliated with Alcoholics Anonymous, but you'll find a strong AA influence at this upbeat site: ***www.sobercity.com***

For help with a gambling problem or to find a certified gambling counselor, call the National Council on Problem Gambling twenty-four-hour hotline at 1-800-522-4700, or go to the Web site: ***www.ncpgambling.org***

The Gamblers Anonymous Web site has a state-by-state meeting directory as well as a list of questions for anyone who suspects he or she might be addicted to gambling: ***www.gamblersanonymous.org***

For related questions see chapters 1, 8, 9, and 10.

Chapter 12

Life, Liberty, and Medical Miscellany

I know a woman who once called her dermatologist in California from a pay phone in Paris. Oozing poison oak had spread all over both her arms and she was desperate to end the misery—not prolong it. Since she only spoke five words of French, the Parisian pharmacists weren't much help.

She was laughing when she told the story, but she wasn't laughing the day she called her doctor. She needed to know that what she was doing to treat the nasty rash was the right thing, and then she could go on and enjoy the rest of her vacation. It wasn't life or death, it was a nuisance. And, lucky for her, she had a doctor she knew she could reach in an emergency.

I like being that kind of doctor for my radio listeners, the one who can set their mind at ease with a phone call—or give them a good reason why they should call their regular doctor ASAP or get a second opinion. And some of my favorite questions are among those that fall into this chapter— a combination of the "everyday" questions that aren't neatly categorized in a "Cancer" or "Aging" chapter, as well as the truly weird, even disgusting stuff that is what makes medicine so fascinating—and sometimes gives us a good laugh.

Sleep problems. Allergies. Headaches. Health scares. Aching muscles. Sweating. Odors. These topics pop up again and again, and they are impor- tant. But they aren't always on the top of your list when you see your doctor for a regular visit—or you are reluctant to call your doctor for what can seem like a "small" question. Then, too, you may not even realize you have a health issue until a topic is raised on one of my shows. Whatever the circumstance, you have reason to worry, so you call me.

Health issues can aggravate our lives—and sometimes scare us—but usually they don't stop us from living, and they seldom are life-threatening. When it comes to advice, more than anything we just want peace of mind that everything is going to be all right. We want to know when a headache is a sign of a sinus problem and when it is a hint of a possible brain tumor. And how many sleepless nights constitute a problem that needs fixing?

In fact, this chapter—and my show—are a little bit like a new health-care concept that I love and that I hope will flourish: the "group physical."

If images of a room full of naked women or men jump to mind, stop right there. That's not it.

I first heard about these physicals from a friend whose husband uses a health clinic in Palo Alto, California, which is staffed by a bunch of doctors from Stanford University. The friend's husband was overdue for a physical, and when he called the clinic, they said they were booked for the next four months. Sound familiar?

Then they asked if he'd like to participate in one of the clinic's group physicals. If so, he could see his doctor in about six weeks. The guy was curious, so he signed up.

When he told his wife about this appointment, she laughed, because he had no idea what he had signed up for—beyond the fact that they would send him a questionnaire to complete before the date of his physical, and he also had to stop by the clinic in advance, at his convenience, for a few basic tests.

The date for the physical arrived, and the husband's appointment was set for four P.M. Amazingly, he was at the clinic three hours—and not because the doctor was overbooked and he was stuck in the waiting room.

This man and about eight other men of similar age had gotten three solid hours of medical attention from the doctor and his nurse. The physical included private time with the doctor for each of the guys, and when they weren't each with the M.D. they were all together in a room, getting information from the nurse. The husband even got a bunch of small skin lesions removed from his face and came home with some advice for his wife about her toe fungus.

In other words, he got a complete physical as well as access to the questions (and answers) asked by all the other men in the room about everything from cholesterol to snoring to toe fungus—even if a certain medical problem wasn't his problem at the moment. Would he do it again? You bet.

While some folks will never be comfortable talking about their health anywhere but in the privacy of a doctor's office, one on one, I believe most of us are more curious than that. We know we can learn from other people's experiences, good and bad.

While no one visit with a doctor or any one radio show or medical guide can cover every imaginable health question, with these tools we can become familiar with the topics that most people are talking about.

This chapter is an oddball collection of some of those issues. They may have nothing to do with your health at the moment, but they're kind of curious just the same, and they're about subjects that no medical guide should be without. If you don't find the answer you need, call me and we'll talk. But do it from home, not Paris.

Sleeping, Sleep Apnea, Dreams, Night Sweats

Q: I sometimes fall asleep at the snap of a finger when I'm driving my car or when I'm at my desk. I go out with no warning for a few seconds. I have wakened several times just as I was about to hit another car or go off the road. What's wrong with me?

A: These stories always send chills up my spine. When I was in college, I once woke up as I was heading my car toward a telephone pole. I learned my lesson.

You have to make an appointment with a sleep specialist immediately. A seizurelike disorder called narcolepsy causes people to instantly fall asleep. One second they're awake, then bingo—with no warning—they're not. Sometimes there can be a trigger for the sleep attack, such as something that excites the person, or even makes them laugh. What's even weirder is that narcoleptics sometimes can't move when they first wake up in the morning, experiencing a moment or two of paralysis. A spacey or disoriented feeling also can be part of a seizure.

Apnea is another and more common sleep disorder, and its primary symptom is daytime sleepiness. Apnea is at the root of many traffic accidents.

People with apnea are often big snorers. They stop breathing when they snore, which makes their oxygen levels drop.

Check out the sleep disorder information on *www.drdean.healthcentral.com* and other Web sites.

Sleeping while driving isn't healthy for you or others on the road, so please do something about this. Your insurance plan will make you go to a family practitioner, and if he or she won't refer you, you'll have to get pushy. Tell them you've almost killed yourself driving off the road. Tell them you talked to your "cousin" the doctor and throw around words like narcolepsy, apnea, and wrongful-death lawsuit.

Q: Based on some sleep studies, I was diagnosed a couple of years ago with what the doctors call "narcolepsy with a question mark."

I do not have the traditional narcolepsy symptoms of collapsing into sleep. I just have extreme daytime sleepiness, especially when I'm driving. Even if I roll the window down, blast music, and sing, I start to doze. Nothing seems to work.

The doctor prescribed Ritalin, because he thought it would keep my concentration sharp and my energy high, but it isn't doing that. Within an hour of taking it, I feel sleepy. Coffee has the same effect on me. I know that's not normal. What should I do to fix this?

A: No, that's not normal. In pharmacology, that's called a paradoxical reaction—you get an effect that's opposite of what the drug should do. Some people get perked up by barbiturates, which should make them drowsy.

Coffee, like nicotine, is tricky. It has different effects on different people. Some smokers say that nicotine relaxes them, and some will tell you it wires them. Some smokers smoke nicotine in the morning and it gets them going, but the same smoker will smoke in the afternoon and it will calm him down.

QUIZ

On average, how long does it take for a person to fall asleep?
A) three minutes   B) seven minutes   C) nine minutes
D) thirteen minutes
(B: seven minutes.)

The Edell Report
Good Steps For a Good Night

Sleeping poorly is not good for your health. But the remedy may be as simple as practicing what the experts call "sleep hygiene." Here are a few of the basic rules, and you can find a lot more information on the Internet:

- *Don't go to bed until you're sleepy.*
- *Avoid naps.*
- *Get on a schedule, going to bed and waking at the same time every day.*
- *Don't exercise before you go to bed.*
- *Save your bed for sleeping and sex—not for reading, work, or TV.*
- *Don't stay in bed longer than twenty minutes if you can't sleep; get up but try to avoid light.*
- *Avoid caffeine, nicotine, and alcohol four to six hours before bed.*
- *Have a light snack before bed.*

Sweet dreams.

Hyperactive kids have the same paradoxical reaction to Ritalin and caffeine that you have. One of the ways to diagnose hyperactivity in a child is to see if caffeine will calm him or her down. Ritalin will wire a normal adult, make them speedy, but it seems to calm a hyperactive child.

The fact that Ritalin is not having the desired effect on you, and coffee slows you down, makes me question your diagnosis. Narcolepsy can be difficult to spot, and you should consider seeing a neurologist or sleep specialist for another opinion. You and your doctor might consider a new anti-fatigue medicine called Provigil.

You are putting your life on the line by driving when you're sleepy. You need to go back to the doctor for a different treatment or a different medication.

Q: My right arm gets so numb when I sleep at night that it wakes me up. I also have numbness in my right middle fingertip. This has been going on for years, and the doctors just shrug their shoulders. Then, recently, my arm swelled dramatically, and I was also really nauseous. But by the time I reached the doctor, my symptoms were gone. Should I push for some tests or am I being neurotic?

A: Nighttime numbness—especially in a nerve that is already irritated by daytime misuse—is almost always caused by a sleeping position that is compressing a nerve. The pressure leaves the arm temporarily paralyzed.

If you were to train a video camera on yourself all night, I'll bet you'd see yourself frozen in a position that is pinning the arm.

The swelling you describe is a much less common and more serious symptom that could imply a compromise of venous return—blood flow to the heart—in your arm.

Some people—and you may be one of them—have a bony prominence near the rib cage and the collarbone, which pinches and blocks the flow of blood. By taking your pulse with your arm raised in different positions, a doctor can find any spots with impeded blood flow.

Before labeling yourself neurotic, you've got to exhaust all the possibilities, and you haven't done that yet. Try pursuing this with an orthopedist.

Q: My husband gets bad night sweats frequently. What causes them? Is this something we should be worried about?

A: If this is something new, you want to find an explanation for the change. There are many serious illnesses for which night sweats are a symptom, including Hodgkin's disease, lymphoma, HIV, and many other viral diseases.

Lung disease is also marked by night sweats. The lungs are important in getting rid of moisture, and if they aren't able to do a proper job, sweating takes over.

I'm not saying that your husband has any of these conditions, and I don't want to scare you needlessly, but if his body's ability to adjust his nighttime temperature has changed, he should see a doctor.

A weight gain can be the cause of sweatiness. This is the simple physics of the relationship between surface area and volume at work. If we become larger and rounder, the body has less opportunity to blow heat off the surface of the skin, which causes more sweat.

It also could be something as simple as the fact that the room is too hot.

During sleep we don't control the room's temperature or our body's temperature like we do when we're up and walking around. Consider some of these diagnoses and have your husband see his doctor if the cause isn't obvious.

Oh, My Aching Back, Neck, Joints

Q: My husband injured his back nine months ago. The doctors' treatment plan was ten months of injections of sugar water in his back as well as a prescription for painkillers. He is still in pain, and his legs are going numb, and the doctors say nothing is wrong. I don't think he is getting adequate care. Do you?

A: Numbness in the legs can become permanent, so it is cause for immediate action. The sugar water–injection treatment is called prolotherapy, it's controversial, and not all back doctors accept it.

The very high concentration of sugar water is believed to relieve pain because its toxicity to tissue causes the tissue to scar and contract.

But, in his condition, your husband is in desperate need of a second opinion. You have a right to his medical records and X rays. You've got to take these to another orthopedist for a consultation, even if you have to pay for it yourselves.

Numbness has patterns of distribution like a watershed, where rivers drain only a certain part of a mountain range. The area of numbness gives information about the cause of the numbness. If only the hands and feet have numbness—what's called stocking-glove distribution—it is not due to nerve damage, because no individual nerves cover just these areas. The distribution of numbness may be influencing your husband's doctors in their choice of treatment.

However, when the legs go numb, you can't afford to play wait-and-see any longer.

Q: I heard you say that bed rest is now considered bad for bad backs. Is that the case for all back problems? I have periodic lower back pain, and I

The Edell Report
The Wear and Tear Drug for Boomers?

Everyone I know with aching joints keeps asking me where I stand on the supplement glucosamine. Well, it looks promising, but I want to see the results from a large study now under way involving more than a thousand people with osteoarthritis.

As many of you runners know, osteoarthritis is caused by the breakdown of cartilage, and it can affect all large, weight-bearing joints as well as the hands. This study is focusing on knees, and it's randomized, double-blind, and placebo controlled, so it should be the gold standard for glucosamine/chondroitin research. Participants will take glucosamine alone, chondroitin sulfate alone, a glucosamine/chondroitin combo or the placebo. The study, which is being coordinated by the University of Utah School of Medicine and involves nine medical centers around the country, began in 2000, so we should be seeing results sometime very soon. Stay tuned.

want to do what's best for the quickest relief. Also, is it true that the back braces lots of people wear when they do heavy lifting don't work?

A: First, a word of caution: Anyone with back pain needs to know what is causing it; I never recommend self-care for first-time sufferers, because the pain can be an indicator of anything from kidney stones or gallbladder problems to cancer or arthritis. Treatment should begin only after there is a diagnosis of the cause of the pain.

Now to your question. Evidence is confirming that the more you rest a routine aching back in bed, the worse it gets. People who get up and move around do better—and simply walking a lot can be one of the best exercises you do.

Back pain can be extremely complicated, and difficult to treat, and one issue that is getting more and more scientific scrutiny is back surgery. An excellent surgeon I know who operated on football great Joe Montana's back tries to avoid surgery whenever possible. He noticed that most patients say, "Doc, it's OK as long as I sit just like this." Starting from that position of comfort, he teaches the patient to acclimate the back. He teaches the person how to maintain that one pain-free position as he gets in and out of bed, gets up and down from the chair at the kitchen table, stands to wash dishes or eases into the car. Then he helps him slowly strengthen his muscles from those pain-free positions.

"Slowly" is the key word here, because as back-pain sufferers know, suddenly going into deep knee bends or toe touches gets us into real trouble.

In general, back-specific exercises are where most orthopedists should start with treatment today. And surgery is the very last resort, with success highly dependent on the type of problem being corrected. If you are considering surgery, especially something as highly invasive and, thankfully, controversial as spinal fusion, don't do anything until you've read an article by Dr. Jerome

QUIZ

True or False? A survey of orthopedic surgeons recommended hard mattresses for people who suffer from lower-back pain.

(False. Seventy percent of the surgeons questioned recommended a firm mattress, and 95 percent said that mattresses play a key role in managing back pain. Only 9 percent recommended a hard mattress.)

Groopman (see *www.jeromegroopman.com*) that appeared in the *New Yorker* magazine. It shows you just how complex back pain is to both diagnose and treat.

As for back braces, research shows that while workers say they feel better when they wear them, there is no reduction in injury.

Q: I have a carpal tunnel problem. The chiropractor says that a protruding disk in my neck is causing all the pain. Can you explain this in more detail? And does this sound right?

A: A disk in your neck can cause pain in your arm, but it doesn't cause carpal tunnel syndrome. Tweaking your neck left and right all day long won't fix carpal tunnel syndrome, either.

Your first step is to get a correct diagnosis from an orthopedist. If you do have carpal tunnel syndrome, ask a hand surgeon about splints, exercises, steroid injections to relieve the inflammation as well as newer, less-invasive surgeries.

Q: I've been addicted to computer chat rooms for the past year. I prop my left elbow on the table when I type, and now I have tingling around my left pinky and ring finger. Will changing my position with my keyboard help? I now have it sitting on a little beanbag table on my lap.

A: The position you've used was probably compressing the ulnar nerve (known more commonly as the funny bone) as it passes across your elbow. Just sitting in a chair in a certain position, or even lying in bed with our elbows pressed flat, can put pressure on the ulnar nerve and cause the pinky and the pinky side of the ring finger to tingle.

QUIZ

What's the most important treatment for a muscle sprain?
A) a compression bandage   B) rest   C) ice   D) stretching
E) elevation
(*C: ice; it should be applied immediately, because cold constricts blood vessels, which controls bleeding and reduces swelling. Rest, compression, and elevation are also beneficial.*)

Adjust the keyboard so that it's more ergonomically appropriate (you can find guidelines about this on the Internet) and if you haven't already done too much damage, the change in position will make the tingling subside. You want to support the forearm itself, and not press against your elbow. There are fancy ergonomic chairs that hold your arms in the right position as long as you don't press your elbow against the chair.

If you have a permanent injury, you'll need to see an orthopedist who can diagnose and treat nerve damage.

The Ups and Downs of Blood Pressure

Q: I had a recent experience related to hypertension. I had two doctor's appointments, one in the morning and one in the afternoon. When the first doctor took my blood pressure, it was 130/80. When the second doctor took my blood pressure it was 170/105. Can blood pressure really fluctuate that much in a day?

A: Which doctor did you like more? I'm not being funny. There is a reaction called white-coat hypertension, meaning that because of tension or worry a patient's blood pressure rises just by being in the room with the doctor. And yes, blood pressure certainly can fluctuate that much in a day.

Dismissing white-coat hypertension as a temporary reaction is dangerous. Because your blood pressure is showing this sensitivity to stress, you need to keep on top of it. It's easy to track by yourself. Go buy your own blood pressure cuff and learn to use it, so you can see what your pressure is at home.

Then talk to your doctor about what action you can take to lower it. He or she may mention a major new study of eight hundred adults, who were generally overweight and had "above-optimal" blood pressure readings. Research found that you can lower your blood pressure without medication by making a variety of specific changes in your day-to-day habits.

According to a report in the *Journal of the American Medical Association,* the habits and changes that are most beneficial are 180 minutes of moderately intense exercise each week, a loss of at least fifteen pounds—if you are overweight—reduced salt consumption, no more than one alcoholic drink per day for women and two for men, and a reduced-fat diet that emphasizes fruits and vegetables.

How high is high blood pressure? The borderline used to be 120/80, but some doctors now think even that is too high, while others feel that's OK. There are no absolutes here. Ask your doctor what he or she thinks your target should be. Some experts say that if a person's readings are inconsistent they should wear a monitor for 24 hours to see what their blood pressure is when they aren't in the doctor's office.

Please don't take your situation lightly. High blood pressure has no symptoms, so it's often ignored. But it's a potential killer, and is often a primary cause of heart attacks and strokes.

Q: I have tried about nine different medications prescribed by my cardiologist to treat my high blood pressure. Either the drugs don't help, or they have disabling side effects.

So, the cardiologist suggested I try biofeedback or yoga, which appeals to me because I have had good results with biofeedback in the past. But today I received a letter from my HMO saying, "We have determined the service is not covered by the member's benefits plan." Isn't the HMO's decision a bad one, even for them? Drugs for the rest of my life are going to cost a whole lot more money than biofeedback.

A: First, I have to ask an obvious question: Did you use all the medications correctly? What doctors call "lack of compliance" is a huge issue, and one reason medications don't always have the impact that they should.

In addition, some side effects of medications will disappear over time. Is it possible you and your doctor gave up too early on one of the drugs?

Now, to your question: I used to fantasize about HMOs focusing on prevention, because keeping people healthy is cheaper than treating them when they're sick. All that most managed-care companies can see is that biofeedback for a month would cost more than a bunch of pills, even though the biofeedback might eliminate the problem. Many medical choices are penny wise, pound foolish.

Unfortunately, many HMOs are so up to their ears in day-to-day management that they don't take time to develop solid preventive programs.

I also used to dream that doctors would have the last word. What's wrong with that? After all, your doctor knows enough to understand the benefits that biofeedback and yoga could give you. The doctor is trying to do the best for you. So, go through the appeals process if you have the time and the energy. Give them a run for their money.

At the same time, do what you can to take care of your own health. Your blood pressure might improve if you lose a few pounds (if you've got some to spare), get some exercise, and lower the sodium in your diet.

I have no objection to you trying to lower your blood pressure without drugs. Some of these techniques would be the same ones I would recommend to prevent high blood pressure in the first place.

Fight for what you want, but not at the expense of your health. If biofeedback or yoga classes will help you, you might have to pay for them.

Some health plans do cover these options, but, of course, when we are choosing a plan, we can't always anticipate what kind of care we will need—and we may not be willing, or able, to pick the more expensive and comprehensive plan.

Allergies, Rashes, and Mold

Q: I used to get poison ivy every time I went fishing. Once when I had it all over my arm, a friend of mine, who is an elderly Indian man, brought me a little twig with the bark peeled off, and he told me to chew it into a paste and swallow it. I did what he said, and he then told me that I had just swallowed the root of poison ivy. Well, that was forty years ago. I still fish all the time, and I have never had another case of poison ivy. Did this work, or have I just managed to avoid poison ivy all these years?

A: I've heard stories like this before, and they scare me. I suppose that this could desensitize some individuals to the allergen in the poison ivy, but when it fails, it can kill you. It's a very dangerous thing to do. You were lucky. It's also possible the twig you chewed was not poison ivy.

The mucous membranes in your mouth do not respond to poison oak/ivy like skin does. In most people who are sensitive to it, poison ivy or poison oak would cause swelling and fatal choking when it touched their lips and mouth. Some individuals have died just from inhaling the smoke of burning poison ivy or poison oak.

Desensitization is an old Native American idea, and we have tried to use the concept to fight poison ivy and poison oak allergies by developing allergy shots in a series of gradually increased doses, but the results are very inconsistent.

The reaction to poison oak, which is on the West Coast, and poison ivy, which is on the East Coast, is your basic allergy, and people are sometimes surprised to learn that late in life they can become allergic to substances that never bothered them before.

Repeated exposure to the irritant is what makes the body sensitive to it. For example, someone who has been enjoying strawberries for forty years can become allergic to them in middle age. Poison ivy and poison oak can do that, too.

Once, I could walk through the stuff stark naked and not have a problem. But nowadays I'm not so lucky and I make sure I'm covered with pants, a long-sleeved shirt, and protective lotion.

Q: I am a healthy thirty-eight-year-old in agony with poison oak that started on one thigh and then spread to the other. After five days of misery, I called my doctor, who wrote me a prescription for prednisone. The dose is three 20 mg. tablets for the first two days, two tablets for the second two days, and one tablet for the last four days. The pharmacist said this is a very powerful dose. Is it too much, and what could I have done to prevent this?

A: I think you were talking to an inexperienced pharmacist. You've been given the recommended dosage of prednisone—which really is a miracle drug for the short haul. Unfortunately, when used for a long time, this form of cortisone has serious side effects, including thinning bones, stretch marks, buffalo hump, and a swollen, balloon face. People who are on long-term cortisone for arthritis, autoimmune disease, or to prevent transplant rejection are, unfortunately, familiar with these effects.

I do question if the prednisone will do you a lot of good five days into the outbreak. That's pretty far along in the inflammatory response to poison oak. However, since you've started it, it can't hurt to finish the prescription. In general, sooner is better when attacking poison oak and poison ivy with medica-

---

QUIZ

At what age are you most prone to allergies?
A) 0–3   B) 4–7   C) 7–19   D) 19–35
E) age isn't a factor
(A: 0–3, unless there's a family history of allergies, then it's 0–7.)

tion. But most of the time it will go away on its own, after plenty of gross ooz-ing and itchiness.

Contrary to popular myth, poison oak blisters do not weep and spread to new sites, and scratching doesn't spread it either. Any new blisters that pop up are occurring wherever the toxin touched the skin—blistering can take days to appear and may not occur in all spots on your body at the same time.

You can have fresh poison oak toxins under your fingernails and on your clothing, and you can get it from your pets, if they have had contact with it and then rub against you.

Essentially, the weepy, itchy, horrible rash is an allergic reaction to the toxin in the plant. Touching almost any part of the plant can mean trouble for some of us. But not everyone is sensitive to it.

If you are exposed to poison oak, poison ivy, or poison sumac, your best chance of avoiding the rash is to wash with soap and water and rinse with lots of cool water as soon as possible—preferably within fifteen minutes, according to the experts at the University of California at Davis. Also, put any clothes that were exposed through the wash several times before wearing them again. If your dog comes in contact with the plant, make sure he gets a bath—and wear gloves while you're doing that.

Q: Is it ever possible that exercise is bad for you? I break out in a rash every time I run, and while it goes away pretty quickly, it's very aggravat-ing. This happens at all times of the year.

A: There is such a thing as an allergy to exercise. I have it, but in my case it's all in my head. But American long-distance runner Deena Drossin has the real thing, and it's serious enough that she carries an EpiPen when she runs, just in case she needs to immediately treat a severe reaction.

You are right to be suspicious and concerned. Rarely, some people who seem to have acute asthma or who break out in hives or have some other skin reaction can actually be allergic to exercise and can have the same reaction that some folks have to peanuts or bee stings. Other symptoms can include the swelling of your hands, feet or face. However, the reactions are almost always mild, and there's only one known death linked to this disorder.

If you eat certain foods or take aspirin or anti-inflammatory drugs before exercising, those could be aggravating your situation. Seafood, celery, wheat and cheese have been identified as possible troublemakers.

To start, make an appointment with an allergist. If you don't get any answers there, see a dermatologist.

Q: I'm twenty-four and I've been playing tennis since I was ten years old. Just this year I have started breaking out in blisters on my arms and legs when I sweat during a game. I get hundreds of watery blisters. They don't hurt or itch at all, so I didn't even see them until my girlfriend pointed them out. What's going on?

A: I think you are having a reaction to the sun. Because you are sweating as you run around in the sun, you're assuming the blisters have something to do with the sweat. Sweating is not known to cause blisters, but the sun surely can. And certain medications like tetracyclines, as well as skin lotions, oils, sunscreens, even citrus and vegetables, can cause a skin reaction when you go out in the sun.

Did you ever hear of grocers' dermatitis? People who regularly handle everything from celery and parsley to carrots and citrus can be afflicted. And after Club Med organized a contact sport using an orange as the ball, it became known as Club Med dermatitis. The orange was passed body-to-body among scantily clad beachgoers without the use of hands. The combination of sun and citrus oils caused attacks of blisters all over those bodies.

The easy way to test your photosensitivity is to cover up with long sleeves and pants. You are sure to sweat, but you won't be exposed to the sun. If you still get blisters, we've got to look for another cause, and you'd want to see a dermatologist.

Q: I make breakfast every day in a diner. I had a bad cut on my hand and started wearing latex gloves with powder in them. Over six months I used about one hundred pairs every three or four days. Then my hands began getting really red and kind of itchy, and all of a sudden, there are millions of little lines and cracks all over my palms. The pharmacist said my hands probably got sensitized to the latex. Could that be right?

A: It's possible. Latex allergy is very common now. We never knew that before the latex era, but since hospital workers, dentists, and food handlers all now wear latex, we're seeing that it is an incredibly common allergy. We're also seeing it in people who use latex condoms.

To actually develop an allergy, you have to be around the thing you are allergic to, so that is why it is understandable that you went for a while without having any problems. And when you wear latex gloves a lot, you can get a superficial fungal infection of the skin because of so much contact with sweat. That much moisture alone could cause an irritation, or perhaps a mild infection. So it could be as simple as that.

If you do have an allergy to latex, there are alternatives such as gloves made out of polyethylene or some other material. Treat your hands with a hydrocortisone cream. The lines, which were caused by the inflammation, will go away.

Again, this is not necessarily an allergy. Remember that pharmacists are not dermatologists. Though they know a hell of a lot more than what we use them for, diagnosing a rash can be quite tricky.

Q: I had an anaphylactic reaction to hair dye, and my throat closed up. And when I am around perfume and cleaning fluid, I begin to cough and wheeze. Does this mean I suffer from multiple chemical sensitivity (MCS)?

A: No. If you go into anaphylactic shock from hair dye, and if perfume makes you cough and wheeze, you have asthma and/or allergies. That is not MCS.

You have diseases that we can treat pretty effectively. But study after study has shown that there is no such thing as MCS. When we put people in a room and—without telling them—pipe in these supposedly sickening chemicals, they don't get sick.

DID YOU KNOW?
BOTOX FOR YOUR ELBOW

If you are considering surgery for your tennis elbow, ask your doctor about trying Botox shots first. One small study found that 75 percent of the patients who received either one or two shots had good to excellent results two years after the treatment. The other test group in the study had surgery, and 85 percent of that group reported good to excellent results two years later as well. With both treatments, it took more than a year for the majority of the patients to see the best results.

Chemicals, and phobias about chemicals, abound in the modern world. Just turn on the TV to see the scare of the day. We're bombarded with messages about sickness caused by chemicals in the environment, and soon some of us succumb and start to feel sick.

Near my home, the federal government built housing for people who supposedly were chemically sensitive. All the two-by-fours were wrapped in foil, and plans specified concrete and other hypoallergenic materials. I told the head of the project that he wasn't solving the problem, that scientific evidence had determined that this is all psychological. The guy said, "We don't care about the evidence." I am still amazed by that comment. Your government dollars at work.

A few months after the project was completed, the tenants were sleeping in their cars, because they thought the new apartments had chemicals in them. Sleeping in cars? Think about all the fumes and plastics and "stuff" that builds up in cars, yet these people thought they felt better sleeping in them. That just doesn't make sense.

See related MCS question in chapter 8.

DID YOU KNOW?
BLACK CATS AND ALLERGIES

Black cats might indeed bring bad luck if you're an allergy sufferer.

One study found that dark-colored cats are the worst offenders when it comes to causing more wheezing, sneezing, and overall misery to people unlucky enough to have allergies.

While the reason is unclear, researchers at Long Island College Hospital in New York speculated that darker cats may produce more of an allergen called "Fel d 1" in their skin and saliva than do lighter-colored felines.

If you have a cat of any color and suffer from allergies, you need to see an allergist about possible remedies.

Q: First, I read about the real Erin Brockovich testifying before a California state senate committee about toxic mold dangers. Then I got a notice from my insurance company that my policy no longer covers mold claims. How can I protect myself from this?

A: Erin Brockovich became famous because of a toxic-waste case, but I don't know how she became an infectious diseases expert.

Unfortunately, toxic mold may be the next new health panic that is not supported by evidence. The toxic mold story is the following: There is a very unusual species of mold, stachybotrus, that one study claimed might have the ability to release spores in high amounts that could be toxic in the lungs of young children and infants.

That study has since been discredited, but not before the next great American health freak-out was launched.

People become easily confused on this subject, especially if they have ever gone to an allergist and been tested for molds, spores and fungi, etc. There are people who are allergic to mold, but it is not a toxic thing—it's an allergy. And those people have hay fever and other more commonly known maladies. They respond to household mold the way they might respond to dust.

If you have a moldy house, it's because dampness exists—you have a water leak, or your basement does not have a proper vapor barrier, or your house was built incorrectly. Or you may be living on the side of a cliff where there is a spring or other source of water. That is a problem that should be fixed; dampness is not a good thing.

But the idea that your fatigue, concentration problems, and lumbago are due to mold, and you deserve millions of dollars, is preposterous. To lawyers mold is gold, and millions already have been paid out. That's why, if you are a homeowner, your insurance company may have already sent you a special notice that mold is no longer covered by your policy. This reminds me of the days when women with breast implants were in court making claims about a disease that never existed. Billions of dollars were paid out during that panic.

I put mold in the same category as multiple chemical sensitivity (see previous question), which has already been proven to be a psychosomatic illness.

The "research" behind the mold "epidemic" is junk science at its best. There is no hard evidence that mold causes the problems you hear about. But lawyers will keep this ball rolling as long as they can.

See more allergy questions in chapter 1.

The Edell Report
Freshen the Air with Real Flowers

When the kitty litterbox gets out of hand, do you open up a pine or lemon air freshener to battle it out with the box?

If so, you may be creating indoor air pollution that is damaging your lungs. The same hazardous reaction that occurs outdoors between the ozone layer and pine forests appears to occur indoors with air freshener products.

When pinene—a substance emitted by evergreen forests—meets the ozone, tiny particles form. These submicron particles are small enough to be inhaled and they are regulated by the Environmental Protection Agency, because they aggravate heart and lung disease.

Indoors, in a laboratory, an observant scientist noticed that a white message board in the room was getting dingy. He examined it under a microscope and found a thin coat of submicron particles was being produced by limonine gas, from citrus products, in reaction to ozone.

This led to an experiment. Researchers sprayed a coffee table with a lemon-scented wax and exposed it to ozone. The tiny, penetrating particles began forming within thirty minutes.

More research is needed to understand the health implications, but I hate air fresheners, especially in cars, and this is just one more reason to avoid them.

Organ Transplants and Donations

Q: I am under pressure from my husband to see if I would be approved as a liver donor for his stepmother. I am not close to this woman and neither is he, but he seems to feel some obligation toward her, and he can't be a donor himself. I love my husband, but I'm very concerned about putting our family in jeopardy since we have two teenagers. What are the risks involved with this surgery?

A: Your husband has put you on the spot, and I don't blame you for being upset. Many facts should be considered before you make this decision, but the bottom line is: It's your body and you should not do this unless you are totally convinced it is the right thing to do. Don't feel guilty saying no.

Living-donor liver transplants are an amazing thing—and they are becoming more common every day, which is fortunate, since lots of folks with hepatitis C eventually need this surgery, and it works with children, too. The success rate is very high, but this is major surgery involving a vital organ, and there are risks for both the recipient and the donor.

Donors don't have to be related, but your blood type has to be compatible. If that were the case, and you were to volunteer as a possible donor, you would have to go through a variety of screening tests before it was determined that you were the right donor. Some facilities also have age limits for the donor, so that could be a factor, too.

The actual surgery involves the removal of about half of the donor's liver, and the donor's portion of the surgery normally lasts about five hours. The donor is usually hospitalized for about five to seven days, and it typically takes about six weeks to two months for a full recovery. As I said, this is major surgery.

The liver is a fascinating organ and a resilient one. In successful surgeries, the donated portion of the liver doubles in volume within two weeks and reaches 100 percent volume within the first sixty days. The donor's liver regenerates quickly at first, reaching about 75 percent of its size within three months. But then the regrowth slows down, and it takes more than a year to return to its original size—and women see slower regrowth than men.

Again, you alone can make this decision. Make sure you know about all the risks. Good luck.

Q: I'm an extremely healthy fifty-seven-year-old man. I've never been sick a day in my life. I would like to donate one of my kidneys while I'm still alive. I called a couple of nephrologists and they seemed uninterested. Why is that?

A: Putting your own health at risk to give a body part to a stranger is such an unusual act of such extreme generosity that I can see why people might be suspicious or guarded. However, there is a better way to go about this, and you may be successful in finding a good home for your kidney.

What you want to do is called a "nondirected donation," and there's a lot of information on the specifics of this process at the National Kidney Foundation Web site (*www.kidney.org*), including a directory of transplant centers around the country. Basically, once you've done the research and became totally familiar with what's involved, you can call these centers and ask to talk to the kidney transplant coordinator. He or she can tell you if that center accepts nondirected donations.

One big thing you need to know is that donors are never financially compensated for their organs. You would be responsible for any travel expenses (if the surgery was occurring in another city or state) and time lost from work.

Your desire to give is a wonderful thing, and I urge you to pursue this, if you can afford to. The need is great.

Q: With so many men dealing with prostate problems, what are the chances of doing prostate transplants?

A: This is not something we are going to see in the near future.

Two major factors for successful transplants are the body's acceptance of the new organ and the mechanics of removing and replacing the organ.

At this point, I don't think we would have trouble with acceptance, but the anatomy of the prostate makes for a daunting mechanical challenge. The prostate is wrapped around the outlet of the bladder and has hundreds of nerves and connections.

Because the prostate is not a necessary organ—sorry guys, but we can live without it—overcoming the complexities of the surgery is not as pressing as is the search for other medical solutions. Simply removing a sick prostate is a satisfactory solution.

Medical Practices, Records, Insurance, Etc.

Q: I just found out that my girlfriend pays extra money every month so she can talk to her doctor whenever she wants to. She is a lawyer, so she has a good income and good insurance, but I know she's paying a lot to do this. What do you know about this?

A: Welcome to the troubled world of modern medical practices. "Boutique medicine," "concierge," or "retainer" practices have sprung out of a desire by many doctors to have smaller practices that allow them to spend more time with patients and avoid the hassles of insurance paperwork. But they are highly controversial.

Boutique practices require a membership or retainer fee from patients who receive, in return, such things as same-day appointments, twenty-four-hour, seven-day-a-week access to doctors, and other conveniences. The membership fee varies, but I've heard of amounts ranging from $1,500 to several thousand dollars—and that's an annual fee. What the fee covers varies with the practice. It may include an annual screening and a plan for preventive care, but generally it does not cover lab tests, prescription costs, specialists, or hospitalization, and patients are encouraged to keep some insurance.

Within some medical practices, patients have been dropped if they chose not to become members, although most doctors who move into boutique practices try to find new doctors to take over their existing clientele—those patients who choose not to move with the doctor.

Some opponents of this service call it "pay for privilege" health care, and while that may be an accurate description, I'm not going to beat up on any doctor who wants to provide a better level of care and has patients who are willing to pay for it. That's capitalism. I've seen too many folks who are more than willing to pay $40,000 to $50,000 for an SUV, or $3 a day for a latte, but who resist paying for the cost of modern medicine and keep pining for the "good old days." The "good old days" are long gone.

Q: My insurance company won't pay for a routine sigmoidoscopy, so I want to ask my doctor if he'll write down that I've had some bleeding. What do you think?

A: In the short term, you might get away with this, but think of the long term. You will have this symptom on your medical records forever, and that could affect your future insurance coverage.

Beyond your individual dilemma, your question reflects the larger social problem that would require a person to ask this of his doctor in order to get the care he wants. Insurance companies want doctors to practice cookbook medicine. In other words, to treat patients according to a recipe. Well, some of us cook quickly and some of us cook slowly. In a doctor's office, the test that's appropriate for one might be inappropriate for another.

But be careful about pushing your doctor to make up a symptom to justify a test. And don't be surprised if your doctor says no. Of course, if you do fib about some bleeding, then the insurance company is obligated to do the test.

Q: Last year I had a stroke and was hospitalized. When I saw my medical records, I was shocked and upset to see that I am described as an alcoholic. This isn't true. How can I get my records changed? Should I ask my doctor to write in there that I'm not an alcoholic?

A: No. A note like that will only bring attention to the error.

You should get the statement expunged. In some states—I know California is one—you have a right to your medical records. The hospital might give you the runaround and attempt to blow you off with just a summary, but insist on finding the place in the records that has the damning note.

Unless you are a regular patient, how would the doctor even have that fact or make that judgment? There aren't any tests for alcoholism. There's no way of knowing for sure, unless the patient admits the fact.

You can imagine the complexity of record keeping in a hospital. Amazingly, it's not all computerized, but that's another story. Usually, after examining you and taking your history, the doctor goes into a corner someplace and dictates through a phone line to the medical records department.

Doctors are often rushed, and they talk fast and zip over things. Very easily, "no history of alcoholism" can be heard as "alcoholism." The doctors are supposed to sign off on the reports, but you can be sure they don't sit and read every page. They just cross their fingers and hope. And that's the story of how mistakes end up in medical records.

The doctor should be very willing to have the error corrected. If you have a good relationship with the doctor, just request the change. If not, ask, "What evidence do you have that I'm an alcoholic? Correct that report or I'll sue you."

However, should you be an alcoholic in complete denial about your condition, this last comment would be unwise.

I am a bit curious about what you actually saw, because doctors don't usually use the word "alcoholic" in medical records. We have special lingo for sensitive situations. For instance, the doctor might have simply noted "ETOH," the scientific notation for alcohol, or scribbled something like "patient has odor like alcohol." The note could even have referred to a family history of alcoholism. So, start by asking him just what is in the file.

Q: Some of the doctors listed in the directory provided by my insurance company are board certified and others are not. Is this important when picking a pediatrician?

A: Yes. Board-certified physicians have passed rigorous examinations by other physicians in addition to completing medical school and residency. You want a board-certified pediatrician.

Some insurance lists are outdated, and some older doctors with decades of experience may be practicing from an era when board certification was not well established. So, if you're interested in a doctor who's not listed as certified, double-check with another source to verify the doctor's credentials.

Q: Where can I find statistics on complications and outcomes of various surgeries? With cataract surgery, for example, what are the chances of a poor outcome?

A: The simplest questions are sometimes the toughest and most important ones to answer.

You can find this kind of information in medical journals or online by doing a search on the specific type of surgery. You also can contact a university medical center or just ask your doctor.

Research is done to analyze and monitor data on the complications and outcomes of surgeries. However, so many variables are involved that statistics alone are not usually useful in assessing specific surgeries and the doctors who perform them.

For example, some of the best surgeons have statistically poorer results than their less-talented colleagues. Why? Because the best doctors often handle the most dire and toughest cases.

Also, a very good doctor working with mostly socially disadvantaged patients is going to have poorer results because of the generally poor health in this population.

And the complication rate that is the norm for some types of surgery would be outrageous for other types. We recently reported that stomach stapling has a 41 percent rate of long-term complications. This would be intolerable in obstetrics or orthopedics.

Finally, a doctor can do a perfect surgery and get a bad outcome. In some situations, the doctor does everything right, and still the patient hemorrhages. It's not the doctor's fault, but it will show up on the statistics as a preventable error.

I applaud you for being a good health consumer. The information that will be most valuable to you is your own surgeon's experience and success rate. It is fair to ask the surgeon how many such operations he or she has done and, using cataract surgery, for example, what percentage of the patients had 20/20 vision after surgery.

A surgeon goes into cataract surgery, by the way, not knowing if removing the cataract will solve the problem or if the retina is damaged in some way that surgery can't fix. So we cross our fingers and operate. Ninety-five percent of the time it works.

When the Bugs Are Biting

Q: Why do I attract more mosquitoes than my husband does? When we went to Tahiti, I got about forty bites within a few days, and he had about six. And he does not use repellent.

Also, is it true that vitamin B makes you smell bad to mosquitoes?

A: No objective evidence that I know of backs up the vitamin B anecdotes, although I have heard them, too.

When I was traveling in Africa, my companions were getting bitten like crazy, but I was the lucky guy, like your husband, whom the mosquitoes kept away from.

Scientists have discovered that three chemicals in human skin are attractive to mosquitoes. People with the combination of these three particular chemicals are bitten with much more frequency than are the folks without it.

Primary prevention is the best defense against these critters: Mosquitoes particularly favor arms and legs, so cover up with loose, light-colored clothing, and go scent-free.

In other words, don't use any perfumes, or lotions or shampoo that contain them. I wouldn't even trust products that are labeled "unscented." Mosquitoes can smell the carbon dioxide on your breath, they can smell when a woman is ovulating, so sniffing out an unscented moisturizer is a cinch for them.

Also, taken prophylactically, the antihistamine loratadine, which is Claritin, inhibits the size of the bites. If you are the type who gets huge welts when you are bitten, this will prevent them.

Finally, mosquitoes are at their worst from dusk to dawn. If you've ever spent time in the south, you'll notice that folks sitting out on the porch will

DEAN'S LIST: BE SAVVY ABOUT THE INTERNET

I love what the Internet offers health consumers. And I hate what the Internet offers health consumers. So here are a few of my guidelines for sorting the good stuff from the bad:

1. Consider the source of the information; if it's a known university medical center or a government agency, you're on safe ground. If it's a nonprofit organization, be careful. Most are excellent, but there are a few groups with an obvious bias toward one type of treatment or a controversial diagnosis. When in doubt, see who is operating the Web site by clicking on the "About Us" button or study the board of directors or staff list. If there are no medical doctors on the board of a health-related site, be very cautious. And even if there are, keep your eyes open.

2. If the Web site's URL ends with ".com," that means it's a business. It may be a good business (the Mayo Clinic Web site ends with a .com, and it's a great site), but many health-oriented Web sites that have a ".com" in their name want to sell you something. And many times that product is a supplement or a treatment scam. If a site is primarily used to sell a product, please don't use that site for any health advice!

3. Many excellent government-operated sites have links to other health Web sites for a related topic. In general, that's a good way to find additional reliable information.

4. If a product is only sold on the Internet, please beware. There's a reason you can't find it in retail stores in your community.

5. Finally, when in doubt about information from one Web site, double-check it against another Web site that is unrelated to the first.

pick up and move inside as the sun goes down because "the mosquitoes are beginning to bite."

Q: I was stung on the top of my foot by a yellow jacket. I tried a paste of papain, containing meat tenderizer and a little water, on the area and it worked. I put it on, and it immediately took the pain away. My foot didn't swell up. Will this work for all bites?

A: I don't know—and I'm not sure this solution would even work again on a yellow-jacket bite. I say this because a yellow jacket will inject various amounts of venom when it stings, and you can get various reactions.

I play a lot in the country, so I'm stung all the time and I've been stung by yellow jackets; there can be a big, big swelling or nothing. So I don't know, as an individual, if I put something on it, whether the results will be consistent from bite to bite.

But your home remedy is known, and the thought behind it is that the papain, which is a protein-dissolving enzyme, dissolves the protein-based toxin produced by the injecting insect.

Now, there are doctors who do not believe this at all. They'll say it's worthless, because the papain does not penetrate into the skin and tissues where the toxin is. Some doctors will say that this is just an old wives' tale.

I've not seen good enough studies to prove this, one way or another. I have no objections to you trying this, because if it does work, it's going to take years for the scientists to find out that it's true. So you've beaten the system.

And if your solution doesn't work all the time? Well, you haven't hurt yourself either, unless, of course, you have one of those severe bee allergies and are sitting around putting meat tenderizer on your wound when you should be going to the emergency room or giving yourself an epinephrine injection to save your life. Then your home remedy could be a negative.

I was once so stupid. I was outside in a bathing suit at my country place, digging with a pick ax, trying to dig some little steps into the riverbank. I got into a yellow jackets' nest, and they attacked me en masse.

Now, smart guy that I am, I started swinging at them with the pick ax instead of running, which is what you are supposed to do, because they won't follow you too far. Well, they won. I was stung all over and I felt like a real fool.

Q: Is there really such a thing as bed bugs? My sister is always claiming she's being bitten while she's sleeping at my parents' house in South Florida. My mom says she's crazy.

The Edell Report
The Hard Facts on Repellents

If you really want to avoid a mosquito bite, don't waste your money on gimmicks and repellent wanna-bes. The bottom line is that you will get the best, long-lasting results with a repellent that contains DEET—and the more DEET the better. But if you must go natural, think soybeans.

The results of a repellent study published in the New England Journal of Medicine *also found that:*

- *A product with 23.8 percent DEET had a protection time of about three hundred minutes.*
- *A soybean oil-based product kept the mosquitoes at bay for about ninety-five minutes.*
- *A repellent with a smaller amount of DEET, 4.75 percent, still provided protection for about eighty-eight minutes.*
- *A treatment using a chemical called IR3535 repelled the critters for about twenty-three minutes.*
- *Repellent-doused wristbands did not work at all.*
- *All other botanical-based repellents, including citronella, eucalyptus, peppermint, lemongrass, and geranium, worked for less than twenty minutes.*

Now, are you ready for a picnic?

A: I have no intention of getting in the middle of a family argument, but bed bugs are real, and they do bite, and one species prefers the tropics—so your sister may be on to something. She needs to look for proof of her claim—if the bugs do exist—and the bed sheets should answer the question.

Bed bugs love blood, and while their bites are often painless, they may spend several minutes nibbling on a human, and small, brownish-bloody spots on the sheets are a fairly common indicator of their presence. When they aren't eating, they usually hide in the mattress, bed frame, bed linens or pajamas, and other protected spots.

The bugs are tiny, wingless, and oval-shaped, and they are brown unless they've just finished eating, when they turn red from all the blood they've consumed. They have resurfaced around the United States in the past few years, and some experts think this is linked to an increase in international tourism—the bugs arrive in luggage. In general, they are difficult to eradicate, because they can go months without eating. The good news: They do not transmit diseases. I know, not great news. But it's the best I can do.

Can You Hear Me?

Q: My father-in-law has a problem with tinnitus. I looked it up on *www.drdean.healthcentral.com* **yesterday and found an article by a doctor who has successfully treated people with lidocaine. How common is this treatment?**

A: Tinnitus, a ringing in the ears, is extraordinarily common and can be caused by many different ear diseases, so diagnosis is extremely important.

As for treatment, your father-in-law should show the article to his ear, nose, and throat doctor and see what he thinks. If you aren't satisfied with the response, you can always call the doctor who did the original research; he or she may know other doctors who have either participated in the studies with them or who have written them letters about it, and they may be able to help you.

Lidocaine is a prescription drug used for other purposes. This is an off-label use, but it seems fairly safe. We often don't have any specific cure or treatment for ringing in the ears. It depends on the cause. For a full list of treatment options, from biofeedback to "retraining," check out the Frequently Asked Questions page at the American Tinnitus Association Web site (*www.ata.org*).

A lot of us from the rock 'n' roll generation are going to wind up with this ailment as we grow older, because we went to too many loud rock concerts without earplugs.

Q: My eighteen-year-old daughter went to a shooting range, and the earphones she was told to wear to protect her ears didn't fit her properly. When she came home, she said that her ears were ringing, and four months later they're still ringing erratically. What can we do to heal them or restore them back to normal?

A: She's got to find out what's going on right away. Have the doctor check to see if she ruptured an eardrum or see if anything else is wrong.

Tinnitus is a ringing in the ears like she is experiencing (see previous question). Most of the time it lasts for a couple of days and then it heals. But we think it's similar to radiation, in that your lifetime exposure to loud noises determines your hearing loss as you age, and it is a very subtle thing indeed. In other words, the amount of noise that most of us would find obnoxious in this day and age can be damaging on a cumulative basis.

Sometimes we make the mistake of assuming that because two things happen together that it's cause and effect, but she could have something else going on.

There are a variety of inner-ear disorders and diseases where ringing in the ear is a symptom.

Q: I did a deep-ear cleaning with a Q-tip because I had a lot of wax. I think I pushed a plug of wax further in. I bought a kit at the drugstore, and I put drops in my ear for five days and irrigated with warm water to soften the wax according to the instructions, but nothing happened. Should I just let it loosen by itself?

A: The rule is never, ever poke a cotton-tip applicator or anything else beyond the opening of the ear canal. If you can picture the twists and turns of the ear canal, this is like trying to clean a big, curvy pipe with a toilet plunger. Poking and prodding will not pull anything out; it only packs in the wax more deeply.

You've done everything you can do. Go to a doctor for a quick and easy professional irrigation, and to be sure your eardrum is not punctured. Don't fool with it anymore.

Head Injuries and Headaches

Q: I was hit with full force in the skull a couple of weeks ago. For about three days, I was in a daze with severe headaches and nausea. I went in and had an MRI done, but it didn't show anything. Is that normal?

A: That is normal. It wouldn't show anything, even with a full-blown concussion, unless you fractured your skull or you had bleeding or some other physical sign of trauma.

Your injury puts you in an awkward category of people who are caught in the middle. You had a head blow that doesn't technically render you unconscious, though it came close, and yet you can suffer some of the same effects.

Post-concussion syndrome is a neurological no-man's-land. You could wind up with chronic symptoms, but they might not be documentable on a test. Although some doctors keep thinking they're coming up with ways of finding answers, it's a real problem.

You were smart to go to the doctor; headaches and nausea from a head injury should always be taken seriously.

Q: I've been diagnosed with ocular migraines. I don't have headache pain, like with regular migraines, but my vision gets weird. I see what I call a glassy streak. What can you tell me about ocular migraines?

A: Many patients with migraines report visual distortions or nausea before the headaches set in. Some folks get these premonitions, but not the headache. The visual distortion comes in lots of different forms, and artists with migraines have painted what they see as shimmering, zig-zaggy images.

If visual distortion happens without the headache, that's called an ocular migraine. Along with the visual disturbance, the symptoms people report include paranoid feelings and spaciness. Sometimes they experience the nausea, but not the debilitating pain that is common with regular migraines.

I don't ordinarily advocate treatment with standard antimigraine drugs for ocular migraines. It's most important that you have a good doctor who made this diagnosis, because it's very often missed.

Q: For more than twenty years, I had severe headaches where most of the pain was under one or both of my eyes. I talked to different doctors about this, usually during the course of my annual physical or during treatment for the occasional sinus infection, and it was usually chalked up to

---

QUIZ

What percentage of your brain is water?
A) 15 percent   B) 33 percent   C) 65 percent
D) 80 percent
(D: 80 percent.)

sinus headaches. And, often, sinus medications seemed to take care of the problem. However, my allergist finally sent me to a neurologist when a scan of my sinuses came back clear. And, within less than two minutes, the doctor said he was certain I suffered from migraines. Since then, I've gotten excellent results from Imitrex. My question is: Why wasn't this diagnosed earlier?

A: Aren't headaches crappy? And isn't it infuriating to think you went so long without knowing what was wrong? But, believe it or not, you're not alone. Many different head-pain syndromes have been wrongly blamed on the sinuses.

In one small study, a whopping 96 percent of the people who had self-diagnosed "sinus" headaches actually met the criteria for a migraine headache, based on migraine guidelines from the International Headache Society. Apparently, one of the things that has prompted the wrong diagnosis are symptoms that can occur with both migraines and sinus headaches, especially pain in the sinus areas.

So, anyone who thinks they are in the same situation should challenge their doctor on the point. And see a neurologist if you haven't already.

Imitrex is one of several treatments now used on migraines, and Botox shots are another—early studies are showing good results.

Q: I am constantly going to the doctor with a bad case of sinusitis. It's very debilitating, and I am so tired of dealing with it. Is there something more that my doctor could be doing to keep this from coming back again and again?

A: Good question—and you are not alone. Chronic sinusitis affects more people than arthritis, asthma, and congestive heart disease.

Your sinuses are hollow spaces in the interior of your skull. If your skull were solid bone, your head would be very heavy. It's like a construction technique: When you build a bridge, you don't make it out of solid steel; you have beams and girders and shapes and hollow spaces.

These hollow spaces in your skull are lined with mucous membrane. They secrete stuff all the time, and drain. When you get a blockage of the opening, stuff backs up, and you can get an inflammation or an infection—germs love places that are warm, wet, and dark. So the blockage usually precedes sinusitis (by the way, "-itis" means inflammation).

Many people think they have sinusitis, a sinus infection, or sinus headaches, and they don't (see previous question). It's very important to get this diagnosed by someone who is skilled in this, because there may be something

DEAN'S LIST: IS IT A MIGRAINE?

Migraine headaches are different from other headaches, because there are other symptoms besides the pain. If the following symptoms precede or accompany a headache, make an appointment with a neurologist:

1. Nausea and/or vomiting
2. Pain on only one side of the head
3. Visions of flashing lights, zigzag lines, or temporary loss of vision before the actual headache sets in
4. Sensitivity to bright lights or noises
5. Frequent urination
7. Tingling in face or hands
8. Speech difficulty
9. Weakness of arm or leg
10. Confusion
11. Abdominal pain and diarrhea
12. Movement aggravates the headache

else going on. It's very easy to say you've got sinus problems. We all think we know what that is, but it's a lot trickier making the diagnosis. Sinusitis's specific symptoms include repeated infections, persistent congestion, headaches, and facial pain. And the inflammation can lead to polyps.

Fungus is getting a lot of scrutiny as one of the primary causes of sinusitis, and one study at the Mayo Clinic found fungus in the mucus of 96 percent of the patients studied. It is suspected that an immune system response to various fungi causes the inflammation.

If you have it, one of the things to do is try to prevent routine swelling in your nose, which can block the opening of these sinuses. It can be very beneficial to get any allergies under control, because your sinuses can get blocked up during hay fever season or whenever your nose is reacting strongly to everything from dust to ragweed. If you've got sinusitis, you are more prone to sinus infections if your sinuses get blocked.

In general, a doctor's first treatment goal is to keep the passages open, and approaches may include inhaled antibiotics, steroids, antihistamines, and decongestants. Patients with asthma often have sinus problems, too, and the FDA has approved an asthma medication, Singulair, for allergies, which some doctors are using for sinus problems as well. In severe cases, surgeons may go in and blow out holes in the sinuses to keep them draining, because drainage is everything.

Nose drops can be a very effective tool. It's important to learn how to use them so that the medication gets up into the openings of the sinuses. The more "upside down" your head is right after you use the drops, the better. The drops can help prevent swelling and keep the sinuses open. You can also use antihistamines and decongestants if you feel that the swelling and infection are related to seasonal allergies.

As you can see, this is a complex issue, and I can't say there is immediate relief on the horizon. However, talk to your doctor about a fresh approach to your problem, because it sounds like you need one.

Varicose Veins and Spider Veins

Q: I consulted with a doctor about having spider veins removed from my ankles. He showed me just one before-and-after picture. I requested names of previous patients, because I wanted to ask them how their ankles looked at certain stages and when their marks went away, but the office staff said they don't give out patients' names.

What do you know about these spider vein surgeries? And what kind of a message is the doctor sending?

A: The doctor is sending a message about privacy. You wouldn't want your name given out, would you? People get particularly sensitive about privacy and cosmetic surgery.

However, I know why you're bringing this up, because I've advised listeners many times to ask doctors for other patients to talk to.

When a doctor gets results that really please him, he can ask that patient for permission to put her in touch with other patients. This method of providing references respects privacy, but, of course, the doctor is going to connect you with his most satisfied customers. He's not going to ask for referrals from a disaster case, right? And when he shows you photographs, he's not going to display his mistakes. That said, why don't you ask the staff if they could call a former patient and see if that patient would mind talking to you?

Your call does tell me that something is lacking in your relationship with your doctor, because he should be the one to answer the questions you have about stages of healing. Another patient may have different pigmentation than you do, and her results might not be anything like yours. I do applaud you for asking, though.

In general, spider vein surgery is a quick and simple procedure. I think you'll be very happy with it, but don't expect perfection.

Q: I've had varicose veins for twenty years or so, and I was recently diagnosed with superficial phlebitis (inflammation of a vein). My primary care doctor told me to take ten days off work, use warm compresses, and take Advil. The pain and swelling have gone down, but I'm scared to death it's going to come back.

Yesterday I saw a vascular surgeon to find out about having the veins stripped. He wasn't enthusiastic about that, but he did schedule a vascular reflex test to determine if the veins are functioning correctly. Is there anything else I can do to avoid more problems?

A: Ask your doctor about endovenous treatment—a relatively new, minimally invasive procedure for varicose veins that's normally done on an outpatient basis. Doctors use either a laser or a radio-frequency device to seal the veins shut. For you to be a candidate, your varicose veins must be caused by an "incompetent" saphenous vein, the main vein running the length of the inner leg.

The body has superficial veins and deep veins, and phlebitis in the deeper veins can be dangerous. It can cause an embolism or clot that can go to the heart and into the lungs.

So, the vascular surgeon is doing the right thing with a vein assessment.

Compression sclerotherapy also may be a solution for you if your varicose veins are small to medium in size. The doctor injects a liquid, usually highly concentrated salt water, into the vein. The vein goes "Ouch!" and it contracts. Then it is wrapped very tightly in an ACE bandage. It chokes, then scars, and goes away. Your doctor will know if that will work for your veins.

See more about veins in chapter 7.

Eyes and Eye Surgery

Q: I had LASIK eye surgery in December, and I'm now 20/20 in my right eye and 20/40 in my left. Now I'm a candidate for an enhancement proce-

dure to improve the 20/40. Am I risking my healthy eyes by trying to get them to be perfect?

A: Well, you've already put your eyes at risk once, because all these methods are invasive to the cornea. With LASIK, the doctor actually raises the whole flap of the cornea.

I wouldn't rush into this, because you are 20/20 in your right eye, and you really only need one eye to see clearly. The second eye gives you depth of perception and kind of fills in the visual field, and 20/40 is good enough for that.

Try a pair of temporary glasses to see how much difference 20/30 or 20/20 will make to your left eye. The doctor can make up the glasses for you. They all keep on hand glasses with little slots in them. The doctor will slide sample lenses into the slot so you can see if it makes a big difference. If so, then it might be worth proceeding.

Keep in mind that your vision may continue to change for up to a year. Be patient.

Q: I'm twenty-nine, and I've been wearing glasses since I was three years old. I have a lazy eye and severe nearsightedness. I have one of the worst sets of eyes in my doctor's practice, and I'm sure my lenses could be used for the Hubble space telescope. Is there a safe and practical operation to remedy this?

A: You may be too myopic to be helped by laser surgery, but you might be a candidate for a relatively new, clever use of an old technology, intraocular lenses. They've been around forever, and the procedure has been done millions of times on people with cataracts. Now ophthalmologists are using intraocular lenses to correct extreme nearsightedness.

Watch and wait as the procedure develops and long-term results come in. If it does pan out, lots of people will be able to chuck their glasses. Talk to your ophthalmologist.

Your "lazy eye" may be another matter. It happens when eyes turn in or out, or when one eye is more nearsighted than the other. This makes it impossible for the eyes to work together to focus on the same object and send one image to the brain. The brain hates double images, and since the brain is in charge, it turns off the circuit to one of the wayward eyes. The eye is healthy; the brain just cuts it off because the connection causes double vision.

Patching one of the eyes before a child is five years old may get the eyes to eventually work together. Patching the eye that has not been shut down causes the brain to start up the bad eye again. With both eyes working, a little surgery will align them to focus on the same object.

Much beyond age five, surgery can be used to realign the eyes for cosmetic reasons, but the eye and brain will not be able to reconnect and make a comeback. Peripheral vision may improve, but depth of perception won't be helped.

Q: My adult son has brown eyes, but his irises are changing to a silvery-blue color. This worries him, but his doctor is always really busy, so he asked me to call you. Is this something he needs to address?

A: Being intimidated by your doctor is bad for your health. If the doctor is too busy to answer your son's questions, then the doctor is too busy to have him as a patient, and he should find a different doctor. On the other hand, if your son feels like he's "bothering" the doctor when he calls, your son needs to change his thinking. People have doctors so they can stay well; the doctor wants to keep him well, not have him come into the office when the situation is already out of control.

Now I'll stop the lecture and try to answer the question. All newborn babies have kind of bluish eyes, because the pigment hasn't developed. Soon after birth, we get eye color. On the other end of the spectrum, as we age, the iris can lose its pigmentation and eye color fades again. This is a normal process.

However, some eye diseases are characterized by depigmentation of the iris, and some of these conditions can be serious.

So your son should make an appointment with an ophthalmologist—a medical doctor specializing in eyeballs—to get to the bottom of this. With a couple of quick looks, the doctor will be able to give him an explanation.

And make sure he sees a doctor who will answer his questions.

Q: The cataract surgery I had several years ago resulted in infections, and I haven't been able to see very well since then. My doctor recommends cornea transplants. How safe are they? Right now I don't see well enough to read, and reading is very important to me.

A: This surgery is meant for you. Make sure your library card hasn't expired, because you will need it.

Cornea transplantation is remarkably successful. Because the body does not reject a transplanted cornea as vigorously as it rejects other organs, we can implant corneas from cadavers with consistently positive results.

It is a very delicate surgery, so be sure your surgeon has done many of them. The sutures used for cornea transplants are so fine they actually float in the air like dust. Amazing, huh?

Partly because of the unique features of the eye, ophthalmologists have been responsible for several medical milestones. The first transplantations in the body is one of them. Also, in fighting herpes of the cornea, ophthalmologists were the first specialists to use antiviral drugs.

The Mouth: Taste, Teeth, and More

Q: I am forty years old, and for the last four months, my mouth has been very dry. I feel like I'm losing the surface of my tongue.

I saw a doctor, because I was going through a family trauma. I showed him my tongue, he gave me some blood tests and prescribed medicine for a viral infection. But my tongue is not getting any better, and it feels flat. I do have a tendency to burn it on hot tea in the morning. Could that be a cause?

A: You need to get to the bottom of this problem, but, as you already know, a diagnosis can be tricky.

The dryness could be related to the anxiety and stress from the family troubles you experienced, but we shouldn't assume that. Proper medicine means starting with the most likely cause, then going down a list of possibilities and checking them off until a diagnosis is found.

Dry mouth is a very real symptom, and it can have very real side effects. Tooth decay is one.

An ear, nose, and throat doctor can actually measure your saliva output, so that's where I would start. Then you will have a number showing that you either have enough saliva or you don't.

The most common cause of dry mouth is medication; even over-the-counter drugs can do it. Menopause can cause dry mouth, too, but you are too young for that.

Sjögren's syndrome is a disease whose symptoms include dry mouth. It is an uncommon condition that occurs most often in women who are around fifty years old. Other symptoms are dryness in the eyes and vagina, and also achiness in the joints. You can find more information about the disease from the Sjögren's Syndrome Foundation (*www.sjogrens.org*).

A condition called glossitis is an acute or chronic inflammation of the

DID YOU KNOW?
DO WHAT THE FOOTBALL PLAYERS DO

If you grind your teeth at night—or you wake up with a sore jaw—but you don't want to spend big bucks for a custom-made nighttime sleep guard, head for the sporting goods store. The teeth guards that all football players wear on the field should give you the relief you need. However, you don't need a helmet.

tongue that gives the tongue a smooth appearance. Maybe that's what you mean by "flat." I'm concerned that repeatedly burning your tongue could cause some damage, too.

Pursue this with an ear, nose, and throat specialist who is going to look for some answers for you.

Q: A friend of mine had her tongue scraped by her dentist. The dentist says it reduces bacteria. Is this true?

A: Tongue scraping was in fashion in Victorian times. Yes, bacteria on the tongue are the most common cause of bad breath, and scraping can remove the debris. It's worth a try if you're having a problem.

Before you go for a scraping, though, just try brushing your tongue. It will probably net the same result. It also will make you gag, giving you a preview of what happens during a scraping.

Q: Sometimes, when I sneeze or cough hard, a small white glob comes flying out of my nose or mouth. And I can see these little white specks (slightly larger than a pinhead) on the back of my throat. One time I smushed it between my fingers and it had a terrible smell. Is this serious?

A: I call these things "sneeze nuggets," but they have a real name: tonsil-loliths. They are kind of gross, but generally nothing to worry about. They exist because you still have tonsils, which is where these calcified deposits first form in little pockets. The deposits usually have bacteria in them, and that's why they have the awful odor. But your breath is probably not affected by them. Next time you see an ear, nose, and throat doctor, ask about these. One way to get rid of them is to have a tonsillectomy, but I wouldn't do that. Some folks have success with a Water Pic to wash them out, and you also could try a warm saltwater mouthwash several times a day, or buy a special saltwater mouthwash called Alkalol.

Q: I'm confused about fluoride, and I want to do the right thing for my family. Should they be taking tablets? We live in a rural area, and our water comes from our well.

A: First, it certainly is possible that your well water has fluoride in it naturally, and you should have it tested if you are curious. And if not, you may still be getting enough. The water that irrigates crops can contain fluoride, and so can your toothpaste. Fluoride is good for your teeth, period. But it is possible to get too much.

Some people give their kids fluoride in vitamins, toothpaste, water, etc. The harm is that it can stain your teeth permanently. And too much in an adult can make bones brittle. Don't listen to the fluoride foes who claim every disease known to man from cancer to Alzheimer's is caused by fluoride. It's a good example of how some people managed to miss so much about health and science in the entire twentieth century.

Q: I have horrible, constant burning in my mouth twenty-four hours a day. I can't even lie down to sleep, because my mouth burns even worse. I've slept sitting up for the last two years, and I've had enough of that. What kind of doctor should I see?

A: It sounds to me like you have acid reflux—which is more formally known as gastro-esophageal reflux disease (GERD). Your stomach acid is coming back up through your esophagus, and the acid washing over your vocal cords would burn. It also would give your voice the rough sound that I hear.

Besides heartburn, acid reflux can cause many mouth, throat, and even lung disorders. Make an appointment with an internist or gastroenterologist, because there are prescription drugs and over-the-counter antacids that might help you. Lifestyle changes can have an impact, too. Ask the doctor about avoiding certain foods, sleeping with a different type of pillow, and losing weight—if you have a weight problem.

If none of this works, there are two endoscopic surgeries that are very effective and much less invasive than past techniques. Previously, surgery to

DID YOU KNOW?
YOUR TEETH AREN'T KILLING YOU!

Mercury poisoning is a frequent topic on my radio show, and one particular call makes me crazy. The mercury in the fillings in your teeth is not poisoning you, and beware of anyone who says otherwise. We all have mercury in our bodies from different sources, mostly food. Yes, we can ingest high levels of mercury from eating lots of contaminated fish. That mercury is methylmercury. Fillings are a mix of metallic mercury and silver, and they do not emit enough mercury to harm you; anyone who argues otherwise is trying to sell you something—probably lots of new fillings. If your fillings are the only worry you have in your life, you have a good life. Mercury fillings are ugly, and there are more attractive restorative materials, but for price and longevity, the amalgam fillings have withstood the tests of time and science.

repair an incompetent esophageal sphincter, which is what causes acid reflux, could only be done by cutting open the patient.

Now, by going inside with just a scope, doctors have successfully stopped reflux by putting a stitch in the opening from the esophagus to the stomach. They are also using radio frequency to correct the problem.

There are many potential causes of a burning mouth, including vitamin deficiency, dental materials, and hormones. And there is actually something called burning mouth syndrome, but nighttime is not usually an issue with that problem. The fact that lying down worsens the situation makes me think that GERD should be at the top of a list of possible diagnoses.

Q: I took antibiotics for a week, and now I've got this metallic taste in my mouth. I looked at my tongue in a mirror, and it looks kind of blackish-and-white. Should I be worried?

A: All the germs in your mouth are locked in a struggle to make a living off the territory there. The regular, healthy germs in your mouth constantly battle it out with the bad ones. Taking antibiotics can upset the balance, providing weapons to the bad germs for an enemy takeover against the healthy ones.

I think that your tongue is temporarily overrun with germs that produce black pigment. These aren't harmful germs, and, in my experience, the good guys will regain this turf now that you've stopped taking the antibiotics.

Antibiotics kill lots of germs besides the ones we're sending them in to attack. Aside from the germs that made us sick, they also kill the beneficial germs. This is why it is so important for people only to take antibiotics when they are really needed.

Miscellaneous: Peeing in the Shower and More

Q: I have never bought underarm deodorant in my life, because I never sweat under my arms. My feet are dry as bones, and my hands are like sandpaper. I only sweat on my forearms and chest. Do I have something seriously wrong with me?

A: The simple answer is that we all differ in the number and location of our sweat glands. Also, the climate we grew up in affects how we respond to temperature. For instance, natives of tropical climates don't sweat excessively, but people who move to the tropics from somewhere else can be nasty sweaters.

You are an efficient sweater. So, while you're not seeing it, you are definitely sweating and sweating plenty. Sweat that evaporates as soon as the body produces it means that the body's thermostat is working perfectly. You never see or feel the dampness. That is very efficient.

People with sweat pouring off them have very inefficient thermostats. That's not the best way to cool the body—but if you are a professional basketball player, you may not have much choice.

When we block sweat from one site on the body, the sweat will come out in another place. For example, sweaty palms or excess underarm sweat can be corrected by an operation or an injection of Botox.

However, the trade-off is that the patient will then sweat more from the chest, the forehead, the feet or someplace else on the body. You, by contrast, don't have sweaty hands or armpits, but you do sweat on your chest and arms.

Sweat itself doesn't have a bad odor. That comes from the bacteria that are gobbling the debris on the skin. Antiperspirants stop sweat, and there's nothing wrong with them, but some people who don't need antiperspirants buy them anyway, because most Americans are paranoid about natural body smells.

Finally, at the risk of repeating myself for the millionth time: The aluminum in deodorants or antiperspirants does not cause breast cancer. This is an Internet/urban myth that won't die.

Q: I was a pilot in the navy a long time ago, and, in those days, I had mild problems with motion sickness. As I've aged, it's gotten worse.

My balance is thrown off. Sometimes, when I am lying down, just raising my head is enough to make me feel nauseated. I am planning a trip to Cuba with four friends, and this is very disruptive. What can I do?

A: You probably have a condition called benign positional vertigo, which is curable, so don't give up on your trip.

Make an appointment with an ear, nose, and throat doctor and tell him or her that your "cousin" the doctor thinks you have benign positional vertigo. That way we can spare you unnecessary tests and at the same time keep the doctor who examines you from having his feathers ruffled.

Benign positional vertigo seems to be caused by little calcifications that stimulate the tiny hairs in the inner ear when you move your ear. The doctor can remedy this just by rotating your head in a special manner. It's the simplest thing. You lie down, and the doctor twists your head one way and then the other, those calcifications move out of the way, and, *hasta luego*, you're off to Cuba.

Q: Should you keep a cut bandaged, or should you let it air out, especially at night? My mother is always smacking bandages on every little thing.

A: A small cut that is exposed to air closes within a couple of hours, sealed by the body's own juices. When you bandage a cut and remove the bandage the next day, the cut is still gaping open. So, for minor cuts, I favor air when cleanliness can be maintained.

But if the wound gets dirty and you get an infection, the worst thing you can do is let the cut dry out. You want to keep it a little bit wet, so it can drain and heal. And, of course, if it's a major wound, do what you're told by the doctor or nurse. Don't go unwrapping a stitched-up incision just because Dr. Dean likes air.

The Edell Report
When the Nose Knows

I love body smells, and I love what research tells us about them.

One of my favorites is a study that found that family members can tell each other by smell alone—but only if they're genetically related. Mothers are very good at detecting their birth children by smell, but not their stepchildren. Children are quite good at distinguishing their brothers and sisters over stepsiblings.

Thirty-four pairs of siblings (thirteen full siblings, ten half siblings, and eleven stepsiblings) were given a clean T-shirt to wear for three nights. The kids were all using the same unscented soap. At the end of the three nights, each shirt was put into a container with a small opening in the top for smelling. Each mother was given two shirts and asked which smell she preferred, and which she thought was from her own child. Psychologists at Wayne State University in Detroit, Michigan, conducted the study.

The biological mothers knew which belonged to their child twenty-seven times out of thirty. Stepmothers were wrong five times out of seven. Because the mothers had all been living with their children, results mean they must be using smell to recognize their children's genes, really, because what we smell like is a genetic thing.

Another fascinating bit of research looked at beauty and smells. Men were given the T-shirts of women, and the more beautiful women had smells that were preferred by the men. That's weird, isn't it?

Finally, odor often plays a role in the diagnosis of illness. Stale beer hints of tuberculosis, an ammonia smell is often linked to kidney failure or a bladder infection, and maple syrup tells a doctor the patient could have . . . maple syrup urine disease. And what odor says you are normal? Good old sweat.

DEAN'S LIST: WHAT'S IN MY MEDICINE CABINET?

First of all, I'm not a serious pill popper, so my medicine cabinet may appear rather sparsely stocked. I make no apologies for that. I think our society has been trained to self-medicate, and most of us spend way to much money on over-the-counter drugs we don't need.

Second, my supplies aren't kept in the bathroom, because that's too warm and damp a place to store most medications.

Third, the traditional medicine cabinet is often not a safe place to store dangerous substances if you have young children, so be careful.

Fourth, "house" brands now exist for many drugs, and they can save you lots of money.

Finally, what follows are my personal preferences and I haven't included prescription medications. To make sure you have everything you need to care for your family, ask your doctor for his or her advice.

1. ACETAMINOPHEN: Safest all-around pain reliever.
2. ASPIRIN OR IBUPROFEN: Good when there's inflammation *and* pain, such as arthritis or menstrual cramps. But be careful because these commonly cause stomach upset and bleeding.
3. TUMS: Great for occasional heartburn, and also a good, cheap source of calcium if you need more in your diet. If you need something stronger for your heartburn, see a doctor first.
4. ASSORTED BANDAGES: Be careful with that paring knife!
5. DIPHENHYDRAMINE: An antihistamine pill good for mild allergies and as a sleep aid. As a lotion, it soothes bug bites and rashes.
6. ANTIBIOTIC OINTMENT: I don't keep antiseptics around for cleaning wounds because soap and water work just fine. But if further protection from germs is necessary, dab on a bit of ointment and cover with a bandage.
7. OXYMETAZOLINE NASAL SPRAY: A stuffy nose is one of the most bothersome symptoms of colds and allergies, and this is the quickest, most direct way to relieve congestion.

8. PSEUDOEPHEDRINE HYDROCHLORIDE (decongestant): For those really bad colds.

9. DENTAL TAPE: I floss every morning because my dentist will get mad at me if I don't.

10. IMODIUM (LOPERAMIDE): A classic treatment for diarrhea that's always in my suitcase when I'm headed on vacation.

11. CORTISONE CREAM: works on a variety of rashes.

12. SUNSCREEN AND DEET (bug repellent): My wife and I spend a lot of time in the country.

13. ZILACTIN: It burns going on, but it keeps canker sores from being irritated by the foods I love to eat.

14. MECLIZINE HYDROCHLORIDE (MOTION SICKNESS PILLS): I hate throwing up over the side of a boat if I can avoid it.

15. ACTIVATED CHARCOAL: Find this at the drugstore, to combat poisonings, and while you're at it, experts now recommend that you throw out the ipecac syrup, if you still have it. It turns out that ipecac, which makes you vomit, doesn't work, and may actually be harmful. And some folks with eating disorders may abuse it. So, if your child consumes some poison, go to the phone first, and call poison control. Then administer the activated charcoal.

IF I WAS ON A DESERT ISLAND AND COULD ONLY TAKE ONE THING:

My pharmacology professor in medical school, after quizzing the entire class, voted for codeine. Why? Codeine is a very powerful painkiller; it will stop diarrhea in its tracks; it's a strong sedative; and it's the best cough medicine to be had. However, it is an opiate and you need a prescription. I don't recommend it on a weekly basis.

Q: What causes irritable bowel syndrome? A couple of my relatives have IBS, but when I asked them what caused it, they said that it was usually food, and they said it's more complicated than that.

A: IBS is a confusing and frustrating ailment. Most people have chronic diarrhea, some have constipation, but all suffer from extreme bowel discomfort with cramping and bloating. Unfortunately, some folks are so afraid they will lose control of their bowels unexpectedly that they no longer leave the house. IBS is also one of the biggest causes of lost days at work.

The cause, or causes, of IBS has been the subject of long-running debate within the medical community, and some doctors feel it is largely a psychosomatic condition due to stress, anxiety, and other emotional disorders—all of which can affect bowel function.

However, most doctors consider it a real condition that is probably caused by nerve connections between the brain and gut that don't work quite right. In fact, the gut has its own independent nervous system, and certain messages from the brain might irritate it, as well as gas or certain foods. The result often is painful bowel contractions. Sometimes these contractions stop the passage of the stool, and other times they rush everything out of the body.

Many people get some relief by experimenting with their diet, and avoiding those foods that seem to aggravate the condition. A wide range of foods can create excess gas that is usually caused by bacteria working on undigested carbohydrates, such as beans. In fact, one small study about IBS raised the possibility that excess bacteria in the small intestine is a cause.

Among the most frequently mentioned problem foods are chocolate, caffeinated and carbonated beverages, dairy products with lactose, sorbitol and manitol sweeteners, and gas-producing vegetables, like cabbage, beans, and broccoli. Fructose is a major troublemaker in our diet and can be found in everything from diet sodas to cookies. But it also occurs naturally in honey, many berries, and other fruits.

You can find a lot more information about IBS at the National Institute of Diabetes & Digestive & Kidney Diseases Web site. See our Resource List on page 583.

Q: How can I get my doctor to stop for thirty seconds and listen to me? I have a chronic foot problem called plantar fasciitis and every time I see my doctor, it's a wham-bam appointment. He wants to give me cortisone shots, and that's not what I want to do.

My general practitioner, who is awesome, has told me about other things that will help, like "Cathy, get up and move." He's right, because exercise has really alleviated my symptoms.

I'm in my mid-thirties, I don't want to have cortisone shots from now until I die. Is my only option a new doctor?

A: Some very good doctors are just hard to connect with. Others throw up barriers on purpose, because they're forced by the system to get rid of you in four minutes flat.

Before we talk about how to make the most of your people skills, I want to respond to what you said about cortisone and the pain in the bottom of your foot.

Plantar fasciitis is an inflammation of the tissue in the sole of the foot that connects to the heel bone, and it can be effectively treated with cortisone shots. These are shots that you don't need to worry about, because the cortisone is injected locally. They are mixed with a substance that prevents the rest of the body from absorbing it and applies the medication right where you want it.

This is different from your taking cortisone pills or getting a cortisone shot in your butt, which I would object to, because it's a steroid and it will go all through your body.

However, if you absolutely don't want medication, there are alternatives,

---

DID YOU KNOW?
IT MAY PAY TO SPLIT THE PILL

If you take a lot of medications, and some of them come in the form of hard pills, ask your doctor if you are a candidate for pill splitting. It's easy to do, and it may save you money every month. This is how this works: The doctor writes a prescription for a pill that is twice the dosage that you normally take. Usually, the higher-dosage pill is only modestly more expensive than the lower-dosage pill. Then, every time you need to take that medication, you take a half pill instead of a whole one. This does not work for any "gel" capsules, where cutting the pill is impossible to do accurately.

---

from orthotics in your shoes to night splints and stretching programs. So you're on the right track.

One way to expand communications is to get some information on treatment options from the Internet, print out what you find, and say, "Hey, Doc. Look at this. Is this worth a try?"

The doctor may be offended, but he may also feel like he can save face by focusing with you on a study from an orthopedic journal. Or, you can just smile during your next visit, look him straight in the eye, and say, "I'm not leaving this exam room until you answer my questions."

Sometimes, no matter what you do, it's not a match, and you just have the wrong doctor. At least your situation isn't urgent, so you have time to get recommendations from your general practitioner if you decide to make a change.

Q: My wife gave birth to our daughter twenty-one years ago, and when the nurse brought the baby into the room, my wife said, "This baby doesn't look anything like mine." But the nurse insisted the baby was ours, and that was the last we thought about it until recently, when three lawsuits were settled out of court for baby-switching at that hospital.

DID YOU KNOW?
BAD HABIT OR SOMETHING MORE?

This is a topic usually reserved for bad teen movies, but here we go: nose picking. Yes, there are researchers who've looked at this behavior, and when it reaches the level of a disorder, it has a very fancy name: "rhinotillexomania." Beyond that, here are a few facts you may or may not choose to remember: A survey of 200 adolescents found that "almost everybody does it," and the median frequency was four times a day. A survey of adults found that of the 254 who responded, 91 percent were current nose pickers. One respondent admitted to spending more than two hours a day taking care of business. We will leave it at that.

DID YOU KNOW?
SOCCER FANS, BEWARE:
WATCH AT YOUR OWN RISK

Watching a great soccer match may be good for you. Or maybe not.

It seems that deaths from heart attacks in France dropped by about 33 percent for men on the day that France beat Brazil for the World Cup in 1998. About 26 million French television viewers saw the game.

But Swiss researchers found that during very exciting penalty shoot-outs, heart attacks skyrocketed in their country. Tennis, anyone?

Our daughter has a different blood type than my wife and me. What's the next step to confirming whether she is our daughter?

A: Let's not be too hasty here. After all, you have spent twenty-one years telling your child that you love her and that she means the world to you, right? I would first be clear about what your goals are in pursuing this.

A child easily can have a different blood type than her parents. Secondly, we now have DNA testing, which is 99.9 percent accurate. No one uses blood typing anymore to determine paternity.

If after twenty-one years you suspect that your poor daughter is not your daughter, talk to your doctor about getting a DNA test. I don't think a different blood type alone is reason to be suspicious, though. But you want to be careful about the message you are sending to your child if you have this test done. Will she think you'd feel differently about her if she isn't your natural daughter? Maybe you can mention what's been going on at the hospital in a casual family setting and see if your daughter is even aware of the lawsuits—or if she is curious to know more.

You have some difficult decisions to make for you and for your daughter. Good luck.

Q: If you urinate when you're taking a hot shower, do toxic fumes get into your lungs? I'm thinking that maybe the heat vaporizes the urine.

A: I like your scientific approach to what's probably one of the most common secret human vices.

The answer to your question is that this practice is not at all dangerous. In fact, urine usually contains few if any germs.

Vapors or smells that a substance emits are not the molecules of the substance itself, unless we're talking about a pure, organic liquid, like alcohol. The smell of urine is not urine, but the smell of alcohol is actually alcohol itself.

The vapor in the shower is water vapor. This works like the boiling process does. When we boil a liquid, water vapor forms, and whatever else was in the water gets left behind as a crystalline deposit in the pot. If you boiled a pot of urine—this is probably more than anybody wants to think about—only water would rise from it, and crystals of uric acid would be left at the bottom of the pot.

DID YOU KNOW?
KNOW WHAT YOU EAT

Is it possible to have bloody-looking stools that aren't bloody? Does your urine tell you what you had for dinner? The answer to both questions is yes, especially when beets and asparagus are on the menu. One acquaintance had a full series of tests done after she thought she saw blood in her stools. The doctor forgot to ask her if she had eaten beets until *after* all the tests came back negative. As for asparagus, 50 percent of us are harshly reminded that we consumed the vegetable when we urinate, because of a distinctly sulfurous odor to our urine. Don't worry, you're not sick. It's just that the amino acids in asparagus break down differently in different bodies. It's genetic.

DID YOU KNOW?

What does the expiration date on your prescription meds really mean? Often, not much. Should you throw out the drugs? Not necessarily.

Ninety-six different drugs, which had been stored unopened in their original containers, were tested by the U.S. Department of Defense/FDA Shelf Life Extension Program. The test found that 84 percent had remained stable more than four years after the original expiration date. And some drugs remain potent for more than twenty years.

One notable exception was the epinephrine in EpiPen injections. These had lost potency only ten months after the expiration date.

When in doubt about your own medications, ask your doctor.

Q: I've seen an ad that says that airlines don't change pillows between flights and that I need to buy a travel pillow to avoid spreading colds. Does this mean I can catch head lice from an airplane pillow, too?

A: Here are a bunch of reasons why you should pick something else to worry about:

Lice really are not the type to hide in clothing, seat cushions, or pillows. They much prefer to jump from body to body. Their most common mode of transportation is from hair to hair. They might use an inanimate object as a landing platform, but they don't like to stay there.

See more about lice in chapter 5, on page 255.

More Resources

Also see lists at the end of each chapter.

General Information

The Agency for Healthcare Research and Quality: *www.ahcpr.gov*
Centers for Disease Control and Prevention: *www.cdc.gov*
Current information on clinical research studies: *www.clinicaltrials.gov*
Health & Human Services Office for Civil Rights (for information on privacy protection for health information): *www.hhs.gov/ocr/hipaa*
The Mayo Clinic: *www.mayoclinic.com*
National Institutes of Health: *www.health.nih.gov*
U.S. National Library of Medicine and the National Institutes of Health: *www.medlineplus.gov*
The American Council on Science and Health: *www.healthyfactsandfears.com*

Medical and Dental Associations

American Medical Association: *www.ama-assn.org*
The American Academy of Sleep Medicine: *www.aasmnet.org*
American College of Emergency Physicians: *www.acep.org*
American Academy of Physical Medicine and Rehabilitation: *www.aapmr.org*
American Academy of Periodontology: *www.perio.org*
American Dental Association: *www.ada.org*
The Society of Chiropodists and Podiatrists: *www.feetforlife.org*

Disease

Note: Thousands of organizations are dedicated to diseases, and only a few are covered in this list. For diseases not mentioned here, go to www.rarediseases.org or search the Internet using the name of the disease. Also consult the lists at the end of each chapter in this book.

ALS Association: *www.alsa.org*

American Brain Tumor Association: *www.abta.org*

American Cancer Society: *www.cancer.org*

American Heart Association: *www.americanheart.org*

American Tinnitus Association: *www.ata.org*

Chrohn's and Colitis Foundation of America: *www.ccfa.org*

Cystic Fibrosis Foundation: *www.cff.org*

Huntington's Disease Society of America: *www.hdsa.org*

Juvenile Diabetes Research Foundation: *www.jdrf.org*

Muscular Dystrophy Association: *www.mdausa.org*

National Heart, Lung, and Blood Institute: *www.nhlbi.org*

National Hemophilia Foundation: *www.hemophilia.org*

National Institute of Diabetes & Digestive & Kidney Diseases: *www.niddk. nih.gov*

National Kidney Foundation: *www.kidney.org*

National Organization for Rare Disorders: *www.rarediseases.org*

The National Parkinson Foundation: *www.parkinson.org*

Miscellaneous

American Chronic Pain Association: *www.theacpa.org*

American Foundation for the Blind: *www.afb.org*

Family Violence Prevention Fund: *www.endabuse.org*

National Headache Foundation: *www.headaches.org*

The National Institute of Environmental Health Sciences: *www.niehs.nih.gov*

National Sleep Foundation: *www.sleepfoundation.org*

United Network for Organ Sharing: *www.unos.org*

The U.S. Health & Human Services Organ Donation Web site: *www.organ-donor.gov*

Index